Diagnostic Techniques and Therapeutic Strategies for Parotid Gland Disorders

Mahmoud Sakr
Alexandria University, Egypt

A volume in the Advances in Medical Diagnosis, Treatment, and Care (AMDTC) Book Series

IGI Global
PUBLISHER of TIMELY KNOWLEDGE

Published in the United States of America by
IGI Global
Medical Information Science Reference (an imprint of IGI Global)
701 E. Chocolate Avenue
Hershey PA, USA 17033
Tel: 717-533-8845
Fax: 717-533-8661
E-mail: cust@igi-global.com
Web site: http://www.igi-global.com

Library of Congress Cataloging-in-Publication Data

Names: Sakr, Mahmoud, author.
Title: Diagnostic techniques and therapeutic strategies for parotid gland disorders / by Mahmoud Sakr.
Description: Hershey, PA : Medical Information Science Reference, [2021] | Includes bibliographical references and index. | Summary: "This book explores diagnostic techniques and therapeutic strategies for parotid gland disorders"-- Provided by publisher.
Identifiers: LCCN 2020009786 (print) | LCCN 2020009787 (ebook) | ISBN 9781799856030 (hardcover) | ISBN 9781799856047 (ebook)
Subjects: MESH: Parotid Diseases | Parotid Gland--pathology
Classification: LCC RC815.5 (print) | LCC RC815.5 (ebook) | NLM WI 230 | DDC 616.3/16--dc23
LC record available at https://lccn.loc.gov/2020009786
LC ebook record available at https://lccn.loc.gov/2020009787

This book is published in the IGI Global book series Advances in Medical Diagnosis, Treatment, and Care (AMDTC) (ISSN: 2475-6628; eISSN: 2475-6636)

British Cataloguing in Publication Data
A Cataloguing in Publication record for this book is available from the British Library.

Table of Contents

Preface

Head and neck surgery has now become a major specialty within the surgical domain and the management of parotid gland disorders encompasses a broad array of both benign and malignant diseases.

The purpose of this book is to provide a comprehensive review of the current knowledge of the pathophysiology, clinical and diagnostic techniques as well as therapeutic strategies of parotid gland disorders. We have endeavored to give some rein to the new developments, which are evidence-based and widely supported in the literature.

Chapter 1 describes, in brief, the three stages of embryological development and congenital anomalies of salivary glands, which include heterotopic glands, aplasia, gland duplication and congenitally atretic, imperforate, ectatic, and duplicated ducts.

The second chapter describes the characteristic histological features (microanatomy) of the parotid gland, including the stroma (connective tissue) and parenchyma (secretory units or acini, myoepithelial cells and ductal units). Electron miscroscopy and the structural changes caused by the effect of aging on salivary glands are also described.

In Chapter 3, the anatomy of the patoid gland is described in detail including arterial supply, venous drainage, innervation and lymphatic drainage. In addition, the surface anatomy and structures that pass through the gland, with special emphasis on the facial nerve, are also described.

Chapter 4 discusses the physiology of the parotid gland, control of saliva secretion and the various functions of saliva. It also addresses some derangements of salivary gland secretion and their management such as hypo- and hypoer-salivations.

Chapter 5 describes the clinical (history-taking and physical examination), laboratory, imaging, endoscopic and histological methods for evaluation of the parotid gland.

In Chapter 6, "xerostomia" (dry mouth) is discussed in detail. Risk factors and causes are mentioned and clinical manifestations, evaluation as well as management of this condition are explored and discussed.

In Chapter 7, parotid injuries and their sequelae (parotid fistula, sialocele, etc) are described, and diagnosis and early adequate management are discussed.

Management options, which include pressure dressings and the use of anti-sialagogues, total parotidectomy, tympanic neurectomy, intra-oral transposition of the parotid duct, radiation therapy, the use of botulinum toxin A, as well as fibrin glue, are all discussed.

Chapter 8 addresses the topic of sialolithiasis (stones), which occurs most commonly (80-95%) in the submandibular gland, and less commonly (5-20%) in the parotid gland. Causes and composition of the stones are described. Evaluation and therapeutic options, which include parotidectomy, external lithtripsy, and interventional sialoendoscopy, are discussed.

In Chapter 9, the different causes (viral, bacterial, granulomatous, autoimmune, etc) and management of salivary gland inflammation (sialadenitis) are discussed. The etiology, pathology, clinical presentation and treatment of sialadenosis (sialosis), a chronic, diffuse, non-inflammatory, non-neoplastic disorder causing diffuse enlargement of salivary glands, usually the parotid glands, are explored.

Chapter 10 comprises a list of the different causes of cystic parotid lesions, whether congenital or acquired, and whether bilateral or unilateral cysts are described. This chapter describes in more detail the etiology, clinical pesentation, evaluation and treatment of "sialocele" and "dermoid cyst of the parotid gland". It also summarizes parotid gland tumors based on the World Health Organization histological classification, which categorizes parotid tumors into benign epithelial tumors, soft tissue tumors, hematolymphoid tumors, and secondary tumors.

Chapter 11 describes benign tumors of the salivary glands, which are known to be varied and named after their cell type. A special emphasis on pleomorphic adenoma and Wharthin's tumor is provided. Pathology, clinical presentation, evaluation and management of all benign tumors of the parotid gland are discussed.

Chapter 12 focusses on the etiology, clinical presentation, assessment, prevention and treatment of "recurrent" pleomorphic adenoma. Treatment options are explored and discussed; these include observation, local excision, superficial parotidectomy, total conservative parotidectomy, total parotidectomy with resection of the involved nerve and immediate nerve graft (any procedure is followed by radiotherapy), and radiotherapy alone.

Chapter 13 addresses the risk factors of cancer of the parotid gland, which represents about 20% of all parotid tumors. In this chapter, characteristic histological features, methods of spread, evaluation and management of the individual types of malignant parotid tumors are discussed.

Chapter 14 focusses on "lymphoma", which accounts for 15% of malignant salivary gland tumors with the parotid gland being the most commonly affected (80%). Hodgkin and non-Hodgkin lymphoma are described and whether lymphoma is "primary" or "secondary" is discussed. Treatment is described in detail; it depends upon stage, overall health, age, and subtype of lymphoma and includes chemotherapy, total or radical parotidectomy, and radiotherapy.

In Chapter 15, carcinoma metastatic to the parotid gland is described with special emphasis on history, physical examination, and investigations, which include fiberoptic naso-endoscopy, fine needle aspiration cytology, computed tomography scan, magnetic resonance imaging and positron emission tomography. Treatment options are explored and discussed including surgery (ablative / reconstructive), radiotherapy, chemotherapy, chemoimmunotherapy. This chapter also addresses complications to avoid; these may be wound-, tumor-, gland- or nerve-related.

In Chapter 16, the history of parotidectomy is provided and indications, contraindications, pre-operative planning and the different techniques of parotidectomy procedures are described. These include different types of parotidectomy (superficial or lateral parotidectomy, radical parotidectomy, and extended total parotidectomy), limited procedures (partial superficial parotidectomy and extra-capsular dissection), and enucleation (extra-capsular, and intracapsular). Indications and contraindicaitons of parotidectomy procedures as well as and post-operative complications are discussed.

The focus in Chapter 17 is on "Frey's syndrome", which results from secondary to sympathetic denervation of sweat glands and reinnervation through the auriculotemporal nerve as a secondary event. The aberrant regeneration theory, which explains the physiopathology of Frey's syndrome, is discussed and the different methods of diagnosis and therapeutic options are discussed.

Chapter 18 focuses is on extra-temporal facial nerve reconstruction. The etiology, consequences, and diagnosis of facial nerve paralysis are described. The goals and limitations of nerve reconstruction, the schedule for facial nerve repair, the principles and methods (techniques) of facial nerve reconstruction, as well as muscle transposition, are all described and discussed.

Finally, the book has been structured in such a way as to facilitate quick reference and serve as a practical manual for the clinicians of many specialties who treat patients with parotid gland disorders.

Acknowledgment

I would like to express my deepest thanks and sincere gratitude to all those who provided support and help in the process of writing, editing, proof-reading, and producing this book. Last but not least, I would like to express my deepest gratitude to my family for their unlimited support and unconditioned love.

Introduction

The human salivary gland system can be divided into two distinct exocrine groups. The major salivary glands, which include the paired parotid, submandibular, and sublingual glands, and the minor salivary glands, which are hundreds of small glands lining the mucosa of the upper aerodigestive tract (Michael, Colin, & Denis, 2012).

Salivary glands can be classified as serous, mucous or mixed (sero-mucous). In serous secretions, the main type of protein secreted is alpha-amylase (ptylin), as enzyme that breaks down starch into maltose and glucose, whereas in mucous secretions the main protein secreted is mucin, which acts as a lubricant (Frederic, Judi, & Edwin, 2012).

In humans, between 0.5 and 1.5 liters of saliva are produced every day (Carolyn, Cathy, Julia, Sivakumar, & Nicky, 2012). The secretion of saliva (salivation) is mediated by parasympathetic stimulation; acetylcholine is the active neuro-transmitter and binds to muscarinic receptors in the glands, leading to increased salivation (Carolyn, 2012; Andrew, 2015).

Thus, the major function of the salivary glands is to secrete saliva, which plays a major role in lubrication, clearance, mastication, digestion, swallowing, immunity, taste, speech and the overall maintenance of homeostasis within the human body (Nanci, 2018). The presence of saliva is also vital to the maintenance of healthy hard (teeth) and soft (mucosa) oral tissues. Severe reduction of salivary output not only results in a rapid deterioration in oral health but also has a detrimental impact on the quality of life for the sufferer.

An understanding of saliva and its role in oral health will help to promote awareness among health care workers of the problems arising when the quantity or quality of saliva is decreased; this awareness and understanding is important to the prevention, early diagnosis and treatment of the condition.

REFERENCES

Andrew, N., & Jo, T. (2015). *Cochrane Database of Systematic Reviews, 10.* doi:10.1002/14651858

Carolyn, A., Cathy, E., Julia, J., Sivakumar, S., & Nicky, P. (2012). *Cochrane Database of Systematic Reviews, 5.* doi:10.1002/14651858

Frederic, M. H., Judi, N. L., & Edwin, B. (2012). Fundamentals of Anatomy & Physiology (9th ed.). San Francisco, CA: Pearson.

Michael, E., Colin, D., & Denis, O. (2012). Saliva and Oral Health (4th ed.). Stephen Hancocks Limited.

Nanci, A. (2018). *Ten Cate's Oral Histology: Development, Structure, And Function* (9th ed.). Academic Press.

Chapter 1
Embryology and Developmental Disorders

ABSTRACT

This chapter describes the embryological development and congenital anomalies of salivary glands. Development of the major salivary glands consists of three main stages. The first stage is marked by the presence of a primordial anlage and the formation of branched duct buds. The second stage is marked by the early appearance of lobules and duct canalization and the third stage by maturation of acini and ducts. The primordial parotid gland is the first to appear, during the sixth gestational week. In addition to heterotopic glands, congenital anomalies include aplasia, gland duplication and congenitally atretic, imperforate, ectatic, and duplicated ducts.

EMBRYOLOGICAL DEVELOPMENT

Development of the major salivary glands is thought to consist of three main stages (Arey, 1974; Gibson, 1983). The *first stage* is marked by the presence of a primordial anlage (from the German verb *anlagen*, to set a foundation) and the formation of branched duct buds resulting from repeated epithelial cleft and bud development (Figure 1). Ciliated epithelial cells form the luminal lining, while the external surfaces are lined by ectodermal myoepithelial cells (Bernfield, Banerjee, & Cohn, 1972).

During the *second stage*, early appearance of lobules and duct canalization take place resulting in the appearance of primitive acini and distal duct regions.

DOI: 10.4018/978-1-7998-5603-0.ch001

The *third stage* of major salivary gland development is marked by maturation of acini and intercalated ducts, and reduced prominence of interstitial connective tissue.

Figure 1. Embryo-logical development of the salivary glands

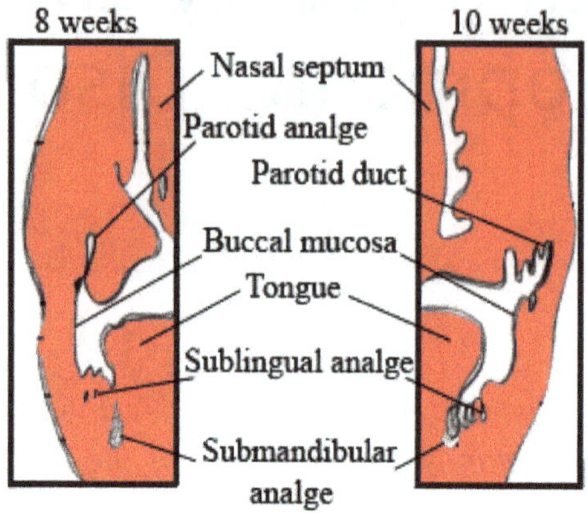

The primordial *parotid gland* is the first to appear, during the sixth gestational week, when oral ectodermal out-pouchings extend into the adjacent mesoderm and serve as the site of origin for growth of glands. After a short journey of dorsal and lateral migration, the parotid gland resides in the pre-auricular region. The facial nerve arbitrarily divides the gland into superficial and deep lobes by the 10th week of gestation. A fully developed capsule from the nearby mesenchyme surrounds the gland by the 12th week (Arey, 1974).

During the sixth week of embryonic life, small buds appear in the floor of the mouth lateral to the tongue and extend posteriorly around the mylohyoid muscle into the submandibular triangle. These buds eventually develop into the *submandibular glands.* A capsule from the surrounding mesenchyme is fully formed around the gland by the third gestational month (Gibson, 1983).

During the ninth embryonic month, the *sublingual gland* anlage is formed from multiple endodermal epithelial buds in the paralingual sulcus of the floor of the mouth. Absence of a capsule is due to infiltration of the glands by sublingual connective tissue. Intra-glandular lymph nodes (LNs) and major ducts also do not generally develop within sublingual glands. Upper respiratory ectoderm gives rise to simple tubuloacinar units. They develop into the *minor salivary glands* during the 12th intrauterine week (Kontis & Johns, 2014).

DEVELOPMENTAL DISORDERS

Aside from *heterotopic* salivary glands, developmental disorders of these glands are rare. Reported congenital anomalies include *aplasia* (absence) (Myers, 1994; Wiedemann, 1997; Kwon, 2006; Karakoc, 2005), gland *duplication* (Codjambopoulo, Ender-Griepekoven, & Broy, 1992), as well as congenitally atretic, imperforate, ectatic, and duplicated *ducts* (Pownel, 1992; Amin, 2001), Agenesis may be associated with abnormalities of the lacrimal apparatus and may also be genetically transmitted (Kwon, Jung, Kim, & Kim, 2006). Agenesis may be partial or total, unilateral or bilateral and may involve more than one salivary gland. Association with *specific syndromes* such as Levy-Hollister syndrome, Down syndrome or Klinefelter syndrome has been reported. The true incidence of parotid agenesis is unknown since most of the cases are asymptomatic. Symptoms include dental caries, thirst, xerostomia and gingival infections. Oral examination reveals absence of the papilla of Stensen's duct. When suspected, magnetic resonance imaging (MRI) is the imaging tool of choice to demonstrate glandular bed being replaced by fat. Congenital parotid fistula is another developmental disorder.

Tumor-like presentations of mal-development include rare *hamartomas* of the *hard palate* (Harada, Morimatsu, Kusukawa, & Kameyama, 1997) and unusual cystic choristomas of the *submandibular gland* (Tang, Glicklich, Siegesmund, Oechler, & McCreadie, 1979), which appear to be a mixture of epithelium of both ectodermal and endodermal derivation. The congenital salivary gland anlage tumor or congenital pleomorphic adenoma (PA) is thought to represent a hamartoma of *minor salivary gland* origin (Dehner et al., 1994).

REFERENCES

Amin, M. A., & Bailey, B. M. (2001). Congenital atresia of the orifice of the submandibular duct: A report of 2 cases and review. *British Journal of Oral & Maxillofacial Surgery*, *39*(6), 48048–2. doi:10.1054/bjom.2001.0672 PMID:11735147

Arey, L. B. (1974). *Developmental Anatomy. A Textbook and Laboratory Manual of Embryology. Revised* (7th ed.). Philadelphia, PA: WB Saunders, Inc.

Bernfield, M. R., Banerjee, S. D., & Cohn, R. H. (1972). Dependence of salivary epithelial morphology and branching morphogenesis upon acid mucopolysaccharide-protein (proteoglycan) at the epithelial surface. *The Journal of Cell Biology*, *52*(3), 674–689. doi:10.1083/jcb.52.3.674 PMID:4109690

Codjambopoulo, P., Ender-Griepekoven, I., & Broy, H. (1992). Bilateral duplication of the submandibular gland and the submandibular duct. *RöFo. Fortschritte auf dem Gebiete der Röntgenstrahlen und der Nuklearmedizin*, *157*(2), 185–186. doi:10.1055-2008-1032994 PMID:1515629

Dehner, L. P., Valbuena, L., Perez-Atayde, A., Reddick, R. L., Askin, F. B., & Rosai, J. (1994). Salivary gland anlage tumor ("congenital pleomorphic adenoma"). A clinicopathologic, immunohistochemical and ultrastructural study of nine cases. *The American Journal of Surgical Pathology*, *18*(1), 25–36. doi:10.1097/00000478-199401000-00003 PMID:8279626

Gibson, M. H. (1983). The prenatal human submandibular gland: A histological, histochemical and ultra-structural study. *Anatomischer Anzeiger*, *153*(1), 91–105. PMID:6837926

Harada, H., Morimatsu, M., Kusukawa, J., & Kameyama, T. (1997). A hamartoma-like mass on the palate? A possible discussion regarding the components of a pigmented naevus and hyperplastic salivary gland. *The Journal of Laryngology and Otology*, *111*(3), 296–299. doi:10.1017/S0022215100137144 PMID:9156075

Karakoc, O., Akcam, T., Kocaoglu, M., & Yetiser, S. (2005). Agenesis of the unilateral parotid gland associated with pleomorphic adenoma of the contralateral parotid gland. *The Journal of Laryngology and Otology*, *119*(5), 409–411. doi:10.1258/0022215053945741 PMID:15949111

Kontis, T. C., & Johns, M. E. (2001). Anatomy and Physiology of the Salivary Glands. In B. J. Bailey (Ed.), *Head and Neck Surgery – Otolaryngology*. Philadelphia, PA: Lippincott Williams & Wilkins.

Kwon, S. Y., Jung, E. J., Kim, S. H., & Kim, T. K. (2006). A case of major salivary gland agenesis. *Acta Oto-laryngolica*, *126*(2), 219–222. doi:10.1080/00016480500314139 PMID:16428204

Myers, M. A., Youngberg, R. A., & Bauman, J. M. (1994). Congenital absence of the major salivary glands and impaired lacrimal secretion in a child: Case report. *The Journal of the American Dental Association*, *125*(2), 210–212. doi:10.14219/jada.archive.1994.0274 PMID:8113532

Pownell, P. H., Brown, O. E., Pransky, S. M., & Manning, S. C. (1992). Congenital abnormalities of the submandibular duct. *International Journal of Pediatric Otorhinolaryngology*, *24*(2), 161–169. doi:10.1016/0165-5876(92)90142-C PMID:1428595

Tang, T. T., Glicklich, M., Siegesmund, K. A., Oechler, H. W., & McCreadie, S. R. (1979). Neonatal cystic choristoma in submandibular salivary gland simulating cystic hygroma. *Archives of Pathology & Laboratory Medicine*, *103*(10), 536–539. PMID:582369

Wiedemann, H. R. (1997). Salivary gland disorders and heredity. *American Journal of Medical Genetics*, *68*(2), 222–224. doi:10.1002/(SICI)1096-8628(19970120)68:2<222::AID-AJMG20>3.0.CO;2-V PMID:9028463

Chapter 2
Histology of the Parotid Gland

ABSTRACT

This chapter describes the characteristic histological features of the parotid gland. The microanatomy of the parotid gland includes the following: stroma (connective tissue) and parenchyma (secretory units or acini, myoepithelial cells, and ductal units). The secretory cells are organized into secretory units or acini, which are lined exclusively by serous cells. Myoepithelial cells are the contractile elements with secretory end pieces and intercalated ducts. The acini are drained by a series of ducts which eventually drain into the major excretory duct (Stensen's duct). Aging of salivary glands show some structural changes, but with no overall change in the amount of saliva secreted with advancing age.

INTRODUCTION

All glands in general are derived from epithelial cells and consist of *parenchyma* (secretory unit and associated ducts) and *stroma* (surrounding connective tissue that penetrates and divides the gland into lobules). The parotid gland (exocrine) secretes saliva via ducts from a flask-like, blind-ended secretory structure called *acinus*. Thus, the microanatomy of the parotid gland includes the following: connective tissue (stroma), secretory units (acini), myoepithelial cells and ductal units as shown in Figure 1.

DOI: 10.4018/978-1-7998-5603-0.ch002

Histology of the Parotid Gland

Figure 1. Microanatomy of the salivary glandular tissue

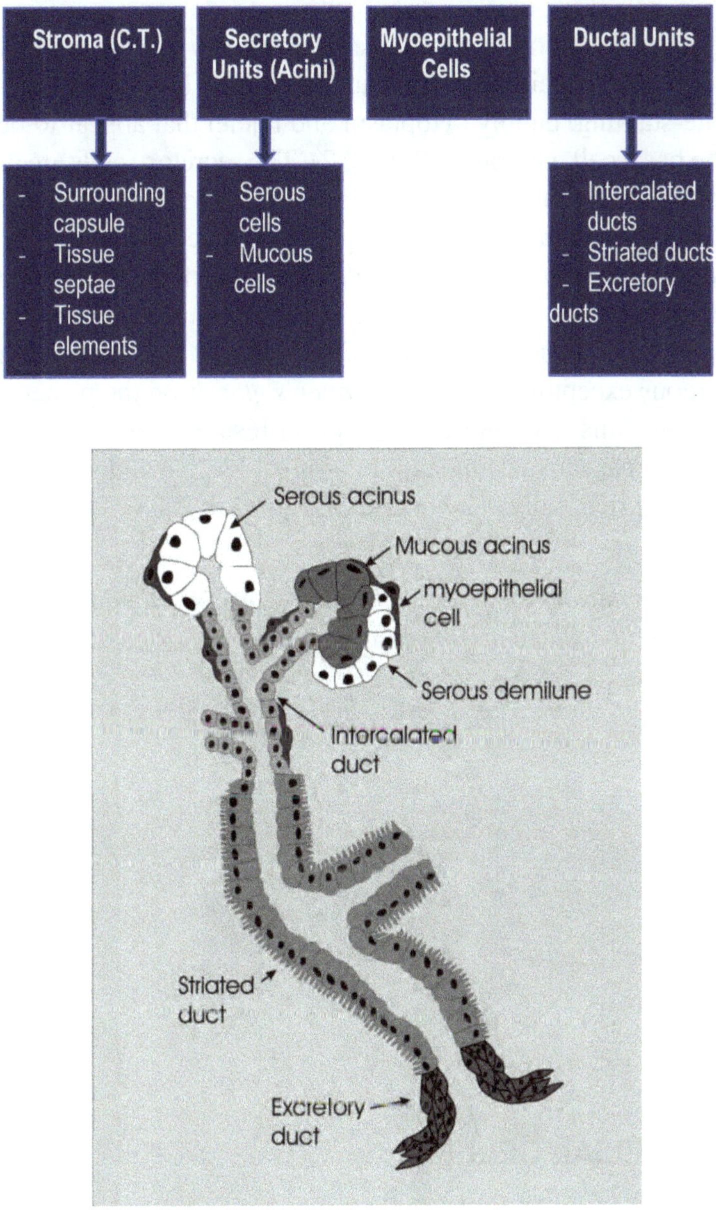

SECRETORY UNIT

The cytoplasm of serous cells contains distinctly *eosinophilic* zymogen granules and their nuclei are spherical in appearance. In contrast, mucous cells have a pale-staining, bubbly cytoplasm and nuclei that appear to be pushed against the basal cell membrane (Figure 2). The secretory cells are organized into secretory units or ***acini***, and they are classified according to the cell types they contain. The acini of the parotid gland are lined exclusively by *serous* cells. The acini of the *submandibular gland* are also mainly serous (90%), but also contain mucous as well mixed acini. The *sublingual gland* is composed primarily of mucous acini. *Minor salivary glands* are either mucinous or sero-mucinous except for the serous *Ebner's glands* on the posterior aspect of the tongue. This histological description results in parotid thin watery, devoid of mucins, saliva, submandibular mixed saliva and sublingual more viscous, mucin rich, saliva (Junqueria & Carneiro, 2003).

Figure 2. Cells of salivary glands under the microscope. Note the differences between serous cells (parotid gland) and mucus cells.

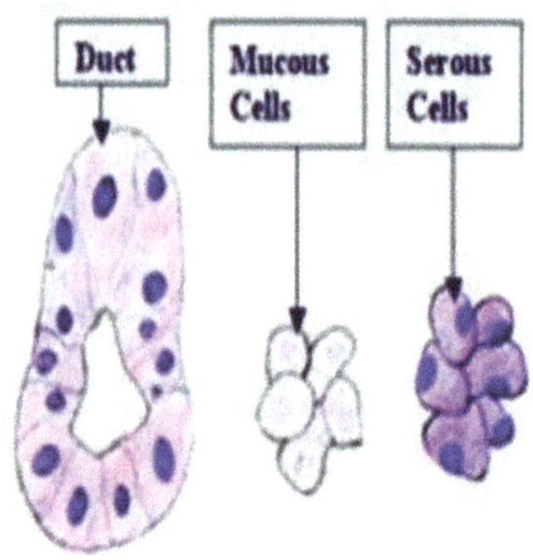

MYOEPITHELIAL CELLS

Myoepithelial cells are the contractile elements with secretory end pieces and intercalated ducts. They are stellate- shaped with numerous branching processes that envelop the secretory end piece. They may be fusiform-shaped with fewer processes. These processes are filled with actin and soluble myosin. Contraction of these processes provides support to the end pieces during active

Figure 3. Duct components: Intra-lobular intercalated ducts comprised of an irregular myoepithelial cell layer lined with squamous or low cuboidal epithelium, drain into the intra-lobular striated ducts lined by a different epithelial arrangement. Striated ducts drain into inter-lobular ducts

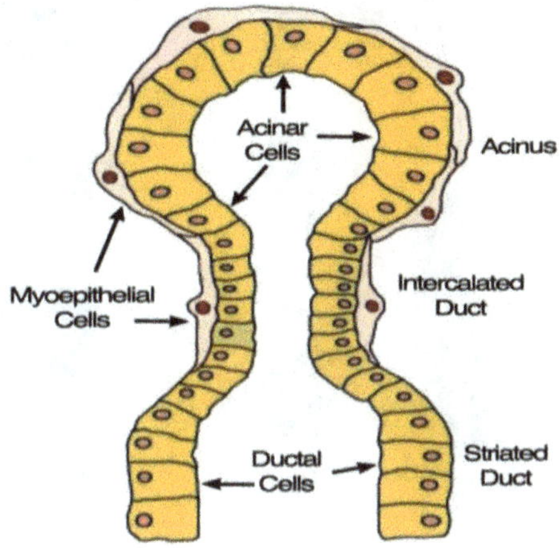

secretion of saliva. Recent advances also suggest that these cells provided signals to the end pieces during active secretion of saliva.

DUCTAL UNIT

The acini are drained by a series of ducts the smallest of which are the intra-lobular intercalated ducts, which are comprised of an irregular myoepithelial cell layer lined with squamous or low cuboidal epithelium, and in turn drain into the striated ducts. The striated ducts are also intra-lobular, but lined by a different epithelial arrangement. Striated ducts drain into the inter-lobular ducts (Figure 3). In the major salivary glands these ducts drain into major excretory ducts (*Stensen's* duct in the parotid gland (Figure 4), *Wharton's* duct in the submandibular gland and *Bartholin's* duct in the sublingual gland) and the epithelium of these ducts changes to squamous as they exit through the oral mucosa. The *minor salivary gland* duct system is simpler than that of the major salivary glands, where the intercalated ducts are longer and the striated ducts are either less developed or not present (Junqueria & Carneiro, 2003).

Figure 4. Microanatomy of the acini and ductal system of the parotid gland

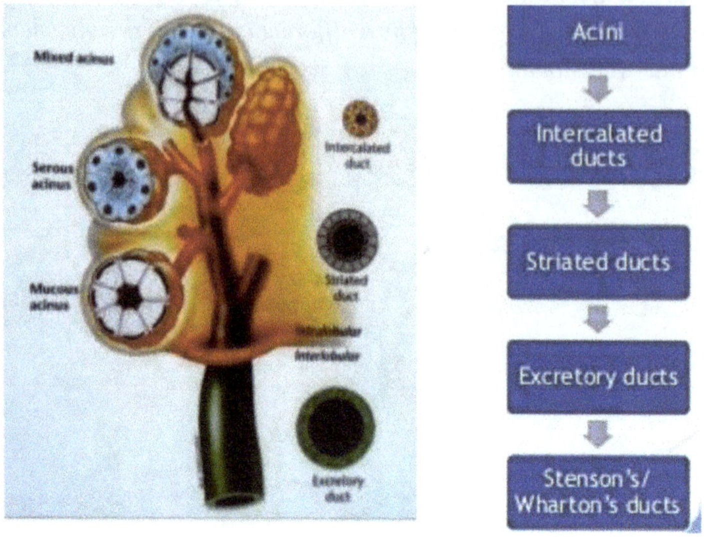

ELECTRON MICROSCOPY (TANAKCHI, 2019)

Acinar Cells

- Numerous cytoplasmic secretory (zymogen) granules in apical portion of cell;
- Extensive rough ER and Golgi;
- Numerous mitochondria;
- Numerous folds are present in basal lamina of acinar cells that are not distended with secretory product;
- Mucous acinar cells have larger, more irregular secretory droplets that are more electron lucent than in serous acinar cells.

Intercalated Duct Cells

- Few special ultrastructural features;
- May have some secretory granules;
- Scant cytoplasm has basal rough ER, apical Golgi and mitochondria;
- Lateral membranes interdigitate with neighboring cells.

Myoepithelial Cells

- Between basal plasma membrane of acinar and intercalated duct cells and basal lamina;
- Flattened and elongated with cytoplasmic processes extending around acinar and intercalated duct cells;
- Long / irregular nuclei;
- Desmosomes attach the myoepithelial cells to acinar and ductal cells.

Striated Duct Cells

- Striations are due to basal vertical folds;
- Numerous mitochondria present.

EFFECT OF AGING

There is no overall change in the amount of saliva secreted with advancing age. However, aging of salivary glands show some structural changes, such as *(Vissink,* 1996; Kim, 1004):

- Decrease in volume of acinar tissue;
- Increase in fibrous tissue;
- Increase in adipose tissue;
- Ductal hyperplasia and dilation.

In addition, there are also some changes in the salivary contents:

- Decrease in concentration of secretory IgA;
- Decrease in the amount of mucin.

REFERENCES

Junqueria, L., & Carneiro, J. (2003). *Basic Histology: Text and Atlas* (10th ed.). New York, NY: McGraw-Hill.

Kim, S. K., & Allen, E. D. (1994). Structural and functional changes in salivary glands during aging. *Microscopy Research and Technique*, *28*(3), 243–253. doi:10.1002/jemt.1070280308 PMID:8068986

Tanakchi, S. (2019). Normal histology. *Pathology Outlines*. http://www. pathologyoutlines. com/topic/salivaryglandsnormalhistology.html

Vissink, A., Spijkervet, F. K., & Van Nieuw, A. A. (1996). Aging and saliva: A review of the literature. *Special Care in Dentistry*, *16*(3), 95–103. doi:10.1111/j.1754-4505.1996.tb00842.x PMID:9084322

Chapter 3
Surgical Anatomy of the Parotid Gland

ABSTRACT

The parotid gland consists of two lobes: superficial and deep with regard to its relation with the facial nerve. It is wrapped around the mandibular ramus and secretes saliva through the parotid (Stensen's) duct. It is a paired organ, weighing 15-30g each. Its superficial lobe overlies the lateral surface of the masseter muscle and is bounded superiorly by the zygomatic arch, while its deep lobe is located in the pre-styloid compartment of the parapharyngeal space between the mastoid process posteriorly, ramus of mandible anteriorly, and external auditory meatus superiorly. Medially, the gland reaches to the styloid process. Inferiorly, the parotid tail extends down to the anteromedial margin of sternocleido-mastoid muscle. Several structures run through the parotid gland, namely, terminal segment of external carotid artery, retro-mandibular vein, parotid lymph nodes, and facial nerve, which soon gives two divisions (temporo-facial and cervico-facial) that give off five branches inside the gland radiating forwards. This chapter explores the surgical anatomy of the parotid gland.

INTRODUCTION

The parotid gland is the largest of the three major salivary glands. It is superficial in location and enclosed by the superficial layer of the deep cervical fascia where it forms the aptly named parotid space. The parotid space is located

DOI: 10.4018/978-1-7998-5603-0.ch003

postero-lateral to the masticator space, lateral to the para-pharyngeal space, and antero-lateral to the carotid space [Figure 1]. In addition to the gland itself, the parotid space contains also the facial nerve, auriculotemporal branches of the mandibular division of the trigeminal nerve, intraparotid lymph nodes (LNs), the external carotid artery (ECA), and the retromandiular vein (Som, 2011; Grossman, 2010; Rastogi, 2012). Although not a true fascial plane, the intraparotid facial nerve separates the parotid gland into superficial and deep portions, an important distinction to make when describing a lesion's location before excision (Kessler & Bhatt, 2018).

Figure 1. The parotid duct dives at an angle of 90° at the anterior border of masseter to pierce the buccal pad of fat, buccopharyngeal fascia, and then buccinators

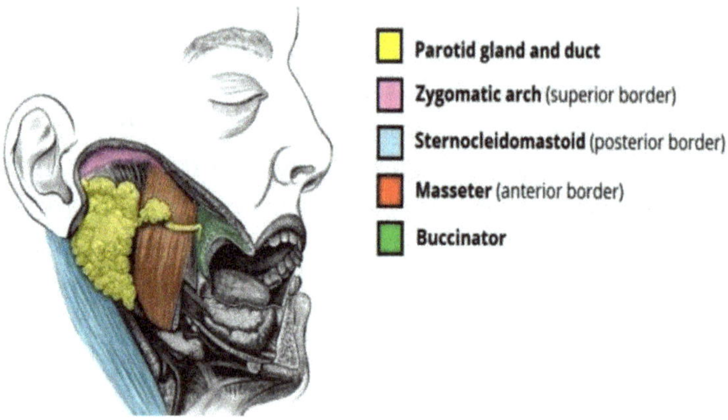

PAROTID FASCIA

The deep cervical fascia continues superiorly to form the parotid fascia which is split into superficial and deep layers to enclose the parotid gland. The thicker adherent, inelastic, superficial fascia extends up to be attached to the zygomatic arch while the thinner deep one is attached to the styloid process, angle and posterior border of the ramus of the mandible and tympanic plate. A portion of the deep lamina thickens to form the stylo-mandibular ligament, which separates the parotid gland from the submandibular gland.

PAROTID DUCT (*STENSEN'S DUCT*, DUCTUS PAROTIDEUS)

The parotid gland drains its serous secretions through the long *Stensen's duct* that arises from the most anterior superficial part of the gland, travels parallel and 1 cm below the zygoma, running on the lateral surface of masseter, just deep to skin, then it finally dives at an angle of 90° at the anterior border of masseter to pierce the buccal pad of fat, buccopharyngeal fascia, then buccinator (Figure 1). It opens in the oral (gingivo-buccal) vestibule opposite the 2nd maxillary molar tooth over the summit of a papilla (Figure 2) (Kontis, 2001; Johns, 1977).

Figure 2. Stensen's duct opens in the oral vestibule opposite the second maxillary molar tooth over the summit of a papilla (arrow)

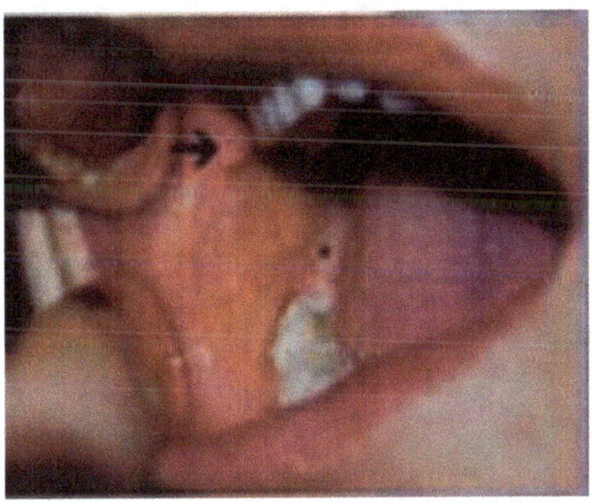

ACCESSORY PAROTID GLAND

Accessory parotid tissue (lobe or gland) may sometimes exist and come to reside over the masseter muscle between the zygomatic arch and Stensen's duct. As proved histologically, this accessory glandular tissue secretes mucous in addition to serous secretions drained through a single short duct that joins the main duct (Frommer, 1977).

SURFACE ANATOMY OF THE PAROTID GLAND

The *anterior* border of the gland corresponds to a line that extends from the ear tragus to the posterior border of the masseter opposite the angle of the mouth, the *inferior* border from there to below and behind the angle of the mandible, the *posterior* border from there to the mastoid process and the *superior* border from the mastoid process to the ear tragus. Surface anatomy of the *parotid duct* corresponds to the middle-third of an imaginary line that extends from the tragus of the ear to the mid portion of the upper lip (Figure 3).

Figure 3. Surface anatomy of the parotid gland (red lines)

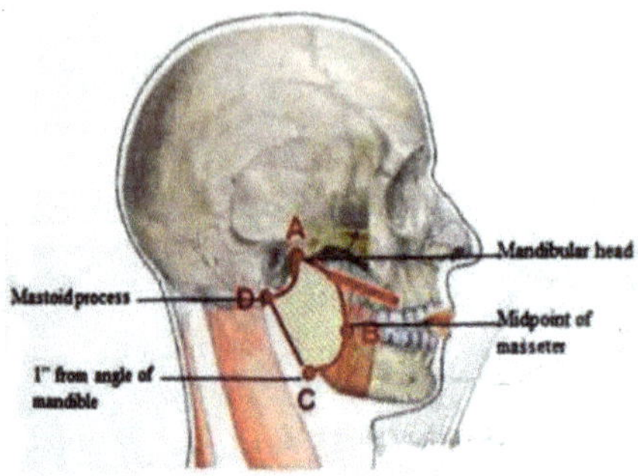

NERVE SUPPLY

The facial nerve (CN VII) exits the skull base through the stylomastoid foramen, which is slightly posterolateral to the styloid process and anteromedial to the mastoid process. The nerve immediately gives off three motor branches for the posterior belly of the digastric, the stylohyoid and the post-auricular muscles. Its main trunk then enters the posterior portion of the gland. Inside the gland, at the pesanserinus (*Latin*: goose's foot), it divides into upper temporo-facial and lower cervico-facial division approximately 1.3 cm from the stylomastoid foramen. The temporo-facial division gives off the temporal, zygomatic and buccal branches, while the cervicofacial gives off the marginal mandibular and cervical branches (Figure 4).

During parotidectomy, the facial nerve must be traced from behind forwards as it emerges from the stylomastoid foramen and enters the parotid gland. The nerve is surrounded by a leash of veins called the neuro-venous plexus

Figure 4. Anatomy of the facial nerve. It divides first into 2 divisions; upper temporo-facial and lower cervico-facial. The upper division gives off the temporal, zygomatic and buccal branches, while the lower gives off the marginal mandibular and cervical branches.

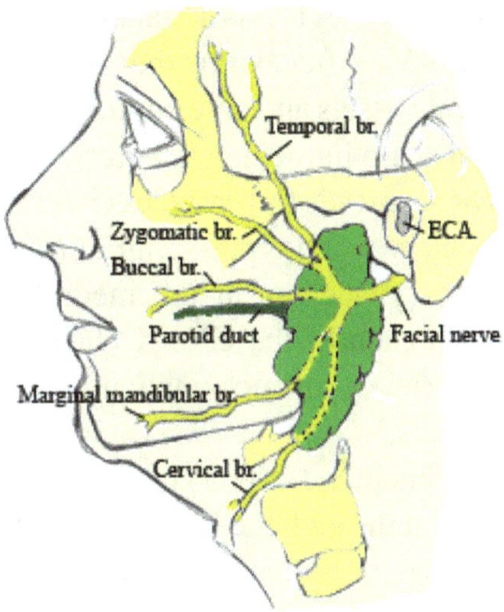

of Patey, which must be followed with fine dissection, preferably under the microscope, to surgically divide the isthmus (between the superficial and the deep parotid lobes).

The *temporal branch* passes with the superficial temporal vessels over the zygoma to supply the frontal belly of occipito-frontalis, orbicularis oculi, corrugator supercilii and anterior and superior auricular muscles. The *zygomatic branch* passes over the periosteum of the zygomatic arch to supply the zygomatic, orbital and infra-orbital muscles. The *buccal branch* travels with the Stensen's duct to supply the buccinator, upper lip and nostril muscles. The *marginal mandibular branch* travels along the inferior border of the parotid gland just deep to the platysma muscle but superficial to the posterior facial and retromandibular veins, to supply the lower lip and chin muscles. Running in the same plane, is the *cervical branch*, which supplies the platysma muscle. All the muscles supplied by the facial nerve are muscles of facial expression.

The *great auricular nerve* (C2,3) is a sensory branch of the cervical plexus that provides general sensation to the parotid gland, the skin of the posterior portion of the ear pinna and the ear lobule. It accompanies the external jugular vein along the lateral surface of the SCM muscle towards the tail of the parotid gland, and there it splits into anterior and posterior branches. It is often injured during parotidectomy leaving the ear lobule senseless. Its harvesting for facial nerve grafting may be needed when the latter is injured or sacrificed.

The *auriculotemporal nerve* (ATN) is a branch of the mandibular division of the trigeminal nerve (CN V). After exiting the foramen ovale, it runs parallel to the superficial temporal vessels and anterior to the external auditory canal to innervate the skin and scalp immediately anterior to the ear.

The *glossopharyngeal nerve* (CN IX) provides visceral secretory innervation to the parotid gland. The nerve carries pre-ganglionic parasympathetic fibers from the inferior salivatory nucleus in the medulla through the jugular foramen. Then, a small branch of the CN IX (Jacobsen's nerve) re-enters the skull through the inferior tympanic canaliculus and into the middle ear to form the tympanic plexus.

The pre-ganglionic fibers then travel as the lesser petrosal nerve into the middle cranial fossa and out through the foramen ovale to synapse in the otic ganglion. Post-ganglionic parasympathetic fibers exit the otic ganglion to join the ATN in the infra-temporal fossa. The ATN enters the substance of the gland from its deep aspect along the neck of the mandible and emerges from the gland just inferior to the root of the zygomatic arch. The ATN so carries fibers that innervate the parotid gland for secretion of saliva (Figure 5).

Figure 5. Parasympathetic innervation of salivary glands

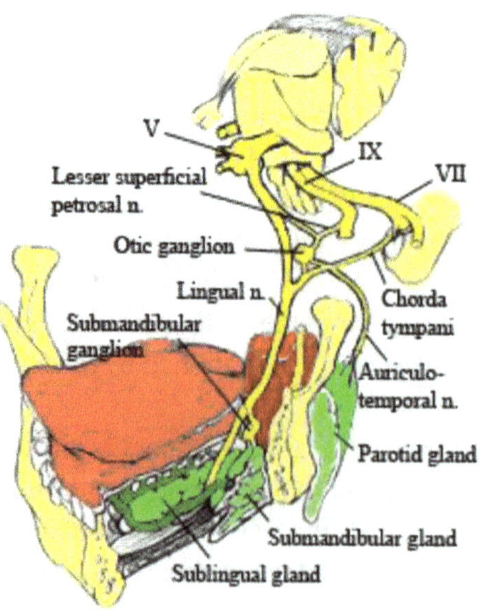

Post-ganglionic sympathetic fibers innervate the salivary glands, sweat glands, and cutaneous blood vessels, mediating vasoconstriction, through the external carotid plexus from the superior cervical ganglion. Acetylcholine serves as the neurotransmitter for both post-ganglionic sympathetic and parasympathetic fibers. This physiologic coincidence allows for the occasional development of "gustatory sweating", also known as *Frey's syndrome*, following parotidectomy (Bhattacharyya & Varvares, 1999).

ARTERIAL SUPPLY

The parotid gland receives its blood supply through branches of the external carotid artery (ECA), mainly through the *posterior auricular artery*. The ECA travels parallel to the mandible under the posterior belly of digastric muscle. It then travels medial to the gland and splits into its two terminal branches; the superficial temporal artery that leaves the superior portion of the gland and the maxillary artery that leaves the medial portion of the gland (Figure 6).

The *transverse facial artery* is a branch of the superficial temporal artery that runs anteriorly between the zygoma and parotid duct to supply it together with the parotid gland and the masseter muscle (Figure 6).

Figure 6. Vascular supply of the parotid gland

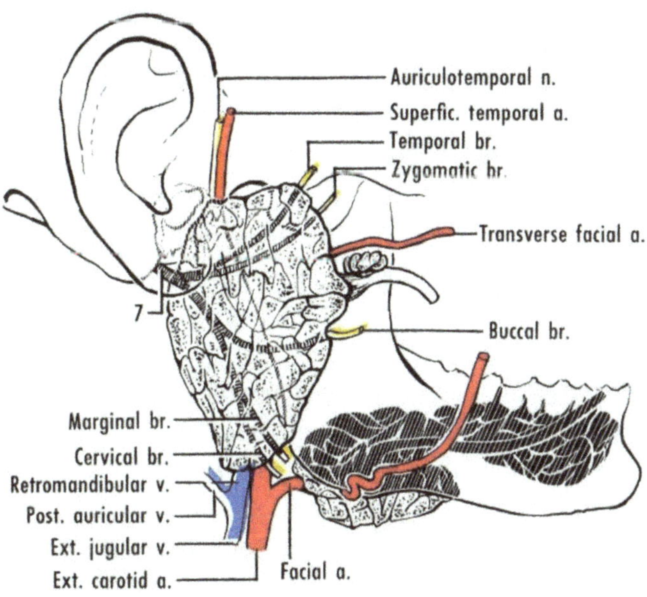

VENOUS DRAINAGE

The *retromandibular vein*, formed by the union of the maxillary and the superficial temporal veins, runs through the parotid gland just deep to the facial nerve. It drains into the external jugular vein as seen in Figure 4 above. There are many variations as regards the surgical anatomy of the retromandibular vein.

LYMPHATIC DRAINAGE

As a result of late encapsulation during embryologic development, the parotid gland, unlike the submandibular and sublingual glands, contains intra-parenchymal lymph nodes (LNs), with salivary gland structures, usually ducts and less frequency acini, in the intra- and peri-parotid lymph nodes. Parotid gland lymph nodes lie in the superficial and partly in the deep fascia over the parotid gland. In addition to the parotid gland, they also drain the temple, side of the scalp, external auditory meatus (EAM), middle ear, upper part of the cheek and parts of the eyelids and orbit.

Ninety percent of the nodes draining the parotid gland are located in the superficial layer between the gland and its capsule (3 to 20 nodes). These drain the parotid gland, EAM, pinna, scalp, eyelids and lacrimal glands. Deep LNs, residing on the lateral wall of the pharynx, drain the parotid gland, external auditory canal, middle ear, nasopharynx and soft palate. Both groups drain into level II of cervical LNs (upper deep cervical LNs) (Netter, 2019).

PARA-PHARYNGEAL SPACE

Tumors of the deep parotid lobe often extend medially into the parapharyngeal space, which is shaped like an inverted pyramid, where the greater cornu of the hyoid bone serves as the *apex* and the petrous bone of the skull base as the *base* as shown in Figure 7.

The parapharyngeal space is bound *medially* by the lateral pharyngeal wall, which consists of the superior constrictor muscles, bucco-pharyngeal fascia and tensor veli palatine. It is bounded *laterally* by the ramus of the mandible and the medial pterygoid muscle, *anteriorly* by the pterygoid fascia and the pterygo-mandibular raphe and *posteriorly* by the carotid

Figure 7. Anatomy of the para-pharyngeal space, which mimics an inverted pyramid

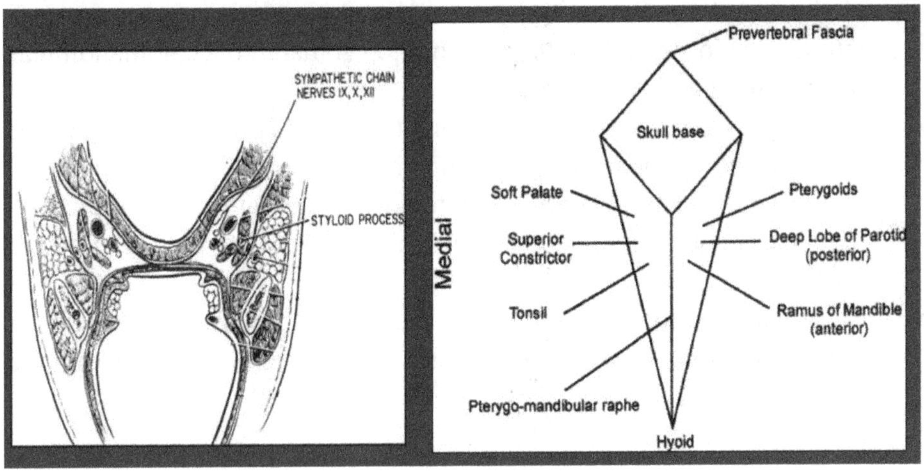

sheath and pre-vertebral fascia (Figure 5) (Drake, Vogle, Mitchell, Tibbitts, & Richardson, 2017).

A line from the styloid process to the medial portion of the medial pterygoid plate divides the parapharyngeal space into pre- and post-styloid compartments. The *pre-styloid* one contains the deep parotid lobe, internal maxillary and ascending pharyngeal arteries, and inferior alveolar, lingual and ATNs. The *post-styloid* compartment contains the internal jugular vein (IJV), carotid artery, vagus nerve (tenth cranial nerve, CN X) all within the carotid sheath as well as the cranial nerves glosso-pharyngeal (CN IX), accessory (CN XI) and hypoglossal (CN XII), and the cervical sympathetic chain. Thus, neurogenic tumors or paragangliomas arising from these nerves lie in this post-styloid compartment (Carrau, Johnson, & Myers, 1997).

Hints and Tips

- The parotid bed is an irregular space located between the ramus of the mandible, the EAM, the mastoid and styloid processes, the digastric, and SCM muscles;
- Structures entering the parotid gland exit from its posterior, superior, inferior, and anterior surfaces. The posterior auricular artery exits from the posterior aspect of the gland. The superficial temporal artery and vein, ATN, and temporal branches of the facial nerve (CN VII) are seen at the superior margin of the gland. Inferiorly, the retromandibular

vein exits the parotid gland. Emanating from the entire facial margin of the gland are the terminal branches of the facial nerve, grouped into five major branches: the temporal, zygomatic, buccal, mandibular (marginal) and cervical branches;

- General sensation to the parotid gland is provided by the great auricular nerve of the cervical plexus. Sympathetic innervation is supplied by the carotid plexus, whereas secretomotor innervation is supplied by the glossopharyngeal nerve (CN IX) and delivered to the gland by the ATN;
- The gland cannot be moved over the deep structures, and becomes more prominent when the patient clenches his teeth by contracting the masseter muscles.

REFERENCES

Bhattacharyya, N., & Varvares, M. A. (1999). Anomalous relationship of the facial nerve and the retromandibular vein: A case report. *Journal of Oral and Maxillofacial Surgery*, *7*(1), 5–76. doi:10.1016/S0278-2391(99)90639-0 PMID:9915401

Carrau, R. L., Johnson, J. T., & Myers, E. N. (1997). Management of tumors of the parapharyngeal space. *Oncology*, *11*(5), 633–640. PMID:9159790

Drake, R., Vogle, A. W., Mitchell, A. W. M., Tibbittis, R., & Richardson, P. (2017). *Gray's Atals of Anatomy* (3rd ed.). Philadelphia, PA: Elsevier.

(2010). Extramucosal diseases of the head and neck. InGrossman, R. I., & Yousem, D. M. (Eds.), *Neuroradiology: The Requisites* (3rd ed.). St. Louis: Mosby; doi:10.1016/B978-0-323-05355-6.00040-9.

Frommer, J. (1977). The human accessory parotid gland: Its incidence, nature, and significance. *Oral Surgery, Oral Medicine, and Oral Pathology*, *43*(5), 671–676. doi:10.1016/0030-4220(77)90049-4 PMID:266146

Johns, M. E. (1977). The salivary glands: Anatomy and embryology. *Otolaryngologic Clinics of North America*, *10*(2), 261–271. PMID:896193

Kessler, A. T., & Bhatt, A. A. (2018). Review of the major and minor salivary glands, part 1: Anatomy, infectious, and inflammatory processes. *Journal of Clinical Imaging Science*, *8*, 47–54. doi:10.4103/jcis.JCIS_45_18 PMID:30546931

Kontis, T. C., & Johns, M. E. (2001). Anatomy and Physiology of the Salivary Glands. In B. J. Bailey (Ed.), *Head and Neck Surgery – Otolaryngology*. Philadelphia, PA: Lippincott Williams & Wilkins.

Netter, F. H. (2019). Atals of Human Anatomy (7th ed.). Philadelphia, PA: Elsevier.

Rastogi, R., Bhargava, S., Mallarajapatna, G. J., & Singh, S. K. (2012). Pictorial essay: Salivary gland imaging. *The Indian Journal of Radiology & Imaging*, *22*(4), 325–333. doi:10.4103/0971-3026.111487 PMID:23833425

Som, P. M., & Brandwin-Gensler, M. S. (2011). Anatomy and pathology of the salivary glands. In *Head and Neck Imaging* (5th ed.). St. Louis: Mosby.

Chapter 4
Applied Physiology of the Parotid Gland

ABSTRACT

The major function of salivary glands is the production of saliva, which performs many functions including lubrication of the food bolus, maintaining the oral cavity pH within 6 to 7, maintaining teeth integrity, fighting bacteria, aiding taste and digestion, and providing a continuous lavaging biofilm for the oral cavity. Saliva is actively produced in high volumes relative to the mass of the salivary glands and is almost completely controlled extrinsically by both parasympathetic and sympathetic divisions of the autonomic nervous system. Some researchers used bilateral tympanic neurectomy for patients with ptyalism (drooling) with good initial results. Others advocated bilateral parotid duct rerouting ± bilateral submandibular gland excision for long-term treatment of drooling. Intra-glandular Botulinum toxin may also have good results for patients with hyper-sialorrhea. Most resting salivary gland flow arises from the submandibular glands and surgery should focus on this gland to control uncontrolled sialorrhea.

CONSTITUENTS (COMPOSITION) OF SALIVA

Saliva contains both inorganic and organic compounds and is characterized by its high volume compared to salivary gland weight, high potassium concentration, and low osmolarity (Figure 1). The large relative volume of

DOI: 10.4018/978-1-7998-5603-0.ch004

saliva production is due to its high secretion rate, which can go up to 1 ml/g of salivary gland/minute.

Figure 1. Constituents of saliva secreted by the parotid gland

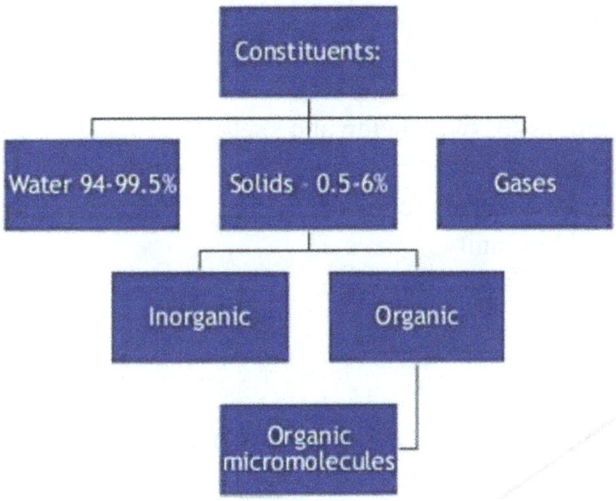

Saliva contains both inorganic and organic compounds and is characterized by its high volume compared to salivary gland weight, high potassium concentration, and low osmolarity. The large relative volume of saliva production is due to its high secretion rate, which can go up to 1 ml/g of salivary gland/minute.

Saliva is mostly hypotonic to plasma due to the fact that reabsorption of Na^+ and Cl^- is greater than the secretion of K^+ and $HCO3^-$ within the salivary ducts.

Several organic compounds present in saliva include α-amylase, lingual lipase, mucus, lysozymes, glycoproteins, lactoferrin, and the IgA secretory piece. Saliva is also comprised of the organic *blood group antigens* A, B, AB, and O. *Kallikrein* is secreted by the salivary glands during increased metabolic activity. Kallikrein enzymatically converts plasma protein into bradykinin, a vasodilator, in order to increase blood flow to the glands. Saliva contains approximately one tenth the total amount of protein as that found in plasma.

FUNCTIONS OF SALIVA

Salivary functions serve to maintain oral health and create an appropriate ecological balance. Salivary components work in concert in overlapping, multi-functioning roles, which can be simultaneously beneficial and detrimental.

Functions of saliva can be summarized as follows:

1. Digestion: Carbohydrates and fats;
2. Lubrication: taste, swallowing and speech;
3. Anti-microbial activity: anti-bacterial and anti-fungal;
4. Buffering activity and clearance;
5. Protection / Immunity;
6. Maintenance of tooth integrity;
7. Taste sensation;
8. Tissue repair.

Digestion of Carbohydrates and Fats

Saliva begins the digestive process. It plays a crucial role in the *digestion of carbohydrates and fats* through two main enzymes. The first is *Ptyalin*, which is an *α-amylase* in saliva that cleaves the internal α-1,4-glycosidic bonds of starches to produce maltose, maltotriose, and α-limit dextrins. This enzyme functions at an optimal pH of 7, but rapidly denatures when exposed to a pH less than 4, such as when in contact with the acidic secretions of the stomach. Up to 75% of the carbohydrate content in a meal, however, is broken down by the gastric enzyme because a significant portion of an ingested meal remains unmixed within the oral region, and thus there is a delay in the mixture of gastric juices with the food bolus.

Starch digestion is not slowed in the absence of ptyalin because pancreatic amylase is identical to salivary amylase and is thus able to break down all carbohydrates when in the small intestine.

The second enzyme is produced by the salivary glands of the tongue (*lingual lipase*), which breaks down triglycerides. Unlike ptyalin, this enzyme is functional within the acidic stomach and proximal duodenum because it is optimally active at a low pH (*John, 2018)*.

Lubrication (Mastication, Swallowing, Speech)

The best lubricating components of saliva are *mucins*: they have the properties of low solubility, high viscosity, high elasticity, and strong adhesiveness.

Any intraoral contact between soft tissues, between soft tissues and teeth, or between soft tissues and prostheses benefits from the lubricating capability of saliva supplied largely by these mucins.

Mastication, speech, and swallowing and traveling of the bolus down the esophagus all are aided by the lubricating effects of mucins.

Anti-Microbial Action (Anti-Bacterial / Anti-Fungal)

Mucins also perform an *anti-bacterial function* by selectively modulating the adhesion of micro-organisms to oral tissue surfaces, which contributes to the control of bacterial and fungal colonization.

Saliva can prevent microbial growth based on the elements it contains. For example, *lactoferrin* in saliva binds naturally with iron. Since iron is a major component of bacterial cell walls, removal of iron breaks down the cell wall, which in turn breaks down the bacteria. Anti-microbial *peptides* such as histatins inhibit the growth of Candida albicans and Streptococcus mutans. Salivary Immunoglobulin A serves to aggregate oral bacteria such as S. mutans and prevents the formation of dental plaque (Allegra, 2018).

Protection / Immunity

The *anti-bacterial properties* of saliva are due to its many protective organic constituents. The binding glycoprotein for immunoglobulin A (IgA), known as the *secretory piece*, forms a complex with IgA that is immunologically active against viruses and bacteria.

Lysozyme causes bacterial agglutination and autolysin activation to degrade bacterial cell walls. *Lactoferrin* inhibits the growth of bacteria that need iron by chelating with the element. *Xerostomia*, (dry mouth), due to lack of salivation, can lead to chronic buccal mucosal infections or dental caries.

As a seromucous coating, saliva lubricates and protects oral tissues, acting as a barrier against irritants. These irritants include, but are not limited to, proteolytic and hydrolytic enzymes produced in plaque, potential carcinogens from smoking and exogenous chemicals, and desiccation from mouth breathing.

Many agents and viruses are actively excreted in Saliva. Mercury poisoning can manifest as stomatitis and lead poisoning by the gingival deposition of lead. The viruses causing rabies and poliomyelitis are excreted into saliva and can be transmitted in this manner.

Buffering Action and Clearance

Saliva also serves as a *protective buffer* for the mouth by diluting harmful substances and lowering the temperature of solutions that are too hot. It washes out foul-tasting substances from the mouth and neutralizes gastric juice to protect the oral cavity and esophagus (Allegra, 2018).

The buffer capacity of both unstimulated and stimulated saliva involves 3 major buffer systems: the bicarbonate, the phosphate, and the protein buffer systems. These systems have different pH ranges of maximal buffer capacity, the bicarbonate and phosphate systems having pH values of 6.1-6.3 and 6.8-7.0, respectively.

Dilution and removal of substances (oral debris, noxious agents) from the oral cavity is referred to as *salivary or oral clearance*. Both the act of swallowing and the salivary flow rate are important to this process, and these are the principal ways by which oral bacteria and injurious, noxious agents are eliminated from the mouth. Accordingly, a high salivary flow rate results in a high clearance and vice versa.

The oral sugar clearance becomes extensively prolonged when the whole unstimulated saliva flow rate is below 0.2 ml/min. Apart from clearing sugars, saliva also clears dietary acids and thereby protects the teeth against erosion.

In general, the higher the flow rate, the faster the clearance and the higher the buffer capacity. Dental caries is probably the most common consequence of hyposalivation. A low flow rate combined with a low or moderate buffer effect clearly indicates poor salivary resistance against microbial attack.

Maintenance of Tooth Integrity

Saliva forms a pellicle on the surface of the tooth to prevent wearing. The film contains mucins and proline-rich glycoprotein from the saliva. The proteins (statherin and proline-rich proteins) within the salivary pellicle inhibit demineralization and promote remineralization by attracting calcium ions *(Nanci, 2003)*.

Demineralization occurs when acids diffuse through plaque and the pellicle into the liquid phase of enamel between enamel crystals. A pH of 5 to 5.5 is the critical pH range for the development of caries. When this occurs, the buffering capacity effect of saliva (increases saliva flow rate) inhibits demineralization. Saliva can then begin to promote the *remineralization* of the tooth by strengthening the enamel with calcium and phosphate minerals (remineralization is the replacement of lost minerals via the organic matrix of the enamel to the crystals) *(Nanci, 2003).*

Taste Sensation

The sense of taste is activated during the initial stage of ingestion of food particles allowing for identification of essential nutrients and of harmful and potentially toxic compounds. Taste is a main stimulant for formation of saliva. On the other hand, presence of saliva in the oral cavity is also essential for taste perception, first of all because food particles need to be in solution in order to stimulate taste receptor cells in the taste buds within the lingual papillae (fungiform, foliate, and vallate papillae) (Nanci, 2003; Matsuo, 2000).

Furthermore, taste sensitivity is related to saliva composition as each receptor cells upper surface is bathed by the oral fluids. The hypotonicity of saliva enhances the tasting capacity of salty foods and nutrient sources. This enhanced tasting capability depends on the presence of gustin, which binds zinc.

Tissue Repair

Saliva can encourage soft tissue repair by decreasing clotting time, increasing wound contraction, production of growth factors and other regulatory peptides *(Mandel, 1987).*

CONTROL FO SALIVA SECRETION

The secretion, blood flow, and growth of salivary glands are mostly controlled by both branches of the autonomic nervous system. Even though the parasympathetic nervous system has more influence on the secretion rate of the salivary glands than the sympathetic system, secretion is *stimulated* by both branches.

Parasympathetic System

Parasympathetic innervation of the major salivary glands follows branches of the facial and glossopharyngeal nerves. Parasympathetic stimulation activates both acinar activity and ductal transport mechanisms, leading to glandular vasodilatation and myoepithelial cell contraction. *Acetylcholine* (ACh) serves as the parasympathetic neurotransmitter that acts on the muscarinic receptors of the salivary glands. The subsequent formation of inositol trisphosphate leads to increased calcium (Ca) concentrations within the cell, released from either intra-cellular Ca stores or from the plasma. This second messenger significantly effects salivary volume secretion. Glandular secretion is sustained by *acetylcholin esterases*, which inhibit the breakdown of ACh. The muscarinic antagonist *atropine*, however, decreases salivation by competing with ACh for the salivary receptor site.

Sympathetic System

Sympathetic supply to the salivary gland is mainly from the thoracic spinal nerves of the superior cervical ganglion. Like parasympathetic innervation, myoepithelial cell contraction also results. Changes in blood flow, however, are biphasic: vasoconstriction due to α-adrenergic receptor activation is followed by vasodilatation due to buildup of vasodilator metabolites. Binding of the neurotransmitter *norepinephrine* to α-adrenergic receptor results in formation of 3',5'-cyclic adenosine monophosphate (cAMP), which then leads to phosphorylation of various proteins and activation of different enzymes. Increases in cAMP result in increased salivary enzyme and mucus content.

Hormones

Within saliva, K^+ concentrations increase while Na^+ concentrations decrease in the presence of anti-diuretic hormone (ADH) or aldosterone. Unlike other digestive glands, however, these two hormones do *not* affect salivary gland secretion rate.

Hormones such as androgens, estrogens, glucocorticoids and peptides also influence salivary composition.

FLOW RATES OF SALIVA SECRETION

The amount of saliva is affected by the total body fluid volume and so dehydration decreases its amount and the so one feels thirsty. In normal circumstances, the minimal total unstimulated salivary flow rate is 0.1 mL per minute, and the minimal stimulated flow rate is 0.2 mL per minute. Maximal stimulated flow rate is 7 mL per minute. The 24-hour volume of salivary secretion has been estimated to be 500 to 1,500 mL. Salivary flow in the unstimulated glands is produced primarily by the submandibular glands (65%), with the parotid, sublingual and minor glands providing 20% and 7% to 8% of the flow, respectively. Once stimulated, the relative contributions of the parotid and submandibular glands are reversed, with the parotid gland supplying greater than 50% of the flow. The minor salivary glands, independent of stimulation, produce less than 10% of the total flow.

The two main *triggers* for salivary production are mastication and gustatory stimuli. Acidic foods are the best stimulus and sweet tastes the least. Olfaction is surprisingly a poor secretory stimulus. The presence of food in the mouth, the act of chewing, and nausea all stimulate salivation, while sleep, fatigue, dehydration, and fear inhibit it. Salivary flow rates are independent of age and flow rates remain constant despite the degeneration of acinar cells during the aging process. *Xerostomia* in the elderly is probably the result of systemic disease or medication side-effects. Salivary gland hypofunction is defined as an unstimulated flow rate less than 0.1 mL per minute or a 50% reduction below basal rates if they have been determined (Kontis, 2001; Holsinger, 2007).

APPLIED PHYSIOLOGY

Hyposalivation

Reduction in salivation (hyposalivation) may be temporary or permanent. Temporary hyposalivation may result from dehydration, fever, or emotional conditions such as fear. Permanent hyposalivation may result from congenital absence (aplasia) or hypoplasia of salivary glands, sialolithiasis, or Bell's palsy.

Xerostomia (Dry Mouth, Pasties, Cotton Mouth)

It results from hyposalivation or aptyalism and may be 1^{ry} or 2^{ry}. The main causes include dehydration due to renal failure, shock, Sjogrin's syndrome, trauma to the gland or ducts, post-radiotherapy, side-effects of some drugs, after smoking marijuana.

Xerostomia is usually not a problem until the flow rate is <0.2 ml/min/gland. Patients suffering from xerostomia can experience difficulty with eating, swallowing, speech, the wearing of dentures, trauma to and ulceration of the oral mucosa, taste alteration, poor oral hygiene, a burning sensation of the mucosa, oral infections including Candida and rapidly progressing dental caries.

Hypersalivation (Pytialism, Sialorrhea, Sialism, Sialosis)

It means excess of saliva secretion and may be *physiological* as in pregnancy or *pathological* as in the following conditions; tooth decay or neoplasm if the mouth or tongue, diseases of the esophagus, stomach or intestine, neurological disorders like cerebral palsy and mental retardation, cerebral stroke, parkinsonism, and nausea and vomiting.

Drooling

It means uncontrolled flow of saliva with inability to retain saliva in the mouth. It occurs in the following conditions; during teeth eruption in children, upper respiratory tract infection or nasal allergies in children, dysphagia, tonsillitis, and peritonsillar abscess.

Paralytic Secretion of Saliva

It results from iatrogenic / traumatic severance of the parasympathetic nerve supply. It leads to increased salivary secretion for 3 weeks (known as paralytic secretion) due to the release of large amounts of adrenalin from the adrenal medulla after denervation. This is followed by reduction in secretion and finally cessation in about the 6th week. Cutting of the sympathetic nerve sully (sympathectomy) does *not* influence paralytic secretion.

Augmented Secretion of Saliva

If the nerves supplying the salivary glands are stimulated twice, the amount of saliva secreted by the second stimulus is larger than that due to the first stimulus. This is explained by the fact that the first stimulus increases excitability of acinar cells. So that when the second stimulus is applied, salivary secretion is augmented.

REFERENCES

Allegra, C. (2018). Saliva. *Flipper e nuvola.*

Holsinger, F. C., & Bui, D. T. (2007). Anatomy, function, and evaluation of the salivary glands. In E. N. Myers & R. L. Ferris (Eds.), *Salivary Gland Disorders* (pp. 1–16). Berlin: Springer-Verlag. doi:10.1007/978-3-540-47072-4_1

John, T. (2018). *Immunity in the oral cavity.* British Society for Immunology, Newcastle University.

Kontis, T. C., & Johns, M. E. (2001). Anatomy and Physiology of the Salivary Glands. In B. J. Bailey (Ed.), *Head and Neck Surgery – Otolaryngology.* Philadelphia, PA: Lippincott Williams & Wilkins.

Mandel, I. D. (1987). The functions of saliva. *Journal of Dental Research, 66*(1_suppl), 623–626. doi:10.1177/00220345870660S103 PMID:3497964

Matsuo, R. (2000). Role of Saliva in the maintenance of taste sensitivity. *Critical Reviews in Oral Biology and Medicine, 11*(2), 216–229. doi:10.1177/10454411000110020501 PMID:12002816

Nanci, A. (2003). *Ten Cate's Oral Histology: Development, Structure, and Function* (6th ed.). St. Louis: Mosby.

Chapter 5
Evaluation of the Parotid Gland

ABSTRACT

This chapter describes the clinical, laboratory, imaging, endoscopic, and histological methods for evaluation of the parotid gland. Diagnostic approaches of parotid gland disorders include clinical evaluation in the form of history-taking (complaints, demographic data, medical profile, medications, and history of the parotid mass itself) and physical examination (intra-oral, extra-oral, and bidigital examination). Laboratory tests entail saliva collection for detection of changes in salivary flow and/or composition. Parotid gland imaging include plain x-ray, sialography, ultrasound (US), computed tomography (CT) scan and CT-sialography, magnetic resonance imaging (MRI), and MR-sialography. Other studies include endoscopy (sialoendoscopy) and parotid biopsy (core-biopsy, frozen-section) and fine needle aspiration cytology (FNAC).

CLINICAL EVALUATION

Despite the availability of modern technology in diagnosis of parotid gland disorders, great care should be taken during history-taking and thorough physical examination as they still play important roles in the clinical diagnosis of the patient.

DOI: 10.4018/978-1-7998-5603-0.ch005

History-Taking

Patients with parotid gland disorders usually *complain of* swelling, pain, xerostomia (dry mouth), foul taste, and occasionally sialorrhea (excessive salivation). Swelling and pain during meals followed by reduction in symptoms after meals may indicate partial stenosis of the duct. *Demographic data* (age / gender) are very important. The autoimmune disorder known as Sjogrin's syndrome, for example, is common in menopausal women while *mumps* usually occurs in children.

Medical profile of the patient may provide helpful clues to diagnosis. Gland dysfunction is often associated with certain systemic disorders such as diabetes mellitus (DM), atherosclerosis, hormonal imbalances and neurological disorders (Graamans, 1991; Mason, 1975). A careful *dietary and nutrition* history should not be neglected, for patients who suffer from chronic dehydration due to bulimia or anorexia or during chemotherapy are at risk for parotitis.

Drug history of the patient should also be considered, for salivary function is often affected by certain drugs such as diuretics and other anti-hypertensive drugs, which may cause xerostomia (Graamans, 1991; Mason, 1975). Since xerostomia is also a debilitating consequence of radiation therapy to the head and neck, history of *prior irradiation* should be sought.

For evaluation of a *parotid mass*, it is important to take history of the parotid mass duration, rate of growth and presence of pain, facial paralysis, cervical lymphadenopathy, eye and joint symptoms and irradiation exposure.

Physical Examination

Initial clinical evaluation involves careful examination of the head and neck regions. Both extra-oral and intra-oral examinations should be carried out in a systematic way to avoid missing any crucial signs. Bimanual palpation (extra-oral with one hand and intra-oral with the palmar aspects of the fingertips of the other) must be also performed to properly examine the submandibular glands.

Inspection

Extra-oral Inspection is performed with the patient facing in front of the examiner, three to four feet away. The examiner should inspect symmetry, color, pulsations, and discharging sinuses on both sides of the patient. Enlargement of the parotid gland may be unilateral or bilateral. *Parotitis* typically presents as pre-auricular swelling, but may not be visible if deep in the parotid tail or within the substance of the gland. Neurologic deficits should also be examined. Facial nerve paralysis in conjunction with a parotid mass, for example, should raise the suspicion of a *malignant* parotid neoplasm.

Intra-oral Inspection is done using a torch or headlight. The orifices of the parotid (Stensen's) ducts are inspected opposite the second upper molar tooth and the two sides compared. Saliva may be seen pouring from the non-affected side only.

Palpation

With the examiner standing in front of or behind the patient, the patient's head is inclined forwards to maximally expose the parotid gland region. Size, tenderness, consistency, mobility, and other features of the parotid gland and associated masses can be easily evaluated with *extra-oral and intra-oral palpation* owing to the superficial anatomical location of the gland.

Auscultation

Rare clinical entities, such as *hemangiomas* and other vascular anomalies, may be identified by auscultation.

LABORATORY STUDIES

Changes in Saliva in Disease

Salivary Flow

Most causes of xerostomia (dry mouth) are systemic in nature, but a significant percentage are idiopathic Dehydration, hospital admission, mental stress, psychopathic emotional states (e.g. depression), fatigue, infection, raised ambient temperature, tranquilizers, ganglionic blockers and light deprivation *decrease* salivary flow. In addition, pernicious and iron-deficiency anemia and loss of salivary tissue (due to irradiation, infection or Sjogren's syndrome) cause decreased flow. After a full-course of radiation therapy flow rates are reduced by 95% or more and this reduction persists indefinitely (Dreizen, Daley, Drane & Brown, 1977). Histopathological studies have shown that the parotid acini and serous cells from the submandibular gland are severely injured, but there is little discernible change in the mucous cells.

On the other hand, cigarette smoking, acute stomatitis, heavy metal poisoning, acrodynia, rabies, ingestion of highly seasoned foods and schizophrenia *increase* the flow. Chewing on one side of the mouth increases the flow on that side.

Salivary Composition

Many diseases affect salivary composition. Primary *aldosteronism* causes a decreased sodium (Na) level with normal potassium (K) content. ANa-K ratio of 0.3 or less is diagnostic, below 0.5 is suggestive and above 1.0 rules out aldosteronism (normal, 1.3) (Lawler, Hickler, & Thorn, 1962). Low Na-K ratios are also found in *Cushing's* disease with a mean ratio of 0.5.24. High ratios occur in *Addison's* disease with a mean ratio of 5.0 (Frawley & Thurn, 1951). In *pregnancy*, the submandibular calcium (Ca) concentration is reduced, whereas the Na concentration is reduced and the K concentration is increased in both parotid and submandibular saliva (Marder, Wotman, & Mandel, 1972).

The salivary glands, like the other exocrine glands, are affected by *cystic fibrosis* (Di Sant' Agnese & Davis, 1976). Total protein, amylase, lysozyme and glycoprotein concentrations are increased in submandibular but *not* in parotid saliva (Mandel, Kutscher, Denning, Thompson, Jr., & Zegarelli, 1967). There is no change in the flow rate in the major glands (Bloomfield, Rush, Allars, & Brown, 1976), but there is a significant reduction in the minor glands (Kurscher, Denning, & Zegarelli, 1968).

Thyroid diseases and their treatment may affect the saliva. The salivary glands concentrate iodine to 40 times the plasma level, regardless of the thyroid-stimulating hormone (TSH) level or the state of thyroid function (Mason, Harden, & Alexander, 1967). *Hyper-parathyroidism* causes an increased amount of Ca and phosphorus (P) in saliva, with the levels paralleling the parathormone levels (Weinberger, Sperling, & DeVries, 1974). In cases of *essential hypertension*, Na concentration and flow rate are decreased (Niedermeier, Dreizen, Stone, & Spies, 1956). In *sarcoidosis*, amylase and kallikrein levels are decreased, whereas albumin and lysozyme concentrations are increased (Bhoola, 1969; Beeley, 1976). *Acute pancreatitis* may cause an increase in the amount of amylase. *Alcoholic cirrhosis* may cause an increased flow rate with increased concentrations of potassium and amylase (Abelson, Mandel, & Karmiol, 1976).

Inflammatory lesions may cause changes in saliva. In acute infections, the Na and K levels approach those of serum (Masson, Heremans, Prignot, & Wauters, 1966). There is also a pronounced decrease in phosphate concentration. Other elements that are increased in amount include glucose, IgA, IgG, IgM, albumin and transferrin, which leak from plasma, and myeloperoxidase, lactoferrin and lysozyme, which are produced by the inflammatory infiltrate. IgG dominates the immunoglobulins, reflecting the normal serum pattern rather than the normal salivary pattern, in which IgA dominates.

Irradiation causes also alteration in the composition of saliva with increased amounts of Ca, Na, chloride, and protein and a decrease in bicarbonate. These changes lead to a significant rise in the number of dental caries.

Numerous systemically administered *drugs* can be detected in saliva, including iodide, heavy metals, thiocyanate, morphine, clindomycin and rifampin (Mandel, 1980). Digitalis toxicity causes greatly elevated levels of K and Ca, and this study can be used to distinguish between toxic and therapeutic doses (Wotman, Bigger, Mandel, & Bartelstone, 1971).

IMAGING STUDIES

For patients with no-specific symptoms (swelling and pain) and unclear physical signs, imaging studies can play an important role in clarifying the etiology of the gland disorder and assist in treatment selection and planning. These include conventional radiology (plain X-ray), sialography, ultrasound (US), computed tomography (CT) scan and CT-sialography, magnetic resonance imaging (MRI) and MR-sialography (Ginat, 2018).

Conventional Radiography (Plain X-Ray)

Conventional Radiography and *Sialography* were widely used in the past but are rarely used nowadays because of their limited value.

For the parotid gland, antero-posterior (AP), tangential, lateral and lateral oblique plain radiographs may be useful in showing calculi, calcifications, soft tissue swellings and bony erosions.

Sialography

The beginnings of the sialographic studies are dated 1902 (White, Pharoah, Wydawnictwo, & Wyd, 2002). Sialography visualizes the ducts and the parenchyma of the salivary gland, after contrast administration into the main salivary duct. For decades it has been the main diagnostic method in the salivary glands (Forman, 1977).

Technique

Initial series of plain films are taken to identify radio-opaque calculi. A sialogogue (lemon juice or citric acid) is given to dilate the duct orifice. The duct is intubated by means of a blunt-tipped slightly angulated, metal cannula or fine thin-walled polyethylene catheter with a tapered end. Approximately, 0.5-1.5 ml of contrast medium (radio-opaque such as Lipiodol Ultrafluid) or a water soluble medium e.g. Hypaue (sodium diatrizoate) is slowly injected by hand until the duct system is filled. To complete examination few drops of lemon juice is given to stimulate salivation. After an interval of 10 minutes, a further plain film is taken, which normally shows most of contrast medium cleared from the ducts. Any filling defect (e.g. stone), retained sections (e.g. chronic sialadenitis), stricture (e.g. inflammation), extravasation (e.g. Sjogrin's syndrome), or irregular borders (e.g. tumor) are noted. Fistulae and abscesses cavities can also be displayed with this technique.

Indications

The main *indications* of sialography include sialolithiasis (or other obstructive disorders), chronic sialadenitis, tumors and duct lesions (Bialek, 2006; Yu, 2008; Forman, 1977; Kalk, 2001; Szolar, 1966; Kalinowski, 2002). It is advised to wait approximately 6 weeks from the moment of inflammatory symptom relief, until sialography (Kalk, Vissink, Fred, Möller, & Roodenburg, 2001). Sialography is also excellent in revealing and localizing calcifications close to salivary ducts (Obaid, Sinha, & Robinson, 2006). It also allows for a high-certainty discrimination of stone location; in the salivary duct or in parenchyma, which is crucial for the choice of the appropriate therapeutic method (Białek et al., 2006). However, it is not a method of choice in salivary gland tumor diagnosis (Yu, 2008; Eyjolsson, 1984; Bryan, 1982; Nixon, 1998). Nowadays, sialography and its modified version, CT sialography, are largely replaced with CT and MRI in salivary gland tumor diagnostics. In suspicion of a malignant tumor, the recommended diagnostic tool is contrast-enhanced MRI (Kalinowski, Heverhagen, Rehberg, Klose, & Wagne, 2002).

The diagnostic reliability of sialography was improved after the introduction of digital *subtraction sialography* (DSS) (Kalk et al., 2002). The use of post-processing enables for a subtraction of a bony background and contrast enhancement of the salivary ducts (Buckenham, George, & McVicar, 1994).

Contraindications

Sialography is *contra-indicated* in case of iodine allergy or acute sialadenitis as it can exacerbate the condition.

Disadvantages

The *disadvantages* of sialography include patient's exposure to ionizing radiation and iodine contrast media, pain during contrast medium injection into the salivary ducts, possibility of calculi dislocation towards the inside of the gland, quality of examination results is operator dependent and movement artifacts (Kaliowski, 2002; Jager, 2000; Necker, 2000). In addition, when interpreting sialography, it should be remembered that air bubbles, injected together with the contrast medium, may simulate the presence of the calculi (Jager et al., 2000).

Complications

Sialography complications include salivary duct perforation, activation of a dormant inflammation, adverse reactions to iodine contrast medium, and bleeding.

Advantages

Sialography requires a lower x-ray radiation dose as compared to CT scan and is more accessible than MRI (Drage, Brown, & Wilson, 2000). Moreover, sialography, owing to its possibilities of a detailed visualization of anatomical and pathological structures of the salivary ducts, plays an important role in the qualification of patients for sialoendoscopic procedures, and in choosing the strategy of the procedure (Hasson, 2007). Despite these advantages, sialography being an invasive investigation has largely been *replaced* by magnetic resonance (MR) sialography.

Ultrasonography (US)

Parotid (and submandibular) glands are examined with US using a 7.5 MHz or higher frequency linear array transducer with patients chin turned away from the side being examined. Both glands have homogenous echo pattern with scattered echogenic steaks produced by branch ducts converging into the main duct. The external carotid artery (ECA) and retromandibular vein can both be seen. Few lymph nodes can by seen within the gland.

Ultrasound (US) remains the initial non-invasive investigation of choice due to its high resolution, easy availability and ability to guide needle biopsy. Ultrasound can detect around 95% of space-occupying lesions of major salivary glands (Gritzmann, Rettenbacher, Hollerweger, Macheiner, & Hubner, 2003). *Color Doppler* can add to the value of US by depicting the blood flow within the lesion.

Computed Tomography (CT)

The parotid gland has low attenuation due to its high fat content and is therefore easily discernible by CT scanning. Computed tomography scanning involves radiation exposure and IV injection of iodinated contrast enhancement, which increases the conspicuity of parotid masses and affords some prediction of their nature. It is useful in situations where magnetic resonance imaging (MRI) is not readily available.

The CT scan should extend from the skull base to the level of the hyoid bone, to demonstrate the facial nerve and to ensure that the parotid tail and the high deep cervical and jugulo-digasric lymph nodes have been included. The parotid duct will be demonstrated on thin sections taken parallel to the hard palate.

The *advantage* of CT imaging is the two-dimensional view of the salivary gland, which can elucidate relationships to adjacent vital structures, differentiate intrinsic from extrinsic disease, and assess the draining cervical lymph nodes.

Differences between intrinsic and extrinsic parotid gland masses, however, are often difficult to assess especially when present in the para-pharyngeal space (Som & Biller, 1979). CT scan is also extremely valuable in defining abscess formation versus phlegmon. In addition, several aspects such as detection of calculus, involvement of mandible and widening of foramina of skull base in case of perineural spread are better seen on CT (Yousem, Kraut, & Chalian, 2000). However, it is *limited* in evaluating the ductal system unless combined with simultaneous sialography (*CT-sialography*) (Quinn Jr., 1976).

CT sialography is an alternative method of increasing conspicuity of parotid masses, but the technique is invasive and is *not* widely practiced as MRI is more beneficial. Presence of metallic dentures / metallic fillings can cause artifacts on CT scanning.

Magnetic Resonance Imaging (MRI)

Magnetic resonance imaging (MRI) gives excellent soft tissue contrast of parotid lesions against a fatty background. It is currently the test of choice in evaluating salivary gland lesions. Not only can it identify and properly size most lesions, but its higher soft tissue resolution allows for better identification of internal tumor characteristics, better definition of tumor margins, and most importantly, identification of perineural spread. In addition, advanced MRI techniques such as diffusion-weighted imaging (DWI) have proven helpful in better characterizing various lesions (i.e., identifying malignant transformation of a pleomorphic adenoma as areas of low apparent diffusion coefficient [ADC] signal in an otherwise hyperintense mass) (Kessler & Bhatt, 2018).

Compared with CT, MRI provides better contrast resolution, exposes the patient to less harmful radiation, reduces artifacts from dental amulgum and yields detailed images on several different planes without patient repositioning (multiplanar imaging). However, *Gadolinium* contrast enhancement decreases the conspicuity of some parotid masses.

MRI is more often used for assessment of para-pharyngeal space abnormalities especially in discriminating between deep lobe parotid tumors and other lesions, such as Schwannoma and/or glomus vagale. Parotid gland masses have low T1 signal, particularly contrasted against the fatty stroma of the parotid. Fat suppressed T1 sequences are superior in determining the extent of invasion. However, MRI is inferior to CT scanning for the detection of early bone erosion and calcification, the presence of which is important in diagnosis of pleomorphic adenoma and sialolithiasis. Chronic inflammation of the salivary glands and calculi are *not* indications for MRI.

MR sialography has been described using heavy T2W1, which contrasts ductal fluid against stroma. It helps in the diagnosis of sialectasis upto some extent.

Figure 1. Algorithm of parotid swelling imaging

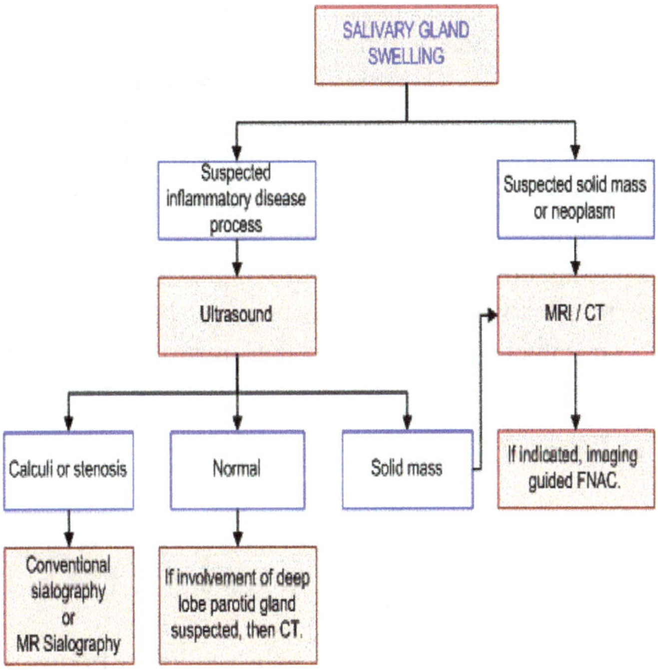

Algorithm of Imaging

An algorithm for imaging of parotid gland swellings, whether cystic or solid, and whether suspected to be inflammatory or neoplastic in origin, is depicted in Figure 1.

ENDOSCOPY (SIALOENDOSCOPY)

Introduction

Sialoendoscopy is a minimally invasive technique that inspects the salivary glands using narrow-diameter, rigid fiberoptic endoscopes, introduced under direct vision through the ductal orifice after its dilatation with a lacrimal probe (Nahlieli & Baruchin, 1997). It is well-tolerated, with minimal complications and has thus opened up a new frontier for evaluation and treatment of salivary gland disorders (Ziegler, Hedemark, Brevik, B., Idris, & Isaksen, 2003).

Direct inspection of the glandular duct and hilum is performed during lavage of the duct. Thus, in one setting, at the time of diagnosis, treatment of benign lesions can be performed (Nahlieli & Baruchin, 2000). Through a CO_2-laser papillotomy, sialolithectomy can be easily performed. Pharmacotherapy and laser-ablation can also be performed. This relatively new technique is an efficient yet simple mode of treatment in the diagnosis and treatment of major salivary gland obstructions, strictures and sialoliths (salivary stones). Depending on the obstruction, sialoendoscopy can be conducted under local anesthesia in an outpatient office or in the operating room under general anesthesia.

Indications

Salivary gland *stones* are one of the major causes of salivary gland infections (sialadenitis). These types of stones can be found in 1.2% of the general population (Rauch, 1970).

The second leading cause of salivary obstruction is from strictures and adhesions, which may result from prior salivary gland infections, including those during childhood such as mumps. Most strictures could be seen in the parotid duct and mostly in the disease process of chronic recurrent sialadenitis.

Technique

Generally, the salivary duct opening needs to be either dilated or incised prior to intra-oral introduction of the endoscope into the gland through its natural orifice in the oral cavity or by a making a small incision in the duct opening. Once the sialoendoscope is in place, saline is utilized to dilate the salivary duct and its branching. Once the endoscopes are introduced into the gland, the internal anatomy is explored either for *diagnosis* or for *treatment* of a specific disease entity.

Instrumentation

The ability to perform this technique is the result of the development of miniaturized endoscopic imaging tools. The majority of sialoendoscopes that are currently in use are of the semi-rigid type, which allows for visualization of the diseased process, but the stiffness allows manipulation and navigation of the internal salivary anatomy.

Multiple types of micro-instrumentation are available by many companies, including grasping forceps, biopsy forceps, drills, needles, laser fibers, and lithotripters. Different practitioners utilize different systems according to the experience and clinical training of the surgeon.

Milestones in Sialoendoscopy

- Konigsberger et al. (1990) and Gundlach et al. (1990) separately performed sialoendoscopy when they introduced an endoscope into the major salivary glands;
- Katz (1991) introduced a 0.8-mm flexible endoscope to diagnose and treat salivary gland stones;
- Nahlieli et al. (1994) used a rigid mini-endoscope to diagnose and treat major salivary gland obstructions.

CYTOLOGY / BIOPSY

Fine Needle Aspiration Cytology (FNAC)

Fine-needle aspiration cytology (FNAC) guided by ultrasound imaging (US) is a widely used diagnostic tool to evaluate both inflammatory and neoplastic lesions of the salivary glands (Forman, 1977; Kalk, 2001; Szolar, 1966). FNAC became popular approximately 40 years ago (Frable & Frable, 1991). It is a minimally-invasive procedure that does *not* require anesthesia (David, Blaney, & Hearp, 2007), well-tolerated, simple, safe and cost-effective (Alphs, 2006; O'Donnel, 2009). Moreover, it can be easily repeated in case of non-diagnostic results, thus improving diagnostic precision (Stewart, MacKenzie,

McGarry, & Mowat, 2000). Furthermore, FNAC allows for improved patient selection for surgery since it can identify disorders such as reactive lymph nodes that might mimic parotid tumors clinically.

Nevertheless, the role of FNAC in the pre-operative evaluation is *not* universally established. At present, the debate focuses on the reliability of FNAC as a diagnostic tool and its usefulness in treatment planning. Although in some Hospitals, FNAC is performed in every case of parotid mass, some authors support the role of cytology only in a selected group of patients with suspected malignancy, metastatic carcinoma or lymphoma (Cohen et al, 2004). However, Butsakis et al stated that pre-surgical FNAC does not impact on the surgical handling of these lesions (Batsakis, Sueige, & El-Naggar, 1992).

At present, there is *no* consensus regarding the effective role of FNAC in the diagnostic work-up of parotid masses (Cohen, 2004; Wong, 2000). In the recent literature, sensitivity ranges from 57% to 98%, specificity from 56% to 100%, and accuracy from 78% to 98% (Frable, 1991; Stewart, 2000; Cohen, 2004; Zurrida, 1993; Jayarans, 1994; Atula, 1996; Cristallini, 1997;

Figure 2. Ultrasound-guided fine needle aspiration cytology

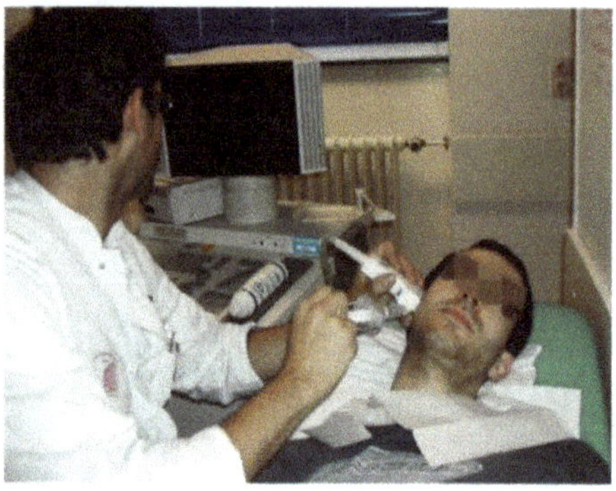

Cajolis, 1997; Al-Khafaji, 1998; Que-Hee, 2001; Bajaj, 2005; Carrillo, 2009). Different causes could account for this variability including the different methods adopted by different authors to classify and diagnose.

Image guidance also improves the yield of FNAC; US guidance (Figure 2) increases the diagnostic accuracy by enabling avoidance of necrotic or cystic regions and by targeting of higher yield areas of the lesion for tissue extraction (McIvor, 1994; Robinson, 1999; Sharma, 2001). Ultrasound guidance also allows the operator to confirm that the needle tip is inserted within the lesion.

Ultrasound Core-Biopsy (USCB)

The perceived and real diagnostic limitations associated with FNAC have led operators to explore alternative biopsy techniques. USCB is a safe and successful technique for the diagnosis of parotid lesions where FNAC is non-diagnostic (Buckland, Manjaly, Violaris, & Howlett, 1999) and is developing into an established technique. The technique (Buckland, 1999; Kesse, 2002) requires an operator, usually a radiologist trained in head and neck US and biopsy techniques. The procedure requires local anaesthetic infiltration, a small skin incision and the use of an automated spring-loaded biopsy device.

Figure 3. USCB undertaken with spring-loaded biopsy automated device, 22 mm throw, 18G-needle (N). Note needle deployed to traverse but not exit the lesion.

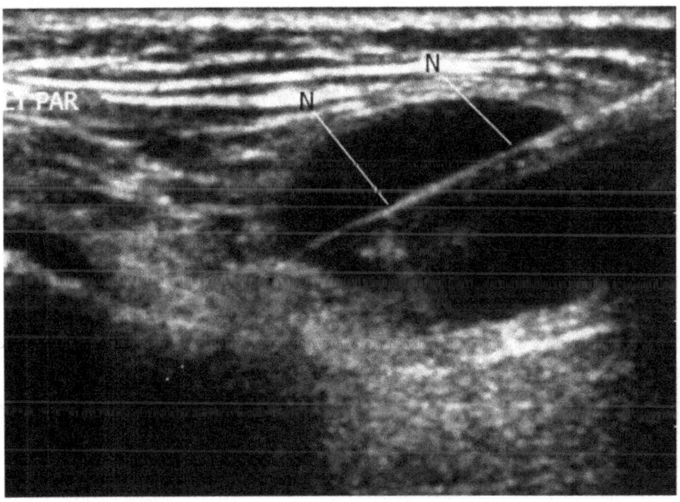

The throw is deployed under US guidance.

Figure 3 shows the biopsy needle within the lesion. The core of tissue is then processed by paraffin section histology. Sections from the core can be used for grading, staging and immunohistochemical analysis, allowing planning of appropriate operative or non-operative management. Figure 4 and Figure 5 show the results of a core biopsy macroscopically and microscopically, respectively. Immunofluorescence analysis is particularly useful for hematological malignancies (Buckland, 1999; Kesse, 2002).

This technique is already well-established in other areas of image-guided biopsy including the breast and abdomen (Zinzani et al., 1998) and is now

Figure 4. Image of biopsy specimen taken in Figure 3. 18G-needle in biopsy tray with overlying needle overlying sheath retracted.

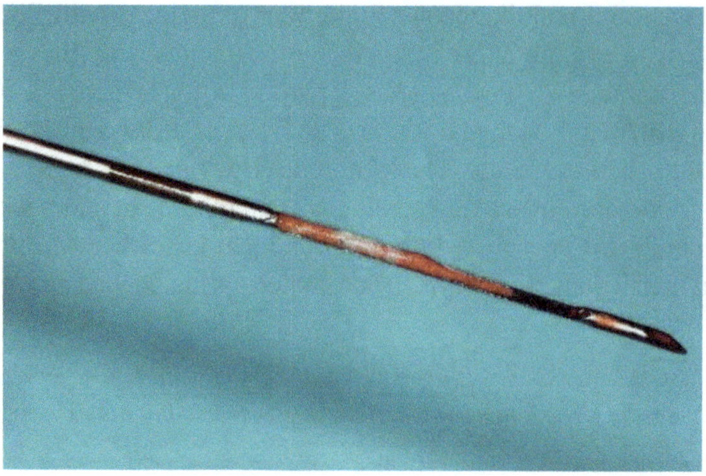

Figure 5. Low power image, H & E stain, of biopsy samples obtained in this case to give an idea of what material is available to the pathologist for reporting and immuno-histochemistry - final diagnosis in this case was B cell non-Hodgkin's Lymphoma

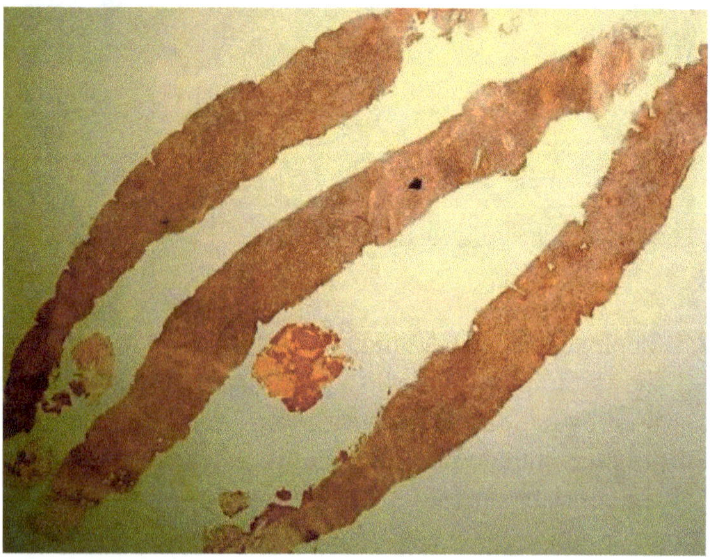

widely accepted by histopathologists and oncologists as a sufficient technique to allow tumor grading and typing (Burke et al., 2011).

A recent meta-analysis incorporates 12 studies and provides substantial evidence supporting the potentially superior diagnostic yield of USCB over FNAC as it showed a higher sensitivity (96%) and specificity (100%) compared to FNAC, a low complication rate (1.6% hematoma rate) and no variation in accuracy between locations (Witt & Schmidt, 2014). The low complication rate is attributed to the ability of US to visualize the vessels and allow the operator to infer the position of facial nerve branches. A systematic observational clinico-pathological study demonstrated USCB of salivary gland lesions to have sensitivity 94%, specificity 100%, accuracy 96%, positive predictive value 100% and negative predictive value 90% (Pfeiffer & Ridder, 2012). A study by Eom et al. (2015) also showed that trainees had a significantly lower accuracy with FNAC than USCB when diagnosing malignant tumors when compared to USCB with lymphomas being diagnosed much more accurately using USCB as reported by Huang et al. (2012).

Despite generally favorable outcomes and diagnostic advantages, USCB is not yet considered the reference standard in parotid lesion biopsy and the optimum technique remains controversial. The potential problems with USCB include possible false negative results, complications of a slightly more invasive technique and tumor seeding. Haldar et al. (2015) described 2 cases which were malignant clinically, on imaging and in the resected specimen, but benign on USCB (false negative). Also, some cases of well-differentiated malignancy require direct histological assessment of the whole excised lesion capsule to demonstrate invasiveness; USCB will miss this. This emphasizes that USCB should not be used alone in parotid lesion assessment.

Intra-Operative Frozen Section (IOFS)

Another salivary gland biopsy technique is intra-operative frozen section (IOFS), which is used in a small number of specialist centers as an alternative to FNAC or where FNAC is not performing well. Results can be telephoned to the surgeon within 20-30 minutes. This is useful where no pre-operative diagnosis is available, for example in deep parotid lesions not amenable to percutaneous biopsy or for lesions that are suspicious on clinical/imaging assessment but benign or considered non-representative on FNAC/USCB. Intra-operative frozen section can be employed to guide further surgical management while the patient is still on the operating table. A meta-analysis published in 2011 looking at data from 13 studies over a 25-year period described 90% sensitivity, 99% specificity and good consistency of results across study centers (Schmidt, Hunt, Hall, Wilson, & Layfield, 2011).

Intra-operative frozen-section (IOFS) *cannot* be recommended as a first-line diagnostic technique, which cannot be widely supported outside dedicated histopathology units. Most pathologists are reluctant to diagnose complex parotid lesions on the table in the absence of further techniques including immuno-fluorescence. The pitfalls and failures outlined above for USCB also apply to IOFS. In general, IOFS can be used as an adjunct to the less invasive options described where diagnostic suspicion and uncertainty remain (Haldar, Sinnott, Tekeli, Turner, & Howlett, 2016).

REFERENCES

Graamans, K., & von der Akker, H. P. (1991). History and physical examination. In A. K. Graamans (Ed.), *Diagnosis of Salivary Gland Disorders* (pp. 1–3). Dordrecht, Germany: Kluwer Academic Publishers. doi:10.1007/978-94-011-3608-2_1

Mason, D., & Chisholm, D. (1975). *Salivary Glands in Health and Disease*. London: WB Saunders.

Dreizen, S., Daley, T. E., Drane, J. B., & Brown, L. R. (1977). Oral complications of cancer radiotherapy. *Postgraduate Medicine*, *61*(2), 85–92. doi:10.1080/00325481.1977.11712115 PMID:834698

Lawler, D. P., Hickler, R. B., & Thorn, G. W. (1962). The salivary sodium-potassium ratio. *The New England Journal of Medicine*, *267*(22), 1136–1137. doi:10.1056/NEJM196211292672207

Frawley, T. F., & Thurn, F. W. (1951). The relation of the sodium-potassium ratio to adrenal cortical activity. In *Proceedings of Second Annual ACTH Conference*. London: Churchill Livingstone.

Marder, M. X., Wotman, S., & Mandel, I. D. (1972). Salivary electrolyte changes during pregnancy-I. Normal pregnancy. *American Journal of Obstetrics and Gynecology*, *112*(2), 233–236. doi:10.1016/0002-9378(72)90121-4 PMID:5008449 di Sant'Agnese, P. A., & Davis, P. B. (1976). Research in cystic fibrosis. *The New England Journal of Medicine, 295*(9), 481–485. doi:10.1056/NEJM197608262950905 PMID:781537

Mandel, I. D., Kutscher, A. H., Denning, C. R., Thompson, R. H. Jr, & Zegarelli, E. V. (1967). Salivary studies in cystic fibrosis. *American Journal of Diseases of Children, 113*, 431–438. PMID:6023475

Bloomfield, J., Rush, A. R., Allars, H., & Brown, J. M. (1976). Parotid gland function in children with cystic fibrosis and child control subjects. *Pediatric Research, 10*(6), 574–578. doi:10.1203/00006450-197606000-00004 PMID:1272635

Kurscher, A. H., Denning, C. R., & Zegarelli, E. V. (1968). Capillary tube test for minor salivary gland secretion in cystic fibrosis of pancreas. *New York State Journal of Medicine, 68*, 2812–2813. PMID:5247015

Mason, D. K., Harden, R., Mc, G., & Alexander, W. B. (1967). The salivary and thyroid glands. *British Dental Journal, 122*, 485–489. PMID:5229415

Weinberger, A., Sperling, O., & De Vries, A. (1974). Calcium and inorganic phosphate in saliva of patients with primary hyperparathyroidism. *Clinica Chimica Acta, 50*(1), 5–7. doi:10.1016/0009-8981(74)90070-9 PMID:4816443

Niedermeier, W., Dreizen, S., Stone, R. E., & Spies, T. (1956). Sodium and potassium concentrations in the saliva of normotensive and hypertensive subjects. *Oral Surgery, 9*(4), 426–431. doi:10.1016/0030-4220(56)90032-9 PMID:13309973

Bhoola, K. D., McNichol, N. W., Oliver, S., & Foran, J. (1969). Changes in salivary enzymes in patients with sarcoidosis. *The New England Journal of Medicine, 281*(16), 877–879. doi:10.1056/NEJM196910162811605 PMID:5812256

Beeley, J. A., & Chisholm, D. M. (1976). Sarcoidosis with salivary gland involvement: Biochemical studies on parotid saliva. *The Journal of Laboratory and Clinical Medicine, 88*, 276–281. PMID:956685

Abelson, D. C., Mandel, I. D., & Karmiol, M. (1976). Salivary studies in alcoholic cirrhosis. *Oral Surgery, 41*(2), 188–192. doi:10.1016/0030-4220(76)90230-9 PMID:1062747

Masson, P. L., Heremans, J. F., Prignot, J. J., & Wauters, G. (1966). Immunohistochemical localization and bacteriostatic properties of an iron-binding protein from bronchial mucus. *Thorax*, *21*(6), 538–544. doi:10.1136/thx.21.6.538 PMID:5339630

Mandel, I. D. (1980). Sialochemistry in diseases and clinical situations affecting salivary glands. *CRC Critical Reviews in Clinical Laboratory Sciences*, *12*(4), 321–366. doi:10.3109/10408368009108733 PMID:7002465

Wotman, S., Bigger, T. J. Jr, Mandel, I. D., & Bartelstone, H. J. (1971). Salivary electrolytes in the detection of digitalis toxicity. *The New England Journal of Medicine*, *285*(16), 871–876. doi:10.1056/NEJM197110142851601 PMID:5112729

Ginat, D. T. (2018). Imaging of Benign Neoplastic and Nonneoplastic Salivary Gland Tumors. *Neuroimaging Clinics of North America*, *28*(2), 159–169. doi:10.1016/j.nic.2018.01.002 PMID:29622111

White, S. C., Pharoah, M. J., Wydawnictwo, C., & Wyd, I. (2002). Radiologia Stomatologiczna. Academic Press.

Forman, W. H. (1977). Subtraction sialography. *Radiology*, *122*(2), 533. doi:10.1148/122.2.533 PMID:319483

Białek, E. J., Jakubowski, W., Zajkowski, P., & Kazimierz, T. (2006). US of the major salivary glands: Anatomy and spatial relationships, pathologic conditions, and pitfalls. *Radiographics*, *26*(3), 745–763. doi:10.1148/rg.263055024 PMID:16702452

Yu, C., Zheng, L., Yang, C., & Shen, N. (2008). Causes of chronic obstructive parotitis and management by sialoendoscopy. *Oral Surgery, Oral Medicine, Oral Pathology, Oral Radiology, and Endodontics*, *105*(3), 365–370. doi:10.1016/j.tripleo.2007.08.008 PMID:18280969

Forman, W. H. (1977). Subtraction sialography. *Radiology*, *122*(2), 536–339. doi:10.1148/122.2.533 PMID:319483

Kalk, W. W., Vissink, A., Fred, K. L., Möller, J. M., & Roodenburg, L. N. (2001). Morbidity from parotid sialography. *Oral Pathology. Oral Radiology and Endodontics*, *92*(5), 572–575. PMID:11709696

Szolar, D. H., Groell, R., Braun, H., Preidler, K., Stiskal, M., Kern, R., ... Stammberger, H. (1966). Ultrafast Computed Tomography and three-dimensional image processing of CT sialography in patients with parotid masses poorly defined by magnetic resonance imaging. *Acta Oto-Laryngologica*, *116*(1), 112–118. doi:10.3109/00016489609137723 PMID:8820361

Kalinowski, M., Heverhagen, J. T., Rehberg, E., Klose, K. J., & Wagne, H.-J. (2002). Comparative Study of MR Sialography and Digital Subtraction Sialography for Benign Salivary Gland Disorders. *AJNR. American Journal of Neuroradiology*, *23*(9), 1485–1492. PMID:12372736

Obaid, H., Sinha, R., & Robinson, L. (2006). Submandibular sialogram performed through a Wharton's duct fistula: Technical adaptation of conventional technique. *European Journal of Radiology*, *60*(1), 56–57. doi:10.1016/j.ejrad.2006.05.015 PMID:16815660

Eyjólfsson, O., Nordshus, T., & Dahl, T. (1984). Sialography and CT-sialography in the diagnosis of parotid masses. *Acta Radiologica Diagnostica*, *25*(5), 361–364. doi:10.1177/028418518402500502 PMID:6507130

Bryan, R. N., Miller, R. H., Ferreyro, R. I., & Sessions, R. B. (1982). Computed tomography of the major salivary glands. *AJR. American Journal of Roentgenology*, *139*(3), 547–554. doi:10.2214/ajr.139.3.547 PMID:6981322

Nixon, P. P., Lancer, J., & Bradley, M. J. (1998). Case Report: Percutaneous Sialography. *Clinical Radiology*, *53*(5), 381–383. doi:10.1016/S0009-9260(98)80015-9 PMID:9630281

Kalk, W. W., Vissink, A., Spijkervet, F. K., Bootsma, H., Kallerberg, C. G. M., & Roodenburg, J. L. N. (2002). Parotid sialography for diagnosing Sjögren syndrome. *Oral Surgery, Oral Medicine, Oral Pathology, Oral Radiology, and Endodontics*, *94*(1), 131–137. doi:10.1067/moe.2002.126017 PMID:12193907

Buckenham, T. M., George, C. D., McVicar, D., Moody, A. R., & Coles, G. S. (1994). Digital sialography: Imaging and intervention. *The British Journal of Radiology*, *67*(798), 524–529. doi:10.1259/0007-1285-67-798-524 PMID:8032804

Jäger, L., Menauer, F., Holzknecht, N., Scholz, V., Grevers, G., & Reiser, M. (2000). Sialolithiasis: MR Sialography of the Submandibular Duct – An Alternative to Conventional Sialography and US? *Radiology*, *216*(3), 665–671. doi:10.1148/radiology.216.3.r00se12665 PMID:10966693

Becker, M., Marchal, F., Becker, C. D., Dulguerov, P., Georgakopoulos, G., Lehmann, W., & Terrwer, F. (2000). Sialolithiasis and Salivary Ductal Stenosis: Diagnostic Accuracy of MR Sialography with a Three-dimensional Extended-Phase Conjugate-Symmetry Rapid Spin-Echo Sequence. *Radiology*, *217*(2), 347–358. doi:10.1148/radiology.217.2.r00oc02347 PMID:11058627

Drage, N. A., Brown, J. E., & Wilson, R. F. (2000). Pain and swelling after sialography: Is it a significant problem? *Oral Surgery, Oral Medicine, Oral Pathology, Oral Radiology, and Endodontics*, *90*(3), 385–388. doi:10.1067/moe.2000.108440 PMID:10982963

Hasson, O. (2007). Sialoendoscopy and Sialography: Strategies for Assessment and Treatment of Salivary Gland Obstructions. *Journal of Oral and Maxillofacial Surgery*, *65*(2), 300–304. doi:10.1016/j.joms.2005.12.052 PMID:17236938

Gritzmann, N., Rettenbacher, T., Hollerweger, A., Macheiner, P., & Hubner, E. (2003). Sonography of the salivary glands. *European Radiology*, *13*(5), 964–975. doi:10.100700330-002-1586-9 PMID:12695816

Som, P. M., & Biller, H. F. (1979). The combined computerized tomography-sialogram. A technique to differentiate deep lobe parotid tumors from extraparotid pharyngomaxillary space tumors. *The Annals of Otology, Rhinology, and Laryngology*, *88*(5 Pt 1), 590–595. doi:10.1177/000348947908800502 PMID:496192

Yousem, D. M., Kraut, M. A., & Chalian, A. A. (2000). Major Salivary Gland Imaging. *Radiology*, *216*(1), 19–29. doi:10.1148/radiology.216.1.r00jl4519 PMID:10887223

Quinn, H. J. Jr. (1976). Symposium: Management of tumors of the parotid gland. II. Diagnosis of parotid gland swelling. *The Laryngoscope*, *86*(1), 22–24. doi:10.1288/00005537-197601000-00004 PMID:1256198

Kessler, A. T., & Bhayy, A. A. (2018). Review of the major and minor salivary glands, part 2: Neoplasms and tumor-like lesions. *Journal of Clinical Imaging Science*, *8*, 1–9. doi:10.4103/jcis.JCIS_46_18 PMID:30546932

Nahlieli, O., & Baruchin, A. M. (1997). Sialoendoscopy: Three years' experience as a diagnostic and treatment modality. *Journal of Oral and Maxillofacial Surgery*, *55*(9), 912–918. doi:10.1016/S0278-2391(97)90056-2 PMID:9294498

Ziegler, C. M., Hedemark, A., Brevik, B., Idris, M., & Isaksen, R. (2003). Endoscopy as minimal invasive routine treatment for sialolithiasis. *Acta OdontoloticaScandanavica*, *61*(3), 137–140. doi:10.1080/00016350310001703 PMID:12868686

Nahlieli, O., & Baruchin, A. M. (2000). Long-term experience with endoscopic diagnosis and treatment of salivary gland inflammatory diseases. *The Laryngoscope*, *110*(6), 988–993. doi:10.1097/00005537-200006000-00020 PMID:10852519

Rauch, S. G. R. (1970). *Diseases of the Salivary Glands* (6th ed.). St. Louis, MO: Mosby.

Konigsberger, R., Feyh, J., Goetz, A., Schilling, V., & Kastenbauer, E. (1990). Endoscopic controlled laser lithotripsy in the treatment of sialolithiasis. *Laryngo- Rhino- Otologie*, *69*, 322–323. PMID:2378659

Gundlach, P., Scherer, H., & Hopf, J. (1990). Endoscopic-controlled laser lithotripsy of salivary calculi. In vitro studies and initial clinical use. *Hals Nase Ohren*, *38*, 247.

Katz, P. (1991). Endoscopy of the salivary glands. *Annales de Radiologie*, *34*, 110–113. PMID:1897843

Nahlieli, O., Neder, A., & Baruchin, A. M. (1994). Salivary gland endoscopy: A new technique for diagnosis and treatment of sialolithiasis. *Journal of Oral and Maxillofacial Surgery*, *52*(12), 1240–1242. doi:10.1016/0278-2391(94)90043-4 PMID:7965326

Frable, M. A., & Frable, W. J. (1991). Fine needle aspiration biopsy of salivary glands. *The Laryngoscope*, *101*(3), 245–249. doi:10.1288/00005537-199103000-00005 PMID:2000011

David, O. D., Blaney, S., & Hearp, M. (2007). Parotid gland fine-needle aspiration cytology: An approach to differential diagnosis. *Diagnostic Cytopathology*, *35*(1), 47–56. doi:10.1002/dc.20581 PMID:17173301

Alphs, H. H., Eisele, D. W., & Westra, W. H. (2006). The role of fine needle aspiration in the evaluation of parotid masses. *Current Opinion in Otolaryngology & Head & Neck Surgery*, *14*(2), 62–66. doi:10.1097/01.moo.0000193184.38310.0a PMID:16552260

O'Donnell, M. E., Salem, A., Badger, S. A., Sharif, M. A., Kamalapurkar, D., Lieo, T., & Spence, R. A. J. (2009). Fine needle aspiration at a Regional Head and Neck Clinic: A clinically beneficial and cost-effective service. *Cytopathology*, *20*(2), 81–86. doi:10.1111/j.1365-2303.2007.00549.x PMID:18241203

Stewart, C. J., MacKenzie, K., McGarry, G. W., & Mowat, A. (2000). Fine-needle aspiration cytology of salivary gland: A review of 341 cases. *Diagnostic Cytopathology*, *22*(3), 139–146. doi:10.1002/(SICI)1097-0339(20000301)22:3<139::AID-DC2>3.0.CO;2-A PMID:10679992

Cohen, E. G., Patel, S. G., Lin, O., Boyle, J. O., Kraus, D. H., Singh, B., ... Shaha, A. R. (2004). Fine-ne.edle aspiration biopsy of salivary gland lesions in a selected patient population. *Archives of Otolaryngology--Head & Neck Surgery*, *130*(6), 773–778. doi:10.1001/archotol.130.6.773 PMID:15210562

Batsakis, J. G., Sueige, N., & El-Naggar, A. K. (1992). Fine-needle aspiration of salivary gland: Its utility and tissue effects. *The Annals of Otology, Rhinology, and Laryngology*, *101*(2), 185–188. doi:10.1177/000348949210100215 PMID:1739267

Wong, D. S., & Li, G. K. (2000). The role of fine-needle aspiration cytology in the management of parotid tumors: A critical clinical appraisal. *Head & Neck*, *22*(5), 469–473. doi:10.1002/1097-0347(200008)22:5<469::AID-HED5>3.0.CO;2-7 PMID:10897106

Zurrida, S., Alasio, L., & Tradati, N. (1993). Fine needle aspiration of parotid masses. *Cancer*, *72*(8), 2306–2311. doi:10.1002/1097-0142(19931015)72:8<2306::AID-CNCR2820720804>3.0.CO;2-E PMID:8402443

Jayaram, G., Verma, A. K., Sood, N., & Khurana, N. (1994). Fine needle aspiration cytology of salivary gland lesions. *Journal of Oral Pathology & Medicine*, *23*(6), 256–261. doi:10.1111/j.1600-0714.1994.tb00055.x PMID:7932245

Atula, T., Greénman, R., & Laippala, P. (1996). Fine-needle aspiration biopsy in the diagnosis of parotid gland lesions: Evaluation of 438 biopsies. *Diagnostic Cytopathology*, *153*(3), 185–190. doi:10.1002/(SICI)1097-0339(199609)15:3<185::AID-DC2>3.0.CO;2-G PMID:8955598

Cristallini, E. G., Ascani, S., Farabi, R., Liberati, F., Macciò, T., Peciarolo, A., & Bolis, G. B. (1997). Fine needle aspiration biopsy of salivary gland, 1985-1995. *Acta Cytologica, 41*(5), 1421–1425. doi:10.1159/000332853 PMID:9305379

Cajulis, R. S., Gokaslan, S. T., Yu, G. H., & Frias-Hidvegi, D. (1997). Fine needle aspiration biopsy of the salivary glands. A five-year experience with emphasis on diagnostic pitfalls. *Acta Cytologica, 41*(5), 1412–1420. doi:10.1159/000332852 PMID:9305378

Al-Khafaji, B. M., Nestok, B. R., & Katz, R. L. (1998). Fine needle aspiration of 154 parotid masses with histologic correlation: Ten-year experience at the University of Texas, MD Anderson Cancer Center. *Cancer, 84*, 153–159. doi:10.1002/(SICI)1097-0142(19980625)84:3<153::AID-CNCR6>3.0.CO;2-P PMID:9678729

Que-Hee, C. G., & Perry, C. F. (2001). Fine-needle aspiration cytology of parotid tumours: Is it useful? *ANZ Journal of Surgery, 71*(6), 345–348. doi:10.1046/j.1440-1622.2001.02121.x PMID:11409019

Bajaj, Y., Singh, S., Cozens, N., & Sharp, J. (2005). Critical clinical appraisal of the role of ultrasound guided fine needle aspiration cytology in the management of parotid tumours. *The Journal of Laryngology and Otology, 119*(4), 289–292. doi:10.1258/0022215054020421 PMID:15949083

Carrillo, J. F., Ramirez, R., Flores, L., Ramirez-Ortega, M. C., Arrecillas, M. D., Ibarra, M., ... Oñate-Ocaña, L. F. (2009). Diagnostic accuracy of fine needle aspiration biopsy in preoperative diagnosis of patients with parotid gland mass. *Journal of Surgical Oncology, 100*(2), 133–138. doi:10.1002/jso.21317 PMID:19507187

McIvor, N. P., Freeman, J. L., Salem, S., Elden, L., Noyek, A. M., & Bedard, Y. C. (1994). Ultrasonography and ultrasound-guided fine-needle aspiration biopsy of head and neck lesions: A surgical perspective. *The Laryngoscope, 104*(6), 669–674. doi:10.1288/00005537-199406000-00005 PMID:8196441

Robinson, I. A., & Cozens, N. J. (1999). Does a joint ultrasound guided cytology clinic optimize the cytological evaluation of head and neck masses? *Clinical Radiology, 54*(5), 312–316. doi:10.1016/S0009-9260(99)90561-5 PMID:10362238

Sharma, G., Jung, A. S., Maceri, D. R., Rice, D. H., Martin, S. E., & Grant, E. G. (2011). US-guided fine-needle aspiration of major salivary gland masses and adjacent lymph nodes: Accuracy and impact on clinical decision making. *Radiology, 259*(2), 471–478. doi:10.1148/radiol.11101087 PMID:21364082

Buckland, J. R., Manjaly, G., Violaris, N., & Howlett, D. C. (1999). Ultrasound-guided cutting-needle biopsy of the parotid gland. *The Journal of Laryngology and Otology, 113*(11), 988–992. doi:10.1017/S0022215100145785 PMID:10696376

Kesse, K. W., Manjaly, G., Violaris, N., & Howlett, D. C. (2002). Ultrasound-guided biopsy in the evaluation of focal lesions and diffuse swelling of the parotid gland. *British Journal of Oral & Maxillofacial Surgery, 40*(5), 384–388. doi:10.1016/S0266-4356(02)00189-4 PMID:12379183

Zinzani, P. L., Colecchia, A., Festi, D., Magagnoli, M., Larocca, A., & Ascani, S. (1998). Ultrasound-guided core-needle biopsy is effective in the initial diagnosis of lymphoma patients. *Haematologica, 83*, 989–992. PMID:9864918

Burke, C., Thomas, R., Inglis, C., Baldwin, A., Ramesar, K., Grace, R., & Howlett, D. C. (2011). Ultrasound-guided core biopsy in the diagnosis of lymphoma of the head and neck. A 9 year experience. *The British Journal of Radiology, 84*(1004), 727–732. doi:10.1259/bjr/60580076 PMID:21427181

Witt, B. L., & Schmidt, R. L. (2014). Ultrasound-guided core needle biopsy of salivary gland lesions: A systematic review and meta-analysis. *The Laryngoscope, 124*(3), 695–700. doi:10.1002/lary.24339 PMID:23929672

Pfeiffer, J., & Ridder, G. J. (2012). Diagnostic value of ultrasound-guided core needle biopsy in patients with salivary gland masses. *International Journal of Oral and Maxillofacial Surgery, 41*(4), 437–443. doi:10.1016/j.ijom.2011.12.005 PMID:22204925

Eom, H. J., Lee, J. H., Ko, M. S., Choi, Y. J., Yoon, R. G., Cho, K. J., ... Baek, J. H. (2015). Compari.son of fine-needle aspiration and core needle biopsy under ultrasonographic guidance for detecting malignancy and for the tissue-specific diagnosis of salivary gland tumors Am*erica.n. Journal of Neuroradiology, 36*(6), 1188–1193. doi:10.3174/ajnr.A4247 PMID:25678480

Huang, Y. C., Wu, C. T., Lin, G., Chuang, W. Y., Yeow, K. M., & Wan, Y. L. (2012). Comparison of ultrasonographically guided fine-needle aspiration and core needle biopsy in the diagnosis of parotid masses. *Journal of Clinical Ultrasound, 40*(4), 189–194. doi:10.1002/jcu.20873 PMID:21953076

Haldar, S., Mandalia, U., Skelton, E., Chow, V., Turner, S. S., Ramesar, K., ... Howlett, D. (2015). Diagnostic investigation of parotid neoplasms: A 16-year experience of freehand fine needle aspiration cytology and ultrasound-guided core needle biopsy. *International Journal of Oral and Maxillofacial Surgery*, *44*(2), 151–157. doi:10.1016/j.ijom.2014.09.025 PMID:25457828

Schmidt, R. L., Hunt, J. P., Hall, B. J., Wilson, A. R., & Layfield, L. J. (2011). A systematic review and meta-analysis of the diagnostic accuracy of frozen section for parotid gland lesions. *American Journal of Clinical Pathology*, *136*(5), 729–738. doi:10.1309/AJCP2SD8RFQEUZJW PMID:22031311

Haldar, S., Sinnott, J. D., Tekeli, K. M., Turner, S. S., & Howlett, D. C. (2016). Biopsy of parotid masses: Review of current techniques. *World Journal of Radiology*, *8*(5), 501–505. doi:10.4329/wjr.v8.i5.501 PMID:27247715

Chapter 6
Xerostomia

ABSTRACT

Xerostomia is most commonly observed in patients treated with certain medications, those subjected to radiotherapy of the head and neck, or in individuals with Sjogren's syndrome. Although it mostly affects geriatric patients, xerostomia can be also observed in young individuals. This condition not only results from the physiological process of aging but is also associated with the number and type of medications administered in the treatment of various systemic conditions. Xerostomia is also a common manifestation in menopausal women due to estrogen deficiency. If it remains untreated, xerostomia can lead to nutritional deficiencies, decreased mood, and finally, depression. Treatment is long-term and requires a high level of patient motivation. Although no standard treatment guidelines are available, many treatment options exist: topical agents to alleviate and/or prevent xerostomia, systemic therapy, or newer devices. While systemic agents (pilocarpine or cevimeline) have been largely studied, new medical devices require large well-designed clinical trials.

INTRODUCTION

Xerostomia (also known as "dry mouth", "mouth dryness" and "oral dryness") is a subjective experience of dryness of the oral cavity resulting from insufficient saliva secretion or a complete lack of saliva (Wiener et al, 2010). Interestingly, patients complaining of xerostomia frequently do not show any objective sign of *hypo-salivation* and their symptoms may be

DOI: 10.4018/978-1-7998-5603-0.ch006

secondary to qualitative and/or quantitative changes in the composition of saliva (van der Putten, 2011; Fox, 1985).

Saliva plays a vital role in maintaining oral health. Its main *component* is water, constituting 99% of its volume. Other components, comprising the remaining 1%, include inorganic salts of sodium, potassium, calcium and magnesium, and organic compounds, such as cholesterol, uric acid and proteins (enzymes) (Ship, 2002; Guzik, 2009). The normal minimal *unstimulated* salivary flow rate (uSFR) is 0.1 mL per minute, and the minimal stimulated salivary flow rate (sSFR) is 0.2 mL per minute. Maximal stimulated flow rate is 7 mL per minute. The 24-hour volume of salivary secretion has been estimated to range from 500 mL to 1,500 mL (Glore, Spiteri-Staines, & Paleri, 2009).

The *principal functions* of saliva include the following:

- Initial digestion of carbohydrates and fats by salivary amylase and lipase, respectively (Guzik, 2009);
- Lubrication, which is essential for taste, swallowing and speech;
- Anti-microbial activity, both anti-bacterial and anti-fungal activity through mucin, lactoferrin and lysosymes;
- Buffering activity and clearance, helping maintaining oral pH within the 6.8–7.2 range; this is achieved by a hydrogen carbonate and phosphate buffering system (Guzik, 2009; Pichór, 2008). Saliva also washes out foul-tasting substances from the mouth and neutralizes gastric juice to protect the oral cavity and esophagus (Guzik & Kamyszm, 2009);
- Protection / Immunity via its anti-microbial properties, formation of sero-mucous coating and excretion of many irritant agents and viruses;
- Maintenance of tooth integrity: Saliva forms a pellicle on the surface of the tooth to prevent wearing. The film contains mucins and proline-rich glycoprotein. The proteins within the salivary pellicle inhibit demineralisation and promote remineralisation by attracting calcium ions (Ship, 2002);
- Modulation of taste sensation by the taste buds within the lingual papillae;
- Tissue repair: Saliva can encourage soft tissue repair by decreasing clotting time, increasing wound contraction, production of growth factors and other regulatory peptides (Mandel, 1987).

In view of the numerous functions played by saliva, any disorders of its secretion are reflected by an array of pathological changes, not only in the oral cavity but also within the alimentary tract (Guzik, 2009; Glore, 2009; Pichor, 2008; Atkinson, 2005; Porter, 2004).

CLASSIFICATION

Based on its *pathogenesis*, xerostomia is classified as true xerostomia (*xerostomia vera, primaria*), resulting from malfunction of the salivary glands, or pseudo xerostomia, also called symptomatic xerostomia (*xerostomia spuria, symptomatica*), in the course of which the patient has a subjective impression of oral dryness despite normal salivary function).

EPIDEMIOLOGY

Xerostomia affects millions of patients throughout the world. The prevalence of xerostomia depends on the population examined (Glore, 2009; Pichor, 2008), and ranges from 5.5% to 46%. Studies have shown differences in the prevalence between the sexes and xerostomia appears to increase with increasing age. The results of several clinical studies suggest that this disorder affects mostly menopausal women (Mirzaii-Dizgah & Agha-Hosseini, 2011), and individuals above the age of 65 years (Pichór & Doboszyńska, 2008). A possible explanation is that older individuals take several xerogenic drugs for their chronic conditions and this may lead to an overall reduction of the unstimulated salivary flow rate (Villa, 2011; Thomson, 2005; Leal, 2010; Astor, 1999; Liu, 2012; Locker, 1993; Thorselius, 2004). Nevertheless, xerostomia is also diagnosed in approximately 20% of 18- to 34-year-old individuals (Glore, "et al"., 2009).

ETIOLOGY

Causes of xerostomia can be classified as *systemic* or *local*. Based on the duration of symptoms, the condition is considered as *persistent* or *periodic*.

It should be remembered that mouth dryness is not always a symptom of true xerostomia. It is frequently a function of the overall status of the patient, resulting from fever, dehydration, cachexia, heatstroke, vomiting or diarrhea (Busato, Ignácio, Brancher, Moysés, & Azevedo-Alanis, 2012).

Moreover, xerostomia is sometimes referred to as *hypo-salivation;* however, these two terms are not synonymous and should not be used interchangeably. Hypo-salivation refers solely to decreased secretion of saliva due to external or internal influences, while xerostomia encompasses the final effect of salivary drainage, i.e. the process of its evaporation, absorption by mucosal membranes, or elimination by swallowing (Guzik, 2009).

Systemic Diseases

Xerostomia is not considered a separate clinical entity, but a disorder of systemic co-morbidities that lead to impaired salivary gland function. It accompanies several disorders such as hypercalcemia, vitamin deficiencies, anxiety, depression, schizophrenia, hyperthyroidism, and Type-1 diabetes mellitus (DM) (Busato, "et al"., 2012). Xerostomia can also be a manifestation of such conditions as Addison-Biermer anemia, Parkinson's syndrome (Guzik, 2009), Alzheimer's disease (Glore, "et al"., 2009), avitaminosis (B_1, B_2, B_6 and B_{12}), or even graft- versus-host disease (Guzik, 2009; Gurvits, 2013).

Endocrine Diseases

Diabetes Mellitus (DM)

Patients with uncontrolled DM often report dry mouth, which is believed to be due to polyuria, dehydration, and autonomic dehydration (Vasconcelos, Soares, Almeida, & Soares, 2010). The prevalence of xerostomia was reported in 14-62% of Type-2 DM patients (Bajaj, 2012; Khovidhunkit, 2009; Busato, 2009), and it was found in 38.5% and 53% of children and adolescents with Type-1 DM, respectively (Busato, 2009; Kosta, 2004).

Ivanowski et al. (2012) reported a close association between *insulin-dependent DM* (Type-1) and enhanced signs of mouth dryness. The authors observed a relationship between elevated salivary urea concentration and xerostomia in the studied subjects as compared to controls without xerostomia. They also documented an association between increased blood glucose concentration and signs of xerostomia.

Thyroid Disease

Mouth dryness is often reported by patients with autoimmune thyroid disease (AITD), including Graves' disease and Hashimoto's thyroiditis (Cooper et al, 2012). AITD is characterized by the presence of serum antibodies against thyroid-specific or thyroid-restricted antigens such as the thyroid stimulating hormone (TSH) receptor, thyroperoxidase (TPO), and thyroglobulin (Tg) (Hutfless, Matos, Talor, Caturegli, & Rose, 2012). The prevalence of AITD has been estimated as 5-15% in women and 1-5% in men. In other words, AITD can be regarded as the most common autoimmune endocrine disease (Cárdenas-Roldán, et al., 2012). A considerable number of patients with primary 2012Sjögren's syndrome (pSS) along with thyroid disease diagnosed by laboratory data and clinical presentation were reported (Karsh, Pavlidis, Weintraub, & Moutsopoulos, 1980). The coexistence of Sjögren's syndrome and thyroiditis is frequent suggesting a common genetic or environmental predisposing factor with similar pathogenic mechanisms. pSS was reported to be 10 times more frequent in patients with AITD, while autoimmune thyroiditis was 9 times more frequent in pSS. Therefore, Sjögren's syndrome should be studied in patients with thyroid disease and vice versa (D'Arbonneau, et al., 2003).

Viral Infections

Human Immunodeficiency Virus (HIV)

Human immunodeficiency virus (HIV) infection is one of the most devastating infections in modern times. Xerostomia can manifest in individuals infected with HIV and in patients with acquired immunodeficiency syndrome (AIDS). Oral manifestations of HIV infection occur in 30-80% of patients (Okoje, Obiechina, & Aken'Ova, 2006). Oral lesions occur early in patients with HIV infection and can predict progression to AIDS. The common HIV-related lesions include oral candidiasis, herpes simplex infection, oral Kaposi's sarcoma, oral hairy leukoplakia, parotid gland enlargement, peri-odontal diseases (linear gingival erythema and necrotizing ulcerative peri-odontitis), human papilloma virus-associated warts, and ulcerative conditions including herpes simplex virus lesions, recurrent aphthous ulcers, neutropenic ulcers, and xerostomia (Nokta, 2008; Reznik, 2005).

Xerostomia can occur due to the side-effects of HIV medications (e.g., didanosine), or the proliferation of CD8 + cells in the major salivary glands (Reznik, 2005). Parotid hypertrophy as a compensative reaction has been also found more commonly in HIV-positive children (Exposito, 2004; Pinto, 2004). In general, the prevalence of xerostomia has been estimated as 1.2-40% of HIV-positive patients (Sharma, 2006; Taiwo, 2006; Freed, 2005; Sontakke, 2011; Pinheiro, 2004). There is a conflict about xerostomia-related HIV medications in the literature; Lin et al. (2003) claimed that xerostomia was not compounded by medications in contrast to other researchers (Reznik, 2005; Pinheiro, 2004).

Jeganathan et al. (2012) reported that the patient's age and duration of HIV infection determine the occurrence of mouth dryness, which in turn is reflected by higher severity of caries and overall deterioration of the quality of life. Chronic inflammation of the salivary glands is observed despite implementation of anti-retroviral therapy, radically inhibiting the secretion of saliva and increasing the dryness of the oral mucosa (Cavasin-Filho & Giovani, 2009).

Hepatitis C Virus (HCV)

The HCV infection is a major health problem among the general population, and its extra-hepatic manifestations have been reported such as Sicca syndrome (Ramos, 2003; Prunoiu, 2008). Several autoimmune and immune complex-mediated disorders have been proposed to be related to HCV infection such as essential mixed cryoglobulinemia, which is frequently associated with Sjögren's syndrome. The association between HCV and Sjögren's syndrome may be related to the close association between HCV infection and mixed cryoglobulinemia, and the salivary gland tropism of HCV (Grossmamm et al., 2010). Although xerostomia has been reported among 5-55% of HCV-infected patients (Ramos, 2003; Grossmann, 2010; Nawito, 2011; Giordano, 2005), some studies did not find any relationship between xerostomia and the presence of HCV infection (de Mattos, 2010; Carrozzo, 2003). Xerostomia is also an adverse event during ribavirin-interferon therapy (Nagao, 2012; Aghero, 2011).

Epstein-Barr Virus (EBV)

Epstein-Barr virus (EBV) is a human herpes virus that establishes long-term latent infection in B-lymphocytes named EBV infectious mononucleosis (EBV-IM) (Arvey, Tempera, & Lieberman, 2013). EBV-IM is a common infection that affects 25-30% of adolescents and adults up to 30 years of age (Hallee, Evans, Niederman, Brooks, & Voegtly, 1974). Association between EBV and autoimmune diseases, such as rheumatoid arthritis (RA), systemic lupus erythematosus (SLE), multiple sclerosis, autoimmune thyroid disease (AITD), inflammatory bowel diseases (IBD), insulin-dependent DM, systemic sclerosis, myasthenia gravis, autoimmune liver diseases, and Sjögren's syndrome have been suggested (Lossius, Johansen, Torkildsen, Vartda, & Holmøy, 2012). It is proposed the inflammatory process in exocrine glands, which culminates in the Sicca syndrome is due to the combined effects of chronic EBV infection and autoimmunity. The mean titer of anti-EBV nuclear-antigen antibodies was significantly higher in Sjögren's syndrome patients than in normal people (Fox et al., 1987).

Cytomegalovirus (CMV)

Cytomegalovirus (CMV) is a common infection with a sero-prevalence among adolescents ranging from 47% to 89% (Stadler et al., 2010). The persistence of CMV with alteration of cell surface expression in certain tissues may initiate tissue destruction that leads to the clinical manifestations of Sjögren's syndrome. Ductal cells of salivary and lacrimal glands are immunologically attacked due to CMV antigenic expression leading to destruction of these ducts and consequently, xerostomia (Burns, 1983). However, no relationship between xerostomia and anti-CMV antibodies was noted (Scully, 1990).

Human T-Lymphotropic Virus Type-1

Human T-lymphotropic virus Type 1 (HTLV-1) is known to cause HTLV-associated myelopathy (HAM)/tropical spastic paraparesis and adult T-cell leukemia (Poetker et al., 2011). It is estimated that 15-20 million persons are currently infected with HTLV-1 worldwide (Proietti, Carneiro-Proietti, Catalan-Soares, & Murphy, 2005). Retroviruses such as HTLV-1 and HIV infect immuno-competent cells, resulting in the destruction or overstimulation of T-cells, and act as potential triggers for autoimmune disease (Manns & Rambusch, 1999).

Bacterial Infections

Actinomycosis

Actinomycosis is an anaerobic bacterial infection affecting men more frequently between the ages of 30-60 years. Approximately, 50% of actinomycosis cases occur in the cervicofacial region, and salivary glands may be involved as well. The organism can colonize inside the ducts of both submandibular and parotid glands and leads to abscess formation and reduction in salivary gland function (Neville, 2009; Mamais, 2011; Sittitrai, 2012).

Autoimmune Diseases

Chronic autoimmune conditions – rheumatoid arthritis (RA), chronic juvenile arthritis, sarcoidosis, systemic sclerosis, and especially Sjogren's syndrome deserve special consideration in relation to xerostomia.

Sjogrin's Syndrome / Miculicz's Disease

A classical triad predominates in *Sjogren's syndrome*; in addition to xerostomia, it also includes dry eye syndrome / kerato-conjuntivitis sicca and polyarthritis (Ramos-Casals, Brito-Zerón, Sisó-Almirall, & Bosch, 2012). The presence of proteins against glandular duct cells, anti-RO/SSA and anti-La/SSB antibodies and rheumatoid factor leads to the destruction of secretory vesicles with associated lymphocytic infiltration (Kobak, Oksel, Aksu, & Kabasakal, 2013). Xerostomia can be also observed in *Mikulicz's disease* (benign lympho-epithelial lesion), which is associated with swelling of the salivary glands as a result of lymphocytic infiltration (Guzik, 2009; Gurvits, 2013).

Rheumatoid Arthritis (RA)

Rheumatoid arthritis (RA) is a systemic disease of connective tissue origin, which affects 1% of the world population. Women are three times more affected than men. RA frequently presents with extra-articular features such as hematological, neurological, and cardiovascular involvement associated with dysfunction of lacrimal and salivary glands. Zalewska *et al.* showed impairment of salivary immunity system of the oral cavity in xerostomic patients with RA (Zalewska, et al., 2013). Secondary Sjögren's syndrome is associated with xerostomia and occurs with autoimmune diseases most frequently with RA (Anurag-Gupta, Epstein, & Sroussi, 2006).

Systemic Lupus Erythematosus (SLE)

Systemic lupus erythematosus (SLE) is an inflammatory connective tissue disease with characteristic auto-antibodies. SLE is much more common in women than men. It may occur at any age, but appears most often in people between the ages of 10 and 50 years. More than 75% of patients with SLE are affected with xerostomia. Coexistence of Sjögren's syndrome and SLE has been reported in one-third of SLE patients. SLE has been shown to be associated with a decreased unstimulated salivary flow rate (Jensen, Bergem, Gilboe, Husby, & Axell, 1999).

Primary Biliary Cirrhosis (PBC)

Primary biliary cirrhosis (PBC) is a cholestatic autoimmune disease predominantly of middle-aged women with progressive destruction of interlobular bile ducts (Anurag-Gupta, Epstein, & Sroussi H, 2006). The most autoimmune disease in PBC patients is Sjögren's syndrome (Karp, Akpek, & Anders, 2010) whose symptoms have been observed in 47-73% of patients (Kumagi, 2012; Selimi, 2012). Xerostomia and dysphagia may be associated with PBC (Mang et al., 1997).

Scleroderma (Progressive Systemic Sclerosis)

Scleroderma is a chronic sclerotic disease with deposition of extra-cellular matrix throughout connective tissue and vascular abnormalities, which leads to tissue hypoxia (Cazal et al., 2008). Fibrosis of capillaries, excretory ducts and acini of salivary and lacrimal glands are associated with xerostomia as oral manifestations of scleroderma (Albilia, Lam, Blanas, Clokie, & Sándor, 2007). Lymphocytic infiltration has been observed among 15% of patients with systemic sclerosis, which is a sign of secondary Sjögren's syndrome (Janin, Gosselin, Gosset, Hatron, & Sauvezie, 1989).

Granulomatous Diseases

Granulomatous diseases such as sarcoidosis and TB may cause salivary gland hypofunction and lead to xerostomia.

Sarcoidosis

Sarcoidosis is a systemic inflammatory disease with unknown etiology characterized by the presence of non-caseating granulomas that can affect any organ (mostly lungs and lymph nodes) (Sekhri, Sanal, DeLorenzo, Aronow, & Maguire, 2011). Coexistence of parotid and submandibular gland swelling and xerostomia has been reported in sarcoidosis patients (Mansour, 2007; Surattanont, 2002; Poate, 2008). Mansour et al. (2007) identified five patients representing both clinical and histological features of Sjögren's syndrome and sarcoidosis, suggesting inclusion of sarcoidosis as diagnostic criteria for Sjögren's syndrome. The salivary glands could be affected by sarcoidosis as well, which was reported in 6% of the case (Mansour, Al-Hashimi, & Wright, 2007).

Tuberculosis (TB)

Tuberculosis (TB) is a chronic bacterial infection, caused by Mycobacterium TB leading to formation of granulomas in infected tissues. The lungs are most commonly affected, but other tissues, including the salivary glands, may be involved. Patients with TB may experience xerostomia and/or salivary gland swelling, with granuloma or cyst formation within the affected glands. Salivary gland enlargement usually presents as part of a characteristic symptom complex, however salivary gland changes have been reported in the absence of systemic symptoms (Babazade, 2012; Grunberg, 2008).

Storage Diseases

Hemochromatosis

Hemochromatosis is defined as a pathological condition with iron overload in vital organs with a hereditary/primary cause (Klopfleisch & Olias, 2012). Organs commonly affected by hemochromatosis are liver, heart, and endocrine glands. Iron deposition in the salivary glands causes hypo-salivation. Patients with normal ferritin level had normal salivary flow rate, whereas those with high levels of ferritin showed decreased stimulatory salivary flow rate (Klopfleisch, 2012; Sanchez-Pablo, 2012).

Amyloidosis

Amyloidosis is characterized by deposition of an extra-cellular protein-like material called "amyloid". Amyloidosis causes various effects on different organs with a variety of extensions. In addition, it may be associated with multiple myeloma and chronic infections. Amyloidosis may be associated with oral involvement in the form of macroglossia (10-40%), oral amyloid nodules, and dry mouth due to amyloid infiltration and destruction of salivary glands (Wey, Chen, Lai, & Chen, 2011). The relationship between amyloidosis and xerostomia has been documented by several authors (El-Fatoiki, 2013; Juusela, 2013; Sowa, 2013).

Others Systemic Diseases

End-Stage Renal Disease (ESRD)

End-stage renal disease (ESRD) represents irreversible loss of the endogenous renal function, which renders the patient permanently dependent upon dialysis or kidney transplantation. ESRD leads to accumulation of certain toxic elements, which affects normal functions of the body, and may have significant complications including cardiovascular disease, immune deficiency, anemia, renal function impairment, and bone disease (Subha, Rajan, Santhi, & Jothimalar, 2012). Xerostomia was found in 28-59% of ESRD patients due to inability of kidneys to reabsorb sodium and the resultant polyuria (Postorino, 2003; Dirschnabel, 2011).

Mouth dryness is also frequently reported by *dialyzed* patients with acute or chronic renal failure. Wilczyńska-Borowska (2005) showed that alkaline pre-dialysis pH of the saliva (8.0) decreases on average to 7.0 within the last hour of the procedure. A highly alkaline pH and decreased clearance of saliva strongly influence the deterioration of oral hygiene. Disorders of saliva secretion and increased pH resulting from elevated urea concentrations induce rapid progression of caries, gingivitis and marginal peri-odontitis.

Ectodermal Dysplasia

Ectodermal dysplasia is a hereditary disease causing anomalies in tissues of ectodermal origin. This results in severe hypodontia and hypoplasia of the alveolar process. The clinical condition is aggravated by a significant xerostomia due to salivary gland aplasia or hypoplasia (Lexner, 2007; Prager, 2006). In a study of 39 patients with ectodermal dysplasia, the salivary flow rate was reduced in 13 (33.3%) patients (Nordgarden, Jensen, & Storhaug, 2001).

Hematopoietic Stem Cell Transplantation (HSCT) and Chronic Graft-Versus-Host Disease (cGVHD)

Chronic graft-versus-host disease (cGVHD) is a multi-organ involvement that occurs post hematopoietic stem cell transplantation (HSCT), with the mouth being one of the most frequently affected sites Noce (Noce et al., 2013). GVHD occurs in 40-70% of patients treated by bone marrow and peripheral blood stem cell transplantation (Nagler, & Nagler, 2004). Oral manifestations are common in patients diagnosed with c GVHD (Noce et al., 2013). Hull et al. (2012) reported that xerostomia as the most common oral symptom in patients with history of HSCT with the majority of patients (53%) having clinical markers of oral cGVHD. Noce et al. (2013) reported that 59.1% of patients diagnosed with cGVHD had salivary gland dysfunction. Boer et al. (2010) showed a decrease in salivary flow rate (16% of patients) and a relation between hypo-salivation intensity and elapsed time after HSCT. There is similarity in oral clinical manifestations of GVHD and Sjögren's Syndrome because of the same autoimmune nature, but differences have also been found. The suggested patho-physiological mechanisms of xerostomia and hypo-salivation observed in GVHD are lymphocytic infiltration, parenchymal destruction, and fibrosis within salivary gland tissue (de la Rosa-Garcia, Bologna-Molina, Vega González, & de Jesus, 2006).

Parkinson's Disease (PD)

Parkinson's disease (PD) is a relatively common, progressive, debilitating, and neurological disorder. Cardinal symptoms are resting tremor, bradykinesia, akinesia, restricted mobility, and postural instability. Levodopa (L-DOPA) has been used as a primary drug for over 30 years. Proulx *et al.* reported that patients with PD produce less saliva than normal. Factors influencing the production of saliva include the use of levodopa and female gender (Proulx, De Courval, Wiseman, & Panisset, 2005). Hyposialorrhea is an early autonomic manifestation of PD (Cersósimo et al, 2009).

The causes and mechanisms of systemic diseases associated with xerostomia are summarized in Table 1. As may be seen, they include neuropathic disorders, immune- and inflammatory-mediated diseases, granulomatous reactions, storage diseases, diseases causing dehydration or alteration in salivary gland structure, as well as genetic disorders.

Table 1. Mechanisms of xerostomia due to systemic diseases (Mortazavi, Baharvand, Movahhedian, Mohammadi, & Khodadoustan, 2014)

Mechanism	Disease
Neuropathic	- Diabetes - Parkinson's disease
Immune- and inflammatory-mediated	- Viral infections (HIV), EBV, CMV, HTLV-1, - GVHD - Rheumatoid arthritis - Primary biliary cirrhosis - SLE - Scleroderma - AITD
Granulomatous Reaction	- Tuberculosis - Sarcoidosis
Storage Disease	- Hemochromatosis - Amyloidosis
Dehydration	- ESRD - Diabetes
Alteration in Salivary Gland Structure	- Scleroderma - Hemochromatosis - Amyloidosis - Actinomycosis - GVHD - CMV infection
Genetic Disorder	Ectodermal dysplasia

HIV: Human immunodeficiency virus, EBV: Epstein-Barr virus, CMV: Cytomegalovirus, HTLV: Human T-Lymphotropic Virus, GVHD: Graft- versus-host disease, SLE: Systemic lupus erythematosis, AITD: Autoimmune thyroid disease, ESRD: End-stage renal disease.

Local Factors

Local factors responsible for mouth dryness include sialadenitis and sialolithiasis, acute infections of the oral cavity and pharynx (e.g. chicken pox, herpetic stomatitis, peri-odontal disease), neoplasms of the mouth, pharynx and esophagus (Pichór & Doboszyńska, 2008).

Xerostomia is a common symptom in patients with *advanced cancer* with prevalence reported of up to 77% of hospital admissions (Jobbins, Bagg, Finlay, Addy, & Newcombe, 1992). Advanced cancer is defined as that which is incurable but is still amenable to life prolonging treatment (Shragge, Wismer, Olson, & Baracos, 2006). Causes in this patient group are numerous and include the consequences of the cancer itself; dehydration and general debility; the effect of cancer treatments; concomitant use of medications such as opioids, anti-muscarinic drugs and diuretics, and pre-existing co-morbidities such as Sjogren's syndrome (Twycross, Wilcock, & Toller, 2009).

In addition, development of xerostomia has been related to cancer therapy. *Chemotherapeutic* agents can change the nature of saliva and the amount produced. This may be temporary with normal salivary flow returning after treatment is completed. Xerostomia occurs also develops after *radiotherapy* to cancers of the head and neck, as it causes lysis of the salivary gland cells (Kakoei, 2012; Perez, 2008; Tribius, 2013).

The list of *internal factors* that can inhibit secretion of saliva includes tobacco smoking, using complete denture prostheses, and mouth breathing due to functional impairment of the upper airways (Pichor, 2008; Hopcraft, 2010). Al-Dwairi and Lynch (2014) studied a group of 130 users of complete denture prostheses and confirmed the association between the occurrence of xerostomia and smoking or female patients' older age.

Aging

Many unfavorable changes develop with time as part of the physiological process of *aging*, including a reduced number of secretory cells within the salivary glands. This condition mainly affects menopausal women (Mirzaii-Dizgah & Agha-Hosseini, 2011) and individuals older than 65 years of age. Contributing factors include the use of certain medications, changes in the body's ability to process medication, inadequate nutrition, and having long-term health problems. An analysis of the etiological factors of xerostomia supports the hypothesis that among older people this condition is not only related to the physiological processes of aging (Ramos-Casals, Brito-Zerón, Sisó-Almirall, & Bosch, 2012), [but also a result of age-related increase in the number of medications used (Kostowski & Herman, 2005). Research conducted at the University of Reims expanded this theory, revealing that the number of drugs administered is more significant than their type (especially with cholinergic and xerogenic drugs) in the etiology of mouth dryness (Desoutter et al, 2012).

Iatrogenic

Iatrogenic causes include mainly medications. Others include intra-operative nerve injury, radiation therapy of cancer of the head and neck, and graft-versus-host disease (GVHD).

Medications

Xerostomia can frequently develop as an adverse effect of certain *medications*. According to literature, more than 500 agents cause or increase mouth dryness as a side-effect (Guzik, 2009; Kostowski, 2005). Interactions between various drug groups also play a role in this process. Chronic pharmacotherapy can be reflected by diminished or even stopped secretion of saliva. This disorder is reversible, and resolves after the therapy is completed.

A subjective feeling of xerostomia may occur in patients taking anti-hypertensive, anti-depressant or immuno-suppressive drugs. The latter cause a decrease in the blood flow through the salivary glands, which may lead to reduced saliva production. This occurs quite often among patients with arterial hypertension, coronary thrombosis, DM and thyroid diseases at the same time, requiring the use of different drugs. The occurrence of dry mouth in this case is connected with the fact that the salivary glands have multiple types of target receptors for a variety of different drugs. The most important among them are anti-cholinergic drugs, which are the main cause of dry mouth. Activation of α-1A, β-1, M3- and H2-receptors occurs on the pathway of cAMP-dependent protein kinase A, while NK-1 and M3R activation is induced on the protein kinase C pathway. GABA and benzodiazepins cause a decrease in saliva production.

Appetite-suppressing drugs may cause a feeling of dry mouth as well. An example of such a drug is sibutramine, which suppresses the re-uptake of serotonin and noradrenaline. It prolongs the feeling of satiety, which causes an intensification of xerostomia (Scully, 2003; Shetty, 2012).

A list of medications, which cause drug-related xerostomia is presented in Table 2.

Table 2. Medications that cause Xerostomia (Kostowski, 2005; Shetty, 2012); Buczko, 2008)

Medications	Examples
Diuretics	Chlorothiazide, hydrochlorothiazide
Anti-depressants	Amitriptyline, imipramine, reboxetine, bupropion hydrochloride
Anti-histaminics	clemastine
Neuroleptics	Derivatives of phenothiazine, butyrophenone, thioxanthene
Bronchodilators	B2-adrenomimetics, inhalatory glucocorticoids, inhalatory cholinolytics (ipratropium)
Anxiolytics	Benzodiazepine derivatives: diazepam, oxazepam, lorazepam
Cholinolytic agents	Atropine, homatropine, scopolamine
Hypotensive agents	Angiotensin-converting enzyme inhibitors: enalapril, captopril, lysinopril, perindopril.
Opioids	Morphine, codeine, methadone, pethidine
Immuno-stimulants	Interferon-alpha (INF-α)
Appetite suppressants	Sibutramine
Anti-migraine drugs	Rizatriptan

Radiation Therapy

The extent of the salivary gland injury caused by radiotherapy is determined by the absorbed dose of radiation, the duration of exposure and the size of irradiated area (Dirix, Nuyts, & Van den Bogaert, 2006). Initial signs of xerostomia, which additionally impair the quality of life in cancer patients, are observed as early as a few days after irradiation. A 60% decrease in the secretion of saliva has been observed immediately after radiotherapy (Kakoei et al, 2012). Initially reversible dysfunction of the salivary glands develops in irradiated patients after receiving a 10 Gy dose. Irreversible impairment of function is associated with doses ranging between 50 and 60 Gy (Perez, 2008). According to Tribius et al. (2013), reducing the dose of radiation to

<26 Gy in patients with epithelial carcinomas of the head and neck attenuated the signs of xerostomia without increasing the risk of treatment failure.

Intra-Operative Nerve Injury

Decreased secretion of saliva, i.e. hypo-salivation, can also result from medical mistakes associated with stapedectomy procedures performed as part of otosclerosis management. An inadvertent injury to the tympanic cord, a branch of the facial nerve (VII) responsible for gustatory and secretory functions, leads to decreased secretion by the submandibular and sublingual glands. According to Mandel (2012), in such cases a subjective impression of mouth dryness appears at rest and is associated with the decreased secretory function of the parotid glands.

Graft-Versus-Host Disease (GVHD)

As mentioned before, xerostomia seen in GVHD results from lymphocytic infiltration, parenchymal destruction, and fibrosis within salivary gland tissue (de la Rosa-Garcia "et al"., 2006).

CLINICAL MANIFESTATIONS

Patients report xerostomia as a distressing symptom with significant impact on the quality of life. Discomfort associated with mouth dryness is the first and most common symptom reported by patients affected by xerostomia. The decreased volume of saliva impairs both the immunological and non-immunological protective barrier; depending on the severity, this can cause the following manifestations (Guzik, 2009; (Busato, 2012; Guvits, 2013):

- Poor nutrition from having problems with chewing and swallowing, with frequent consumption of fluids during meals;
- Predominance of bitter and salty taste;
- *Fetor ex ore*;
- Fissures and ruptures of the lips;
- Burning of the tongue and/or lips (burning mouth syndrome - BMS);
- Dry, pale, ruptured, and lusterless mucosal membranes;
- The presence of "milky" saliva draining from the glandular ducts.

Severe xerostomia can be associated with the development of cervical caries, resulting from the excessive accumulation of dental plaque at normally non-predisposed sites (the front mandibular teeth, the cusps of lateral teeth, or Black class V caries of all teeth), angular cheilitis, and candidiasis (Jańczuk, (2004). Shinozaki et al. (2012) documented an association between fungal infection (candidiasis) and mucosal disorders in patients with oral dryness. They isolated *Candida albicans* and *Candida glabata* from the tongue and angle of the mouth, respectively, in hyposalivation patients. Guobis et al. (2011), postulate an association between mouth dryness and colonization with microorganisms, not only *Candida albicans* but also *Lactobacillus* spp.

Untreated xerostomia leads to many unfavorable changes in the oral cavity, such as sulcation of the tongue and atrophy of the lingual papillae (Guzik, 2009). Moreover, patients suffering from xerostomia experience problems with using complete denture prostheses. Poor retention and displacement of the prosthesis from its location lead to mucosal injury with resultant ulceration (Gajowiak, 2009).

EVALUATION

History-Taking / Questionnaire

Several questionnaires have been proposed to identify patients with xerostomia and hyposalivation. A questionnaire developed by Fox et al. (1987) is most commonly used to take the medical history of patients suspected of xerostomia (Table 3). A positive answer to all the questions was associated with low saliva flow rates. A few years later, Thomson et al created an eleven-item summated rating scale on the severity of chronic xerostomia (Xerostomia Inventory) (Thomson, Chalmers, Spencer, & Williams, 1999). Each response was scored and summed to give a final score. van der Putten et al. (2011) shortened the Xerostomia Inventory and proposed the Summated Xerostomia Inventory-Dutch. Only five items were included. In the questionnaire developed by Sreebny and Valdini (1988), the question "does your mouth usually feel dry" was found to have had a sensitivity of 93%, a specificity of 68%, a negative predictive value of 98%, and a positive predictive value of 54% for hyposalivation. Eisbruch et al. (2003) studied the grade of xerostomia through a validated scale made of three grades. Finally, Pai et al. (2001) proposed an eight-item visual analogue scale with which patients were asked to score their xerostomia.

Clinicians should review the drug history carefully in order to identify medications that can reduce the saliva flow in patients complaining of xerostomia. Finally, a thorough medical history should be obtained in order to identify other known causes of xerostomia such as Sjögren's syndrome, radiation treatment of the head and neck region, and other systemic diseases (particularly hypertension, bronchial asthma, DM, hematological diseases, thyroid diseases, rheumatic diseases, psychiatric diseases, and eating disorders).

Table 3. Structured interview recommended in cases suspected of xerostomia by Fox et al. (1987)

1	Do you experience mouth dryness during the night or upon waking up?
2	Do you experience mouth dryness during the day?
3	Do you keep a glass of water next to your bed?
4	Do you drink fluids while swallowing dry foods?
5	Do you experience mouth dryness during meals?
6	Do you experience problems with swallowing foods?
7	Do you use chewing gum on a daily basis to eliminate a feeling of mouth dryness?
8	Do you use hard fruit or mint candies on a daily basis to eliminate a feeling of mouth dryness?
9	Do you perceive the volume of saliva in your mouth as too small/excessive, or do you just not notice it?
10	Do you need to moisten your mouth frequently?

Oral Examination

A careful oral examination is fundamental to identify clinical signs pathognomonic for hyposalivation. Several helpful signs have been proposed by Osailan et al. (2011): (1) sticking of an intraoral mirror to the buccal mucosa or tongue, (2) frothy saliva, (3) no saliva pooling in floor of mouth, (4) loss of papillae of the tongue dorsum, (5) altered/smooth gingival architecture, (6) glassy appearance to the oral mucosa (especially the palate), (7) lobulated/deeply fissured tongue, (8) cervical caries (more than two teeth), and/or (9) mucosal debris on palate (except under dentures).

Sialometric Tests

Upon documenting the presence of these symptoms, standard sialometric tests are required. The basic tests include determination of stimulated salivary flow rate (s-SFR), unstimulated salivary flow rate (u-SFR), palatal secretion (PAL) and parotid secretion (PAR). These measurements constitute the simplest methods of evaluating the secretory function of the salivary glands.

Very low unstimulated and stimulated salivary flow rates are defined as <0.1 mL/min and <0.7 mL/min, respectively. These values are confirmatory of xerostomia if they co-exist with symptoms specific for this condition (Berti-Couto Sde et al, 2012). It is important to determine both the stimulated and unstimulated volume of saliva, as salivary secretion at rest can be decreased despite a normal volume of stimulated saliva (Glore, Spiteri-Staines, & Paleri, 2009).

Unstimulated whole salivary flow rate is assessed with the patient seated in an upright position. Patients are asked to constantly drain saliva from the lower lip into a graduated container for 15 minutes (draining method) (Navazesh, 1993). Leal et al. (2010) proposed to collect saliva with pre-weighed cotton rolls placed at the orifices of the ducts of the major salivary glands and then reweigh them after the collection time. The saliva can also be collected using a graduated absorbent strip placed on the floor of the mouth (readings at 1, 2, and 3 minutes) (Chen, Wai, Lee, Lake, & Woo, 2005). Other methods to assess the unstimulated whole salivary flow rate include the spitting method and the suction method (Navazesh, 1993; Leal, 2010).

Stimulated salivary flow rate is measured after the patient has chewed an unflavored gum base or paraffin wax (1–2 g) for 1 minute (Navazesh & Kumar, 2008). Otherwise, saliva production can be stimulated with a solution of 2% citric acid placed on the sides of the tongue at intervals of 30 seconds. The saliva is then collected into a graduated cylinder for 5 minutes. Salivary flow (both stimulated and unstimulated) can also be measured selectively from one major salivary gland or minor salivary gland.

The parotid gland secretion is typically collected by using a suction device and placing a cup (the Lashley or Carlson–Crittenden cup) over the Stensen duct (Lashley, 1916). The submandibular gland salivary flow rate can be measured by incannulation of the Wharton's duct (Schneyer, 1955). A similar system to measure the salivary flow rates for both the sublingual and submandibular glands has been developed by Wolff et al. (1997). Minor salivary gland salivary flow can be measured with micropipette and absorbent filter paper (the Periotron® method; ProFlow™ Inc, Amityville, NY, USA) (Eliasson & Carlén, 2010). Flow rates can be calculated in units of μL/min/cm^2 of mucosal area (Smidt, Torpet, Nauntofte, Heegaard, & Pedersen, 2011).

Evaluating Mucosal Dryness

For evaluating mucosal dryness, the modified Schirmer test (also used in ophthalmology), as well as wafer or mirror tests, can be used. The results of the latter test are presented in a three-item scale (Knychalska-Karwan, 1995) as follows:

1. A lack of resistance during the passing of a dental mirror along the oral mucosa;
2. Weak resistance;
3. Considerable resistance during an attempt to pass the mirror.

Augmented Evaluation

In some cases, the evaluation of xerostomia is augmented with a biochemical analysis of saliva, sialography, scintigraphy with technetium-99m (^{99m}Tc), computed tomography (CT) scans or magnetic resonance imaging (MRI) of the salivary glands (Jang et al, 2012).

TREATMENT

Despite a high prevalence and clear impact on patients' quality of life, there is poor recognition of the effect of xerostomia and a lack of evidence regarding the effective management of this condition. Initial aims of management should be to identify the primary cause and treat reversible causes where possible.

Several treatment strategies for the management of xerostomia have been proposed in the past years and they all aim to reduce patients' symptoms and/or increase salivary flow. Easy remedies are proper hydration; increase in humidity at night-time; avoidance of irritating dentifrices and crunchy/hard foods; and use of sugar-free chewing gums/candy (Visvanathan & Nix, 2010). Medications include mucosal lubricants, saliva substitutes, and saliva stimulants.

Patient Education

Education of the patient aims at the implementation of systematic and proper *oral hygiene*. It is important in the prevention and treatment of mouth dryness, and is reflected by excellent therapeutic outcomes. *Avoidance of* dry, acidic and salty foods is recommended, as is the elimination of stimulants, especially tobacco and alcohol (Jańczuk, 2004).

Prevention of Infection and Ulceration

Upon establishing the etiology of the condition, *withdrawing certain groups of medications* or eliminating their interactions, xerostomia therapy focuses on the prevention of candidiasis and ulceration of periodontal and soft tissues. It must be mentioned that antibiotics and antifungal agents cause only temporary improvements, as all xerostomia-related infections tend to recur (Ship, 2002; Guzik, 2009).

SYMPTOMATIC RELIEF (PHARMACOLOGICAL AND NON-PHARMACOLOGICAL)

If further *symptomatic relief* of xerostomia is required, treatment is divided into *non-pharmacological* and *pharmacological* measures, which include *mucosal lubricants, salivary substitutes* (artificial saliva) or *salivary stimulants* that increase the flow if the salivary glands are intact (Sialagogues) (Davies, Broadley, & Beighton, 2002). Non-pharmacological examples include mouth care, ice cubes and chewing gum and candy (Davies et al, 2010).

Systemic Salivary Stimulants

Pilocarpine and Cevimeline

Pilocarpine and Cevimeline are two systemic US Food and Drug Administration-approved sialogogues for treatment of dry mouth. Their effect depends on the presence of functional glandular tissue. Oral pilocarpine is a parasympathomimetic medication with muscarinic action (Taka, 2003; Wiseman, 1995). Cevimeline is a salivary gland stimulant with a stronger affinity for M3 muscarinic receptors (Twabuchi, 1994a; Twabuchi, 1994b;

Weber, 2008; Chambers, 2007). Since cevimeline has a minute effect on M2 and M4 receptors in the lungs and heart, its use is not associated with such adverse events as bradycardia. Pilocarpine and cevimeline provide a similar benefit in patients with dry mouth (Braga et al, 2009). Pilocarpine is typically administered at a dose of 5 mg three times a day for at least 3 months and cevimeline is prescribed at a dose of 30 mg three times a day for at least 3 months (Aframian et al, 2007). Witsell et al. (2004) confirmed the efficacy of cevimeline administered at that dose (30 mg doses three times per day) in patients irradiated with > 40 Gy to the head and neck region. After six weeks of treatment, the mucosal status of these patients returned to its pre-radiotherapy level.

Side effects generally include: excessive sweating, cutaneous vasodilatation, emesis, nausea, diarrhea, persistent hiccup, broncho-constriction, hypotension, bradycardia, increased urinary frequency, and vision problems. Both pilocarpine and cevimeline are relatively *contraindicated* in patients with uncontrolled bronchial asthma or chronic pulmonary disease and in β-adrenergic blocker users, and should be used with caution in patients with active gastric ulcers or uncontrolled hypertension. Pilocarpine is also contraindicated in individuals with narrow-angle glaucoma and iritis, and should be used with caution in individuals with nephrolithiasis or cholelithiasis, chronic pulmonary disease, asthma, or cardiovascular diseases (Wiseman & Faulds, 1995) such as angina and in patients who have had myocardial infarctions (Kostowski, 2005; Buczko, 2008).

Other Systemic Sialagogues

Other systemic sialagogues include Bethanecol, Anethole trithione and Yohimbine). Bethanecol found to increase the stimulated and unstimulated salivary flow rates of patients with xerostomia secondary to radiation, but objective changes in salivary flow rates did not always correlate with symptomatic improvement. It is given in a dose of 25 mg; 3 times daily orally (Gorsky, Epstein, Parry, Epstein & Le en, 2004).

Anethole trithione is a cholagogue that has been shown to improve oral symptoms and increase the salivary flow in patients with xerostomia and hyposalivation (Hamada et al, 1999). It is specifically used to treat Sjogren's associated xerostomia. It increases the number of receptor sites on the salivary acinar cells. Patient's benefits have been reported when Sjogren's patients were administered 25 mg doses 3 times a day. A synergistic effect on salivation has been observed when a combination of pilocarpine and anethole trithione has been administered (Fox, Busch, & Baum, 1987). More studies are necessary to prove the efficacy of this medication.

Patients who were treated with psychotropic drugs (tricyclic antidepressants or neuroleptics) and were suffering from xerostomia benefited from *Yohimbine* use, an alpha 2 adrenoceptor antagonist (Bagheri, Schmitt, Berlan, & Montastruc, 1997).

Intra-Oral Topical Agents

Intra-oral topical agents are among the most common recommended treatments for the management of xerostomia. These include chewing gums, saliva stimulants, and substitutes.

Topical Sialogogue

Satisfactory results were reported using a *topical sialogogue spray* containing a combination of *1% malic acid with xylitol and fluorides* to attenuate the signs of xerostomia in patients treated with antihypertensive and antidepressant agents. However, this has the potential to cause mild enamel erosion. The dissociation of malic acid leads to stimulation of gustatory acid receptors. Although xylitol and fluoride ions do not modulate the secretion of saliva, they reduce the cariogenic and erosive potential of the malic acid (Gomez-Moreno, 2013a; Gomez-Moreno, 2013b).

Salivary Substitutes

In order to improve xerostomia patients' quality of life, various forms of *salivary substitutes* have been introduced. These include gels (Biotene), aerosols (Glandosome spray), lozenges (Saliva Orthana lozenges), oral rinses and chewing gums (Guzik & Kamyszm 2009). Saliva substitutes aim to increase viscosity and mimic natural saliva without altering the salivary flow.

Commercially available *sugar-free chewing gums and candies* can also be used to simulate salivary flow (Furness, Worthington, Bryan, Birchenough, & McMillan, 2011). In particular, chewing gums have been shown to increase saliva secretion and decrease oral mucosal friction (Olsson, Spak, & Axéll, 1991). Jang et al. (2012) studied a group of xerostomia patients who had undergone liver resection and observed that mouth dryness was efficiently alleviated by chewing gum. Clinical xerostomia in those patients had been caused by the administration of opioid analgesics.

Saliva substitutes contain *minerals* (eg, fluoride, calcium, and phosphate ions), which enhance mineralization of the enamel, carboxymethyl-cellulose or hydroxyethyl-cellulose (water-soluble polymers), flavoring agents (to improve the smell of artificial saliva), and preservatives (eg, propyl or methyl paraben) (Visvanathan & Nix, 2010). Other efficacious remedies include muco-adhesive lipid-based bioerodible tablets (Furness, Worthington, Bryan, Birchenough, & McMillan, 2011) or mucin spray, although their efficacy for management of xerostomia remains controversial (Blixt-Johansen, 1992; Duxbury, 1989; van der Reijden, 1996; Sweeney, 1997; Gravenmade, 1993).

Mucin-containing *lozenges* provided benefit for the treatment of xerostomia when compared to a placebo. Other topical agents (toothpaste, mouth rinse, mouth spray, and gel) containing olive oil, betaine, and xylitol may be effective in improving xerostomia secondary to medication use (Ship, McCutcheon, Spivakovsky, & Kerr, 2007). *Herbal rinses* (linseed, hollyhock flower or common marshmallow) have also been reported by several authors to be successfully used in the symptomatic treatment of oral dryness (Guzik, 2009; Guvits, 2013; Jańczuk, 2004).

It is noteworthy that, saliva substitute *spray* containing carboxymethyl-cellulose, (Donatsky, Johnsen, Holmstrup, & Bertram, 1982), xanthan gum-containing spray (Jellema et al, 2001), or buffered Profylin gel (Persson, Lingström, Bergdahl, Claesson, & van Dijken, 2007) did ***not*** seem to improve dry mouth symptoms. Moreover, lemon lozenge use in individuals with xerostomia did ***not*** show any increase in salivary flow when compared to baseline paraffin-stimulated mean flow rate and the gum-stimulated flow rates (Stewart, Jones, Bates, Sandow, Pink, & Stillwell, 1998).

The saliva substitute *Saliva Orthana*, a mucin-containing oral spray, was tested in a double-blind, single-phase, placebo-controlled trial for patients complaining of xerostomia (Sweeney, Bagg, Baxter, & Aitchison, 1997). The results of this study did ***not*** show any significant improvement when compared to the placebo. When *oral lubricants* are considered, the *gel formulation* appears to be the most efficient and appreciated by patients (Furumoto, Barker, Carter-Hanson, & Barker, 1998). Patients taking oral lozenges of anhydrous crystalline maltose showed an increase in saliva production and a decrease in perceived symptoms of xerostomia (Fox, Cummins, & Cummins, 2001). Patients applying the anti-cholinesterase *physostigmine* on the oral mucosa to stimulate salivary production from the minor glands reported great benefit, and this could be a valid alternative to systemic treatment (Khosravani, Birkhed, & Ekström, 2009).

Interestingly, Regelink et al. (1998) reported that saliva substitutes are not effective in patients with reasonable stimulated salivary flow. Jackiewicz-Barańska et al. (2007) examined available preparations and concluded that none of the commercial products are ideal substitutes for human saliva, as none of them contain digestive and bactericidal enzymes or other naturally occurring proteins. In conclusion, artificial saliva is a salivary substitute and is considered a poor substitute for natural saliva (Twycross & Wilcock, 2012).

MODIFICATIONS IN PATIENT MEDICATIONS

Although the evidence available is limited, with patients on medications known to induce salivary gland hypofunction, a treatment alternative includes decreasing the dosage of the medications or potentially replacing the medications with less xerogenic drugs (Sreebny & Valdini, 1987). Studies have shown that xerostomia became more manageable through medication dose reduction and medication replacement (Azodo, 2012; Trindade, 1998). It is worth mentioning that any change in medication should be discussed with the referring physician.

Other Treatment Options

Other remedies have been proposed for the management of xerostomia.

Intra-Oral Electro-Stimulation and Appliances

Intra-oral electro-stimulation has also been tested to increase salivary flow (Strietzel, 2011; Strietzel, 2007). Furthermore, reports have shown that *intra-oral appliances*, such as the saliva stimulation device Saliwell Crown or the electro-stimulating device GenNarino, have been effective in reducing dry mouth and increasing the production of saliva (Alajbeg et al, 2012).

Acupuncture

A novel technique is the use of *acupuncture* in the management of xerostomia associated with irradiation of head and neck malignancies. According to

Simcock et al. (2013), marked alleviation of dryness can be observed as early as after eight acupuncture sessions. The acupuncture-treated group showed improvement when compared to the controls, in whom education regarding oral hygiene was the only form of intervention. However, additional larger studies are necessary to confirm these findings (Blom, 1992; O'Sullivan, 2010).

Radiation Therapy and/or Cytoprotective Agent

Patients who undergo radiation of the head and neck region may benefit from the use of intensity-modified *radiation therapy and/or of amifostine (cytoprotective agent)* (Gu, 2014). *Amifostine* has been found to be useful in the prevention of xerostomia in patients subjected to radiotherapy. It exerts a broad cyto-protective effect on all normal tissues by protecting them against the destruction of DNA by generating free radical scavengers and providing hydrogen ions for the repair of injured molecules. The selective protection of normal tissues is possible due to the associated higher concentration of free thiol as compared to neoplastic tissue. The efficacy of amifostine treatment varies considerably from very high effectiveness to a placebo effect depending on the clinical status of the particular patient. Adverse effects of this agent include hypotension and vomiting (Dwilewicz-Trojaczek, 2004).

Stem Cell Therapy

Finally, although all the aforementioned methods attenuate the signs of hyposalivation, they do not eliminate the underlying problem, e.g. radiotherapy-induced injury to glandular tissue. Pringle et al. (2013) postulated using *stem cell therapy* in such cases. According to this author, recent progress in understanding the cellular turnover of the salivary glands and identification of their stem and progenitor cells constitute a basis for the implementation of this form of therapeutic intervention.

REFERENCES

Wiener, R. C., Wu, B., Crout, R., Wiener, M., Plassman, B., Kao, E., & McNeil, D. (2010). Hyposalivation and xerostomia in dentate older adults. *The Journal of the American Dental Association*, *141*(3), 279–284. doi:10.14219/jada.archive.2010.0161 PMID:20194383 van der Putten, G. J., Brand, H. S., Schols, J. M., & de Baat, C. (2011). The diagnostic suitability of a xerostomia questionnaire and the association between xerostomia, hyposalivation and medication use in a group of nursing home residents. *Clinical Oral Investigations*, *15*(2), 185–192. doi:10.100700784-010-0382-1 PMID:20165967

Fox, P. C., van der Ven, P. F., Sonies, B. C., Weiffenbach, J. M., & Baum, B. J. (1985). Xerostomia: Evaluation of a symptom with increasing significance. *The Journal of the American Dental Association*, *110*(4), 519–525. doi:10.14219/jada.archive.1985.0384 PMID:3858368

Ship, J. A. (2002). Diagnosing, managing, and preventing salivary gland disorders. *Oral Diseases*, *2*(2), 77–89. doi:10.1034/j.1601-0825.2002.2o837.x PMID:11991308

Guzik, Ł., & Kamyszm, E. (2009). Kserostomia – więcej niż suchość w jamie ustnej. *Farmakoterapia*, *6*, 411–414.

Glore, R. J., Spiteri-Staines, K., & Paleri, V. (2009). A patient with dry mouth. *Clinical Otolaryngology*, *34*(4), 358–363. doi:10.1111/j.1749-4486.2009.01930.x PMID:19673984

Guzik, Ł. (2009). Kserostomia – obraz kliniczny i terapia. *Forum of Medical Rodzm*, *4*, 292–296.

Pichór, A., & Doboszyńska, A. (2008). Suchość jamy ustnej – niedoceniany problem kliniczny. *Medical Paliative Practice*, *2*, 26–28.

Mandel, I. D. (1987). The functions of saliva. *Journal of Dental Research*, *66*(1_suppl), 623–626. doi:10.1177/00220345870660S103 PMID:3497964

Atkinson, J. C., Grisius, M., & Massey, W. (2005). Salivary hypofunction and xerostomia: Diagnosis and treatment. *Dental Clinics of North America*, *9*(2), 309–326. doi:10.1016/j.cden.2004.10.002 PMID:15755407

Porter, S. R., Scully, C., & Hegarty, A. M. (2004). An update of the etiology and management of xerostomia. Oral Surg, Oral Med, Oral Pathol. *Oral Radiology, and Endodontology*, *97*(1), 28–46.

Mirzaii-Dizgah, I., & Agha-Hosseini, F. (2011). Unstimulated whole saliva parathyroid hormone in postmenopausal women with xerostomia. *The Journal of Contemporary Dental Practice*, *12*(3), 196–199. doi:10.5005/jp-journals-10024-1034 PMID:22186816

Villa, A., Polimeni, A., Strohmenger, L., Cicciù, D., Gherlone, E., & Abati, S. (2011). Dental patients' self-reports of xerostomia and associated risk factors. *The Journal of the American Dental Association*, *142*(7), 811–816. doi:10.14219/jada.archive.2011.0269 PMID:21719803

Thomson, W. M. (2005). Issues in the epidemiological investigation of dry mouth. *Gerodontology*, *22*(2), 65–76. doi:10.1111/j.1741-2358.2005.00058.x PMID:15934347

Leal, S. C., Bittar, J., Portugal, A., Falcão, D. P., Faber, J., & Zanotta, P. (2010). Medication in elderly people: Its influence on salivary pattern, signs and symptoms of dry mouth. *Gerodontology*, *27*(2), 129–133. doi:10.1111/j.1741-2358.2009.00293.x PMID:20337727

Astor, F. C., Hanft, K. L., & Ciocon, J. O. (1999). Xerostomia: A prevalent condition in the elderly. *Ear, Nose, and Throat Journal*, *78*(7), 476–479. doi:10.1177/014556139907800707 PMID:10429321

Liu, B., Dion, M. R., Jurasic, M. M., Gibson, G., & Jones, J. A. (2012). Xerostomia and salivary hypofunction in vulnerable elders: Prevalence and etiology. *Oral Surgery, Oral Medicine, Oral Pathology and Oral Radiology*, *114*(1), 52–60. doi:10.1016/j.oooo.2011.11.014 PMID:22727092

Locker, D. (1993). Subjective reports of oral dryness in an older adult population. *Community Dentistry and Oral Epidemiology*, *21*(3), 165–168. doi:10.1111/j.1600-0528.1993.tb00744.x PMID:8348792

Thorselius, I., Emilson, C. G., & Osterberg, T. (1988). Salivary conditions and drug consumption in older age groups of elderly Swedish individuals. *Gerodontics*, *4*(2), 66–70. PMID:3209028

Busato, I. M., Ignácio, S. A., Brancher, J. A., Moysés, S. T., & Azevedo-Alanis, L. R. (2012). Impact of clinical status and salivary conditions on xerostomia and oral health-related quality of life of adolescents with type 1 diabetes mellitus. *Community Dentistry and Oral Epidemiology*, *40*(1), 62–69. doi:10.1111/j.1600-0528.2011.00635.x PMID:21883355

Gurvits, G. E., & Tan, A. (2013). Burning mouth syndrome. *World Journal of Gastroenterology*, *19*(5), 665–672. doi:10.3748/wjg.v19.i5.665 PMID:23429751

Vasconcelos, A. C. U., Soares, M. S. M., Almeida, P. C., & Soares, T. C. (2010). Comparative study of the concentration of salivary and blood glucose in type 2 diabetic patients. *Journal of Oral Science*, *52*(2), 293–298. doi:10.2334/josnusd.52.293 PMID:20587956

Bajaj, S., Prasad, S., Gupta, A., & Singh, V. B. (2012). Oral manifestations in type-2 diabetes and related complications. *Indian Journal of Endocrinology and Metabolism*, *16*(5), 777–779. doi:10.4103/2230-8210.100673 PMID:23087863

Khovidhunkit, S-oP., Suwantuntula, T., Thaweboon, S., Mitrirattanakul, S., Chomkhakhai, U., & Khovidhunkit, W. (2009). Xerostomia, hyposalivation, and oral microbiota in type 2 diabetic patients: A preliminary study. *Journal of the Medical Association of Thailand*, *92*, 1220-1228.

Busato, I. M. S., Ignácio, S. A., Brancher, J. A., Grégio, A. M. T., Machado, M. Â. N., & Azevedo-Alanis, L. R. (2009). Impact of xerostomia on the quality of life of adolescents with type 1 diabetes mellitus. *Oral Surgery, Oral Medicine, Oral Pathology, Oral Radiology, and Endodontics*, *108*(3), 376–382. doi:10.1016/j.tripleo.2009.05.005 PMID:19716505

Costa, C.C., Resende, G.B., Souza, J.M., Tavares, S.S., & Almeida, I.C. (2004). Study of the oral manifestations in diabetic children and their correlation variables. *Arquivos Brasileiros De Endocrinologia E Metabolpgia*, *48*, 374-378.

Ivanovski, K., Naumovski, V., Kostadinova, M., Pesevska, S., Drijanska, K., & Filipce, V. (2012). Xerostomia and salivary levels of glucose and urea in patients with diabetes. *Prilozi Makedonska Akademija na Naukite i Umetnostite*, *33*, 219–229. PMID:23425883

Cooper, J. D., Simmonds, M. J., Walker, N. M., Burren, O., Brand, O. J., Guo, H., ... Coleman, G. (2012). Seven n.ewly identified loci for autoimmune thyroid disease. *Human Molecular Genetics*, *21*(23), 5202–5208. doi:10.1093/hmg/dds357 PMID:22922229

Hutfless, S., Matos, P., Talor, M. V., Caturegli, P., & Rose, N. R. (2012). Significance of prediagnostic thyroid antibodies in women with autoimmune thyroid disease. *The Journal of Clinical Endocrinology and Metabolism*, *96*(9), E1466–E1471. doi:10.1210/jc.2011-0228 PMID:21715532

Cárdenas-Roldán, J., & Amaya-Amaya, J. (2012). Autoimmune thyroid disease in rheumatoid arthritis: A global perspective. *Arthritis (Egypt)*, 864-907.

Karsh, J., Pavlidis, N., Weintraub, B. D., & Moutsopoulos, H. M. (1980). Thyroid disease in Sjögren's syndrome. *Arthritis & Rheumatology (Hoboken, N.J.)*, *23*(11), 1326–1329. doi:10.1002/art.1780231118 PMID:7447970

D'Arbonneau, F., Ansart, S., Le Berre, R., Dueymes, M., Youinou, P., & Pennec, Y. L. (2003). Thyroid dysfunction in primary Sjögren's syndrome: A long-term followup study. *Arthritis & Rheumatology (Hoboken, N.J.)*, *49*(6), 804–809. doi:10.1002/art.11460 PMID:14673967

Okoje, V., Obiechina, A., & Aken'Ova, Y. (2006). Orofacial lesions in 126 newly diagnosed HIV/AIDS patients seen at the University College Hospital, Ibadan. *African Journal of Medicine and Medical Sciences*, *35*, 97–101. PMID:17209335

Nokta, M. (2008). Oral manifestations associated with HIV infection. *Current HIV/AIDS Reports*, *5*(1), 5–12. doi:10.100711904-008-0002-8 PMID:18417029

Reznik, D. (2005). Oral manifestations of HIV disease. *Top HIV Medication*, *13*, 143–148. PMID:16377852

Expósito-Delgado, A., Vallejo-Bolaños, E., & Martos-Cobo, E. (2004). Oral manifestations of HIV infection in infants: A review article. *Medicina Oral, Patologia Oral y Cirugia Bucal*, *9*, 415–420. PMID:15580118

Pinto, A., & De Rossi, S. S. (2004). Salivary gland disease in pediatric HIV patients: An update. *ASDC Journal of Dentistry for Children*, *71*, 33–37. PMID:15272653

Sharma, G., Pai, K., Suhas, S., Ramapuram, J., Doshi, D., & Anup, N. (2006). Oral manifestations in HIV/AIDS infected patients from India. *Oral Diseases*, *12*(6), 537–542. doi:10.1111/j.1601-0825.2006.01232.x PMID:17054765

Taiwo, O., Okeke, E., Jalo, P., & Danfillo, I. (2006). Oral manifestation of HIV/AIDS in Plateau state indigenes, Nigeria. *West African Journal of Medicine*, *25*, 32–37. PMID:16722356

Freed, J. R., Marcus, M., Freed, B. A., Der-Martirosian, C., Maida, C. A., Younai, F. S., ... Shapiro, M. F. (2005). Oral health findings for HIV-infected adult medical patients from the HIV Cost and Services Utilization Study. *The Journal of the American Dental Association*, *136*(10), 396–405. doi:10.14219/jada.archive.2005.0053 PMID:16255464

Sontakke, S. A., Umarji, H., & Karjodkar, F. (2011). Comparison of oral manifestations with CD4 count in HIV-infected patients. *Indian Journal of Dental Research*, *22*(5), 732–736. doi:10.4103/0970-9290.93470 PMID:22406727

Pinheiro, A., Marcenes, W., Zakrzewska, J., & Robinson, P. (2004). Dental and oral lesions in HIV infected patients: A study in Brazil. *International Dental Journal*, *54*(3), 131–137. doi:10.1111/j.1875-595X.2004.tb00268.x PMID:15218892

Lin, A., Johnson, D., Stephan, K., & Yeh, C.-K. (2003). Alteration in salivary function in early HIV infection. *Journal of Dental Research*, *82*(9), 719–724. doi:10.1177/154405910308200912 PMID:12939357

Bossola, M., & Tazza, L. (2012). Xerostomia in patients on chronic hemodialysis. *Nature Reviews. Nephrology*, *18*(3), 176–182. doi:10.1038/nrneph.2011.218 PMID:22249779

Cavasin-Filho, J. C., & Giovani, E. M. (2009). Xerostomy, dental caries and periodontal disease in HIV+ patients. *The Brazilian Journal of Infectious Diseases*, *13*(1), 13–17. doi:10.1590/S1413-86702009000100005 PMID:19578624

Ramos-Casals, M., Trejo, O., García-Carrasco, M., & Font, J. (2003). Therapeutic management of extrahepatic manifestations in patients with chronic hepatitis C virus infection. *Rheumatology*, *42*(7), 818–828. doi:10.1093/rheumatology/keg299 PMID:12730523

Prunoiu, C., Georgescu, E. F., Georgescu, M., & Simionescu, C. (2008). Sjogren's syndrome associated with chronic hepatitis C-the benefit of the antiviral treatment. *Romanian Journal of Morphology and Embryology*, *49*, 5575–5562. PMID:19050807

Grossmann Sd, M. C., Teixeira, R., de Oliveira, G. C., Gleber-Netto, F. O., Araújo, F. M. G., & Araújo, F. M. (2010). Xerostomia, hyposalivation and sialadenitis in patients with chronic hepatitis C are not associated with the detection of HCV RNA in saliva or salivary glands. *Journal of Clinical Pathology*, *63*(11), 1002–1007. doi:10.1136/jcp.2010.080036 PMID:20924089

Nawito, Z., Amin, A., El-Fadl, S. A., & El Einen, K. A. (2011). Sicca complex among Egyptian patients with chronic hepatitis C virus infection. *Clinical Rheumatology*, *30*(10), 1299–1304. doi:10.100710067-011-1746-x PMID:21487733

Giordano, N., Amendola, A., Papakostas, P., Cipolli, F., Agate, V.M., & Battisti, E.,…. Nuti, R. (2005). Immune and autoimmune disorders in HCV chronic liver disease: Personal experience and commentary on literature. *New Microbiology*, *28*, 311–317. PMID:16386015

de Mattos, C. S., Teixeira, R., & de Oliveira, G. C. (2010). Detection of HCV RNA in saliva does not correlate with salivary flow or xerostomia in patients with chronic hepatitis C. *Oral Surgery, Oral Medicine, Oral Pathology, Oral Radiology, and Endodontics*, *109*(6), 851–856. doi:10.1016/j.tripleo.2010.02.012 PMID:20451844

Carrozzo, M., & Gandolfo, S. (2003). Oral diseases possibly associated with hepatitis C virus. *Critical Reviews in Oral Biology and Medicine*, *14*(2), 115–127. doi:10.1177/154411130301400205 PMID:12764074

Nagao, Y., Hashimoto, K., & Sata, M. (2012). Candidiasis and other oral mucosal lesions during and after interferon therapy for HCV-related chronic liver diseases. *BMC Gastroenterology*, *12*(1), 155. doi:10.1186/1471-230X-12-155 PMID:23122361

Aghemo, A., Rumi, M. G., Monico, S., Banderali, M., Russo, A., Ottaviani, F., ... Colombo, M. (2011). Ribavir.in impairs salivary gland function during combination treatment with pegylated interferon alfa-2a in hepatitis C patients. *Hepatitis Monthly*, *11*, 918–924. PMID:22308157

Arvey, A., Tempera, I., & Lieberman, P. M. (2013). Interpreting the Epstein-Barr Virus [EBV] Epigenome Using High-Throughput Data. *Viruses*, *5*(4), 1042–1054. doi:10.3390/v5041042 PMID:23549386

Hallee, T. J., Evans, A. S., Niederman, J. C., Brooks, C. M., & Voegtly, J. H. (1974). Infectious mononucleosis at the United States Military Academy. A prospective study of a single class over four years. *The Yale Journal of Biology and Medicine*, *4*(47), 182–195. PMID:4374836

Lossius, A., Johansen, J. N., Torkildsen, Ø., Vartda, F., & Holmøy, T. (2012). Epstein-Barr Virus in Systemic Lupus Erythematosus, Rheumatoid Arthritis and Multiple Sclerosis—Association and Causation. *Viruses*, *4*(12), 3701–3730. doi:10.3390/v4123701 PMID:23342374

Fox, R., Chilton, T., Scott, S., Benton, L., Howell, F., & Vaughan, J. (1987). Potential role of Epstein-Barr virus in Sjögren's syndrome. *Rheumatic Diseases Clinics of North America*, *13*, 275–292. PMID:2827246

Stadler, L. P., Bernstein, D. I., Callahan, S. T., Ferreira, J., Simone, G. A. G., Edwards, K. M., ... Rosenth.al, S. L. (2010). Seropre.valence of cytomegalovirus [CMV] and risk factors for infection in adolescent males. *Clinical Infectious Diseases*, *51*(10), e76–e81. doi:10.1086/656918 PMID:20936976

Burns, J. (1983). Persistent Cytomegalovirus infection-The etiology of Sjogren's syndrome. *Medical Hypotheses*, *10*(4), 451–460. doi:10.1016/0306-9877(83)90011-7 PMID:6308404

Scully, C. (1990). Sjögren's syndrome: No demonstrable association by serology of secondary Sjögren's syndrome with cytomegalovirus. *Journal of Oral Pathology & Medicine*, *19*(1), 43–44. doi:10.1111/j.1600-0714.1990.tb00780.x PMID:2156070

Poetker, S. K., Porto, A. F., Giozza, S. P., Muniz, A. L., Caskey, M. F., Carvalho, E. M., & Glesby, M. J. (2011). Clinical manifestations in individuals with recent diagnosis of HTLV type I infection. *Journal of Clinical Virology*, *51*(1), 54–58. doi:10.1016/j.jcv.2011.02.004 PMID:21388871

Proietti, F. A., Carneiro-Proietti, A. B. F., Catalan-Soares, B. C., & Murphy, E. L. (2005). Global epidemiology of HTLV-I infection and associated diseases. *Oncogene*, *24*(39), 6058–6068. doi:10.1038j.onc.1208968 PMID:16155612

Manns, M. P., & Rambusch, E. G. (1999). Autoimmunity and extrahepatic manifestations in hepatitis C virus infection. *Journal of Hepatology*, *31*(Suppl 1), 39–42. doi:10.1016/S0168-8278(99)80372-9 PMID:10622558

Neville, B. W., Damm, D. D., Allen, C. M., & Bouqout, J. E. (2009). *Oral and Maxillofacial Pathology*. St Louis, MO: Saunders Elsevier.

Mamais, C., Dias, A., Walker, J., & Vydianath, S. R. (2011). Parotid actinomycosis mimicking metastatic lymphadenopathy. *The West Indian Medical Journal*, *60*, 349–350. PMID:22224352

Sittitrai, P., Srivanitchapoom, C., Pattarasakulchai, T., & Lekawanavijit, S. (2012). Actinomycosis presenting as a parotid tumor. *Auris, Nasus, Larynx*, *39*(2), 241–243. doi:10.1016/j.anl.2011.03.011 PMID:21570224

Ramos-Casals, M., Brito-Zerón, P., Sisó-Almirall, A., & Bosch, X. (2012). Primary Sjogren syndrome. *Praxis (Bern)*, *28*(24), 1565–1571. doi:10.1024/1661-8157/a001133 PMID:23184549

Kobak, S., Oksel, F., Aksu, K., & Kabasakal, Y. (2013). The frequency of sicca symptoms and Sjogren's syndrome in patients with systemic sclerosis. *International Journal of Rheumatic Diseases*, *16*(1), 88–92. doi:10.1111/j.1756-185X.2012.01810.x PMID:23441777

Zalewska, A., Knaś, M., Waszkiewicz, N., Waszkiel, D., Sierakowski, S., & Zwierz, K. (2013). Rheumatoid arthritis patients with xerostomia have reduced production of key salivary constituents. *Oral Surgery, Oral Medicine, Oral Pathology and Oral Radiology*, *115*(4), 483–490. doi:10.1016/j.oooo.2012.10.013 PMID:23312539

Anurag-Gupta, B., Epstein, J. B., & Sroussi, H. (2006). Hyposalivation in elderly patients. *Journal - Canadian Dental Association*, *72*, 841–846. PMID:17109806

Jensen, J., Bergem, H., Gilboe, I. M., Husby, G., & Axell, T. (1999). Oral and ocular sicca symptoms and findings are prevalent in systemic lupus erythematosus. *Journal of Oral Pathology & Medicine*, *28*(7), 317–322. doi:10.1111/j.1600-0714.1999.tb02047.x PMID:10432198

Anurag-Gupta, B., Epstein, J. B., & Sroussi, H. (2006). Hyposalivation in elderly patients. *Journal - Canadian Dental Association*, *72*, 841–846. PMID:17109806

Karp, J. K., Akpek, E. K., & Anders, R. A. (2010). Autoimmune hepatitis in patients with primary Sjögren's syndrome: A series of two-hundred and two patients. *International Journal of Clinical and Experimental Pathology*, *25*(3), 582–586. PMID:20661405

Kumagi, T., & Heathcote, E. J. (2008). Primary biliary cirrhosis. *Orphanet Journal of Rare Diseases*, *23*(3), 1. doi:10.1186/1750-1172-3-1 PMID:18215315

Selmi, C., Meroni, P. L., & Gershwin, M. E. (2012). Primary biliary cirrhosis and Sjögren's syndrome: Autoimmune epithelitis. *Journal of Autoimmunity*, *39*(1-2), 34–42. doi:10.1016/j.jaut.2011.11.005 PMID:22178199

Mang, F. W., Michieletti, P., O'Rourke, K., Cauch-Dudek, K., Diamant, N., Bookman, A., & Heathcote, J. (1997). Primary biliary cirrhosis, sicca complex, and dysphagia. *Dysphagia*, *12*(3), 167–170. doi:10.1007/PL00009532 PMID:9190103

Cazal, C., Sobral, A. P. V., Neves, R., Freire-Filho, F., Cardoso, A., & da Silveira, M. (2008). Oral complaints in progressive systemic sclerosis: Two cases report. *Medicina Oral, Patologia Oral y Cirugia Bucal*, *13*, E114–E118. PMID:18223527

Albilia, J. B., Lam, D. K., Blanas, N., Clokie, C. M., & Sándor, G. K. (2007). Small mouths… Big problems? A review of scleroderma and its oral health implications. *Journal - Canadian Dental Association*, *73*, 831–836. PMID:18028759

Janin, A., Gosselin, B., Gosset, D., Hatron, P., & Sauvezie, B. (1989). Histological criteria of Sjögren's syndrome in scleroderma. *Clinical and Experimental Rheumatology*, *7*, 167–171. PMID:2736830

Sekhri, V., Sanal, S., DeLorenzo, L. J., Aronow, W. S., & Maguire, G. P. (2011). Cardiac sarcoidosis: A comprehensive review. *Archives of Medical Science*, *7*, 546–554. doi:10.5114/aoms.2011.24118 PMID:22291785

Mansour, M., Al-Hashimi, I., & Wright, J. (2007). Coexistence of Sjögren's syndrome and sarcoidosis: A report of five cases. *Journal of Oral Pathology & Medicine*, *36*(6), 337–341. doi:10.1111/j.1600-0714.2007.00530.x PMID:17559494

Surattanont, F., Mandel, L., & Wolinsky, B. (2002). Bilateral parotid swelling caused by sarcoidosis. *The Journal of the American Dental Association*, *133*(6), 738–741. doi:10.14219/jada.archive.2002.0270 PMID:12083650

Poate, T., Sharma, R., Moutasim, K. A., Escudier, M., & Warnakulasuriya, S. (2008). Orofacial presentations of sarcoidosis: A case series and review of the literature. *British Dental Journal*, *205*(8), 437–442. doi:10.1038j.bdj.2008.892 PMID:18953304

Babazade, F., Mortazavi, H., & Jalalian, H. (2012). Parotid tuberculosis: A forgotten suspicion (a case report and literature review). *International Journal of Dermatology*, *51*(5), 588–591. doi:10.1111/j.1365-4632.2011.05014.x PMID:22515584

Greenberg, M. S., Glick, M., & Ship, J. A. (2008). *Burket's Oral Medicine*. Ontario: BC Decker Inc.

Klopfleisch, R., & Olias, P. (2012). The Pathology of comparative animal models of human hemochromatosis. *Journal of Comparative Pathology*, *147*(4), 460–478. doi:10.1016/j.jcpa.2012.09.001 PMID:23079103

Sánchez-Pablo, M.-A., González-García, V., & del Castillo-Rueda, A. (2012). Study of total stimulated saliva flow and hyperpigmentation in the oral mucosa of patients diagnosed with hereditary hemochromatosis. Series of 25 cases. *Medicina Oral, Patologia Oral y Cirugia Bucal*, *1*(17), e45–e49. doi:10.4317/medoral.17206 PMID:22157666

Wey, S. J., Chen, Y. M., Lai, P. J., & Chen, D. Y. (2011). Primary Sjogren's syndrome manifested as localized cutaneous nodular amyloidosis. *Journal of Clinical Rheumatology; Practical Reports on Rheumatic & Musculoskeletal Diseases*, *17*(7), 368–370. doi:10.1097/RHU.0b013e31823209ba PMID:21946462

Elfatoiki, F. Z., Funck-Brentano, E., Blanc, F., Clerici, T., & Saiag, P. (2013). Nodular cutaneous amyloidosis associated with Sjögren's syndrome. *Annales de Dermatologie et de Venereologie*, *140*, 378–381. doi:10.1016/j.annder.2013.02.014 PMID:23663711

Juusela, P., Tanskanen, M., Nieminen, A., Kari, K., Suominen, L., Uitto, V. J., & Kiuru-Enari, S. (2013). Xerostomia in hereditary gelsolin amyloidosis. *Amyloid*, *20*(1), 39–44. doi:10.3109/13506129.2013.764284 PMID:23356404

Sowa, T., Komatsu, T., Fujinaga, T., & Kato, T. (2013). A case of solitary pulmonary nodular amyloidosis with Sjögren's syndrome. *Annals of Thoracic and Cardiovascular Surgery*, *19*(3), 247–249. doi:10.5761/atcs.cr.12.01890 PMID:22971705

Subha, P. M., Rajan, P. M., Santhi, S., & Jothimalar, A. (2012). Blood Lead in End-Stage Renal Disease Patients who were on Maintenance Hemodialysis. *Journal of Clinical and Diagnostic Research: JCDR*, *6*, 1633–1635. PMID:23373016

Postorino, M., Catalano, C., Martorano, C., Cutrupi, S., Marino, C., Cozzupoli, P., ... Zoccali, C. (2003). Salivary and lacrimal secretion is reduced in patients with ESRD. *American Journal of Kidney Diseases*, *42*, 722-728.

Dirschnabel, A. J., Martins, A. S., Dantas, S., Ribas, M. O., Grégio, A., Alanis, L., ... Machado, M. A. (2011). Clinica.l oral findings in dialysis and kidney-transplant patients. *Quintessence International, 42*, 127–133. PMID:21359247

Wilczyńska-Borawska, M. I. (2005). The effect of hemodialysis on salivary pH of patients with renal failure. *Czasopismo Stomatologiczne, 7*, 480–485.

Lexner, M. O., Bardow, A., Hertz, J. M., Almer, L., Nauntofte, B., & Kreiborg, S. (2007). Whole saliva in X-linked hypohidrotic ectodermal dysplasia. *International Journal of Paediatric Dentistry, 17*(3), 155–162. doi:10.1111/j.1365-263X.2006.00812.x PMID:17397458

Präger, T. M., Finke, C., & Miethke, R.-R. (2006). Dental findings in patients with ectodermal dysplasia. *Journal of Orofacial Orthopedics, 67*(5), 347–355. doi:10.100700056-006-0619-4 PMID:16953354

Nordgarden, H., Jensen, J., & Storhaug, K. (2001). Oligodontia is associated with extra-oral ectodermal symptoms and low whole salivary flow rates. *Oral Diseases, 7*, 226–232. PMID:11575873

Noce, C., Gomes, A., Copello, A., Barbosa, R., Sant'anna, S., Moreira, M., ... Torres, M. R. (2011). Oral in.volvement of chronic graft-versus host disease in hematopoietic stem cell transplant recipients. *General Dentistry, 59*, 458–462. PMID:22313917

Nagler, R. M., & Nagler, A. (2004). Salivary gland involvement in graft-versus-host disease: The underlying mechanism and implicated treatment. *The Israel Medical Association Journal, 6*, 167–172. PMID:15055275

Hull, K., Kerridge, I., & Schifter, M. (2012). Long-term oral complications of allogeneic haematopoietic SCT. *Bone Marrow Transplantation, 47*(2), 265–270. doi:10.1038/bmt.2011.63 PMID:21441960

Boer, C., Correa, M., Miranda, E., & de Souza, C. A. (2010). Taste disorders and oral evaluation in patients undergoing allogeneic hematopoietic SCT. *Bone Marrow Transplantation, 45*(4), 705–711. doi:10.1038/bmt.2009.237 PMID:19767788

de la Rosa-Garcia, E., Bologna-Molina, R., Vega-González, M., & de Jesus, T. (2006). Graft-versus-host disease, an eight case report and literature review. *Medicina Oral, Patologia Oral y Cirugia Bucal, 11*, E486–E492. PMID:17072252

Proulx, M., De Courval, F. P., Wiseman, M. A., & Panisset, M. (2005). Salivary production in Parkinson's disease. *Movement Disorders*, *20*(2), 204–207. doi:10.1002/mds.20189 PMID:15389996

Cersósimo, M., Tumilasci, O., Raina, G., Benarroch, E., Cardoso, E., Micheli, F., & Pazo, J. H. (2009). Hyposialorrhea as an early manifestation of Parkinson disease. *Autonomic Neuroscience*, *150*(1-2), 150–151. doi:10.1016/j.autneu.2009.04.004 PMID:19419908

Mortazavi, H., Baharvand, M., Movahhedian, A., Mohammadi, M., & Khodadoustan, A. (2014). Xerostomia Due to Systemic Disease: A Review of 20 Conditions and Mechanisms. *Annals of Medical and Health Sciences Research*, *4*(4), 503–510. doi:10.4103/2141-9248.139284 PMID:25221694

Jobbins, J., Bagg, J., Finlay, I. G., Addy, M., & Newcombe, R. G. (1992). Oral and dental disease in terminally ill cancer patients. *British Medical Journal*, *304*(6842), 1612. doi:10.1136/bmj.304.6842.1612 PMID:1628090

Shragge, J. E., Wismer, W. V., Olson, K. L., & Baracos, V. E. (2006). The management of anorexia by patients with advanced cancer: A critical review of the literature. *Palliative Medicine*, *20*(6), 623–629. doi:10.1177/0269216306070322 PMID:17060256

Twycross, R., Wilcock, A., & Toller, C. (2009) Alimentary symptoms. In Symptom Management in Advanced Cancer (4th ed.). Oxford: Palliativedrugs.com Ltd.

Kakoei, S., Haghdoost, A. A., Rad, M., Mohammadalizadeh, S., Pourdamghan, N., Nakhaei, M., & Bahador, M. (2012). Xerostomia after radiotherapy and its effect on quality of life in head and neck cancer patients. *Archives of Iranian Medicine*, *15*, 214–218. PMID:22424038

Perez, C. A. (2008). *Brady's: Principles and Practice of Radiation Oncology* (5th ed.). Philadelphia, PA: Lippincott Williams and Wilkins Company.

Tribius, S., Sommer, J., Prosch, C., Bajrovic, A., Muenscher, A., Blessmann, M., ... Tennstedt, P. (2013). Xerostomia after radiotherapy: What matters-mean total dose or dose to each parotid gland? *Strahlentherapie und Onkologie*, *189*(3), 216–222. doi:10.100700066-012-0257-2 PMID:23354440

Hopcraft, M. S., & Tan, C. (2010). Xerostomia: An update for clinicians. *Australian Dental Journal*, *55*(3), 238–244. doi:10.1111/j.1834-7819.2010.01229.x PMID:20887509

Al-Dwairi, Z., & Lynch, E. (2014). Xerostomia in complete denture wearers: Prevalence, clinical findings and impact on oral functions. *Gerodontology*, *31*(1), 49–55. doi:10.1111/ger.12002 PMID:22957806

Mirzaii-Dizgah, I., & Agha-Hosseini, F. (2011). Unstimulated whole saliva parathyroid hormone in postmenopausal women with xerostomia. *The Journal of Contemporary Dental Practice*, *12*(3), 196–199. doi:10.5005/jp-journals-10024-1034 PMID:22186816

Kostowski, W., & Herman, Z. S. (2005). Farmakologia. Warszawa: Podstawy Farmakologii. Wyd.

Desoutter, A., Soudain-Pineau, M., Munsch, F., Mauprivez, C., Dufour, T., & Coeuriot, J. L. (2012). Xerostomia and medication: A cross-sectional study in long-term geriatric wards. *The Journal of Nutrition, Health & Aging*, *16*(6), 575–579. doi:10.100712603-012-0007-2 PMID:22660000

Scully, C. (2003). Drug effects on salivary glands: Dry mouth. *Oral Diseases*, *2003*(4), 165–176. doi:10.1034/j.1601-0825.2003.03967.x PMID:12974516

Shetty, S. R., Bhowmick, S., Castelino, R., & Babu, S. (2012). Drug induced xerostomia in elderly individuals: An institutional study. *Contemporary Clinical Dentistry*, *3*(2), 173-175. doi:10.4103/0976-237X.96821 PMID:22919217

Buczko, W. (2008). Kompendium farmakologii i toksykologii Mutschlera. Leki wpływające na układ nerwowy, 8, 172-178.

Dirix, P., Nuyts, S., & Van den Bogaert, W. (2006). Radiation-induced xerostomia in patients with head and neck cancer. *Cancer*, *107*(11), 2525–2534. doi:10.1002/cncr.22302 PMID:17078052

Mandel, L. (2012). Hyposalivation after undergoing stapedectomy. *The Journal of the American Dental Association*, *143*(1), 39–42. doi:10.14219/jada.archive.2012.0016 PMID:22207665

Jańczuk, Z. (2004). *Choroby jamy ustnej związane z zaburzeniami wydzielania śliny. W: Choroby błony śluzowej jamy ustnej i przyzębia. Podręcznik dla studentow stomatologii*. Warszawa: Wyd. Lek. PZWL.

Shinozaki, S., Moriyama, M., Hayashida, J. N., Tanaka, A., Maehara, T., Ieda, S., & Nakamura, S. (2012). Close association between oral *Candida* species and oral mucosal disorders in patients with xerostomia. *Oral Diseases*, *18*(7), 667–672. doi:10.1111/j.1601-0825.2012.01923.x PMID:22548381

Guobis, Ž., Kareivienė, V., Basevičienė, N., Paipalienė, P., Niedzelskienė, I., Sabalys, G., ... Gervickas, A. (2011). Microflora of the oral cavity in patients with xerostomia. *Medicina (Kaunas, Lithuania)*, *47*, 646–651. PMID:22370462

Gajowiak, I. (2009). Zastosowanie preparatow adhezyjnych we wspołczesnej protetyce stomatologicznej. *Porad Stomatology*, *6*, 221–228.

Fox, P. C., Busch, K. A., & Baum, B. J. (1987). Subjective reports of xerostomia and objective measures of salivary gland performance. *The Journal of the American Dental Association*, *115*(4), 581–584. doi:10.1016/S0002-8177(87)54012-0 PMID:3477595

Thomson, W. M., Chalmers, J. M., Spencer, A. J., & Williams, S. M. (1999). The Xerostomia Inventory: A multi-item approach to measuring dry mouth. *Community Dental Health*, *16*(1), 12–17. PMID:10697349

van der Putten, G. J., Brand, H. S., Schols, J. M., & de Baat, C. (2011). The diagnostic suitability of a xerostomia questionnaire and the association between xerostomia, hyposalivation and medication use in a group of nursing home residents. *Clinical Oral Investigations*, *15*(2), 185–192. doi:10.100700784-010-0382-1 PMID:20165967

Sreebny, L. M., & Valdini, A. (1988). Xerostomia. Part I: Relationship to other oral symptoms and salivary gland hypofunction. *Oral Surgery, Oral Medicine, and Oral Pathology*, *66*(4), 451–458. doi:10.1016/0030-4220(88)90268-X PMID:3186220

Eisbruch, A., Rhodus, N., Rosenthal, D., Murphy, B., Rasch, C., Sonis, S., ... Brizel, D. (2003). How sho.uld we measure and report radiotherapy-induced xerostomia? *Seminars in Radiation Oncology*, *3*(3), 226–234. doi:10.1016/S1053-4296(03)00033-X PMID:12903012

Pai, S., Ghezzi, E. M., & Ship, J. A. (2001). Development of a Visual Analogue Scale questionnaire for subjective assessment of salivary dysfunction. *Oral Surgery, Oral Medicine, Oral Pathology, Oral Radiology, and Endodontics*, *91*(3), 311–316. doi:10.1067/moe.2001.111551 PMID:11250628

Osailan, S., Pramanik, R., Shirodaria, S., Challacombe, S. J., & Proctor, G. B. (2011). Investigating the relationship between hyposalivation and mucosal wetness. *Oral Diseases*, *17*(1), 109–114. doi:10.1111/j.1601-0825.2010.01715.x PMID:21029258

Berti-Couto Sde, A., Couto-Souza, P. H., Jacobs, R., Nackaerts, O., Rubira-Bullen, I. R., Westphalen, F. H., ... Tolazzi, A. L. (2012). Clinica.l diagnosis of hyposalivation in hospitalized patients. *Journal of Applied Oral Science*, *20*(2), 157–161. doi:10.1590/S1678-77572012000200006 PMID:22666830

Navazesh, M. (1993). Methods for collecting saliva. New York Academy of Sciences, 694, 72-77.

Leal, S. C., Bittar, J., Portugal, A., Falcão, D. P., Faber, J., & Zanotta, P. (2010). Medication in elderly people: Its influence on salivary pattern, signs and symptoms of dry mouth. *Gerodontology*, *27*(2), 129–133. doi:10.1111/j.1741-2358.2009.00293.x PMID:20337727

Chen, A., Wai, Y., Lee, L., Lake, S., & Woo, S. B. (2005). Using the modified Schirmer test to measure mouth dryness: A preliminary study. *The Journal of the American Dental Association*, *136*(2), 164–170. doi:10.14219/jada.archive.2005.0137 PMID:15782519

Navazesh, M., & Kumar, S. K. (2008). University of Southern California School of Dentistry Measuring salivary flow: Challenges and opportunities. *The Journal of the American Dental Association*, *139*(Suppl), 35S–0S. doi:10.14219/jada.archive.2008.0353 PMID:18460678

Lashley, K. S. (1916). Reflex secretion of the human parotid gland. *Journal of Experimental Psychology*, *1*(6), 461–493. doi:10.1037/h0073282

Schneyer, L. H. (1955). Method for the collection of separate submaxillary and sublingual saliva in man. *Journal of Dental Research*, *34*(2), 257–261. doi:10.1177/00220345550340021301 PMID:14367622

Wolff, A., Begleiter, A., & Moskona, D. (1997). A novel system of human submandibular/sublingual saliva collection. *Journal of Dental Research*, *76*(11), 1782–1786. doi:10.1177/00220345970760111001 PMID:9372796

Eliasson, L., & Carlén, A. (2010). An update on minor salivary gland secretions. *European Journal of Oral Sciences*, *118*(5), 435–442. doi:10.1111/j.1600-0722.2010.00766.x PMID:20831576

Smidt, D., Torpet, L. A., Nauntofte, B., Heegaard, K. M., & Pedersen, A. M. (2011). Associations between oral and ocular dryness, labial and whole salivary flow rates, systemic diseases and medications in a sample of older people. *Community Dentistry and Oral Epidemiology*, *39*(3), 276–288. doi:10.1111/j.1600-0528.2010.00588.x PMID:21070322

Knychalska-Karwan, Z. (1995). *Stomatologia Geriatryczna*. Krakow Collegium Medicum UJ.

Jang, S. Y., Ju, E. Y., Kim, D. E., Kim, J. H., Kim, Y. H., Son, M., ... Kim, K. S. (2012). … Kim, K.S. (2012). First flatus time and xerostomia associated with gum-chewing after liver resection. *Journal of Clinical Nursing*, *21*(15-16), 2188–2192. doi:10.1111/j.1365-2702.2012.04132.x PMID:22672009

Visvanathan, V., & Nix, P. (2010). Managing the patient presenting with xerostomia: A review. *International Journal of Clinical Practice*, *64*(3), 404–407. doi:10.1111/j.1742-1241.2009.02132.x PMID:19817913

Davies, A. N., Broadley, K., & Beighton, D. (2002). Salivary gland hypofunction in patients with advanced cancer. *Oral Oncology*, *38*(7), 680–685. doi:10.1016/S1368-8375(01)00133-6 PMID:12167420

Davies, A., Bagg, J., Laverty, D., Sweeney, P., Filbet, M., Newbold, K., ... Mercada.nte, S. (2010). Salivary gland dysfunction ('dry mouth') in patients with cancer: A consensus statement. *European Journal of Cancer Care*, *19*(2), 172–177. doi:10.1111/j.1365-2354.2009.01081.x PMID:19725868

Takakura, A. C., Moreira, T. S., Laitano, S. C., De Luca Júnior, L. A., Renzi, A., & Menani, J. V. (2003). Central muscarinic receptors signal pilocarpine-induced salivation. *Journal of Dental Research*, *82*(12), 993–997. doi:10.1177/154405910308201211 PMID:14630901

Wiseman, L. R., & Faulds, D. (1995). Oral pilocarpine: A review of its pharmacological properties and clinical potential in xerostomia. *Drugs*, *49*(1), 143–155. doi:10.2165/00003495-199549010-00010 PMID:7705213

Iwabuchi, Y., & Masuhara, T. (1994). Sialogogic activities of SNI-2011 compared with those of pilocarpine and McN-A-343 in rat salivary glands: Identification of a potential therapeutic agent for treatment of Sjorgen's syndrome. *General Pharmacology*, *25*(1), 123–129. doi:10.1016/0306-3623(94)90021-3 PMID:7517901

Iwabuchi, Y., Katagiri, M., & Masuhara, T. (1994). Salivary secretion and histopathological effects after single administration of the muscarinic agonist SNI-2011 in MRL/lpr mice. *Archives Internationales de Pharmacodynamie et de Therapie*, *328*(3), 315–325. PMID:7542865

Weber, J., & Keating, G. M. (2008). Cevimeline. *Drugs*, *68*(12), 1691–1698. doi:10.2165/00003495-200868120-00006 PMID:18681491

Chambers, M. S., Jones, C. U., Biel, M. A., Weber, R. S., Kenneth, M., Hodge, K. M., ... Haddad, R. (2007). Open-label, long-term safety study of cevimeline in the treatment of postirradiation xerostomia. *International Journal of Radiation Oncology, Biology, Physics*, *69*(5), 1369–1376. doi:10.1016/j.ijrobp.2007.05.024 PMID:17855005

Braga, M. A., Tarzia, O., Bergamaschi, C. C., Santos, F. A., Andrade, E. D., & Groppo, F. C. (2009). Comparison of the effects of pilocarpine and cevimeline on salivary flow. *International Journal of Dental Hygiene*, *7*(2), 126–130. doi:10.1111/j.1601-5037.2008.00326.x PMID:19416095

Aframian, D. J., Helcer, M., Livni, D., Robinson, S. D., Markitziu, A., & Nadler, C. (2007). Pilocarpine treatment in a mixed cohort of xerostomic patients. *Oral Diseases*, *13*(1), 88–92. doi:10.1111/j.1601-0825.2006.01252.x PMID:17241436

Dwilewicz-Trojaczek, J. (2004). Amifostyna – lek cytoprotekcyjny. *Contemporary Oncology (Poznan, Poland)*, *8*, 101–106.

Gorsky, M., Epstein, J., Parry, J., Epstein, M., Le, N. D., & Silverman, S. Jr. (2004). The efficacy of pilocarpine and bethanechol upon saliva production in cancer patients with hyposalivation following radiation therapy. *Oral Surgery, Oral Medicine, Oral Pathology, Oral Radiology, and Endodontics*, *97*(2), 190–195. doi:10.1016/j.tripleo.2003.08.031 PMID:14970777

Hamada, T., Nakane, T., Kimura, T., Arisawa, K., Yoneda, K., Yamamoto, T., & Osaki, T. (1999). Treatment of xerostomia with the bile secretion-stimulating drug anethole trithione: A clinical trial. *The American Journal of the Medical Sciences*, *318*(3), 146–151. doi:10.1097/00000441-199909000-00009 PMID:10487404

Bagheri, H., Schmitt, L., Berlan, M., & Montastruc, J. L. (1997). A comparative study of the effects of yohimbine and anetholtrithione on salivary secretion in depressed patients treated with psychotropic drugs. *European Journal of Clinical Pharmacology*, *52*(5), 339–342. doi:10.1007002280050298 PMID:9272401

Gómez-Moreno, G., Guardia, J., Aguilar-Salvatierra, A., Cabrera-Ayala, M., Maté-Sánchez de-Val, J. E., & Calvo-Guirado, J. L. (2013). Effectiveness of malic acid 1% in patients with xerostomia induced by antihypertensive drugs. *Medicina Oral, Patologia Oral y Cirugia Bucal*, *18*(1), e49–e55. doi:10.4317/medoral.18206 PMID:22926481

Gómez-Moreno, G., Aguilar-Salvatierra, A., Guardia, J., Uribe-Marioni, A., Cabrera-Ayala, M., Ruiz, R. A. D., & Guirado, J. L. C. (2013). The efficacy of a topical sialogogue spray containing 1% malic acid in patients with antidepressant-induced dry mouth: A double-blind, randomized clinical trial. *Depression and Anxiety*, *30*(2), 137–142. doi:10.1002/da.22017 PMID:23124914

Furness, S., Worthington, H. V., Bryan, G., Birchenough, S., & McMillan, R. (2011). Interventions for the management of dry mouth: Topical therapies. *Cochrane Database of Systematic Reviews*, *12*, CD008934. doi:10.1002/14651858.CD008934.pub2 PMID:22161442

Olsson, H., Spak, C. J., & Axéll, T. (1991). The effect of a chewing gum on salivary secretion, oral mucosal friction, and the feeling of dry mouth in xerostomic patients. *Acta Odontolotica Scandanavica*, *49*(5), 273–279. doi:10.3109/00016359109005919 PMID:1803848

Aframian, D. J., Mizrahi, B., Granot, I., & Domb, A. J. (2010). Evaluation of a mucoadhesive lipid-based bioerodable tablet compared with Biotène mouthwash for dry mouth relief – a pilot study. *Quintessence International*, *41*(3), e36–e42. PMID:20213013

Blixt-Johansen, G., Ek, A. C., Ganowiak, W., Granérus, A. K., von Schenck, H., Unosson, M., & Wiesel, K. (1992). Improvement of oral mucosa with mucin containing artificial saliva in geriatric patients. *Archives of Gerontology and Geriatrics*, *14*(2), 193–201. doi:10.1016/0167-4943(92)90054-8 PMID:15374404

Duxbury, A. J., Thakker, N. S., & Wastell, D. G. (1989). A double-blind cross-over trial of a mucin-containing artificial saliva. *British Dental Journal*, *166*(4), 115–120. doi:10.1038j.bdj.4806731 PMID:2465774

van der Reijden, W. A., van der Kwaak, H., Vissink, A., Veerman, E. C., & Amerongen, A. V. (1996). Treatment of xerostomia with polymer-based saliva substitutes in patients with Sjögren's syndrome. *Arthritis & Rheumatology (Hoboken, N.J.)*, *39*(1), 57–63. doi:10.1002/art.1780390108 PMID:8546739

Sweeney, M. P., Bagg, J., Baxter, W. P., & Aitchison, T. C. (1997). Clinical trial of a mucin-containing oral spray for treatment of xerostomia in hospice patients. *Palliative Medicine*, *11*(3), 225–232. doi:10.1177/026921639701100307 PMID:9205656

Gravenmade, E. J., & Vissink, A. (1993). Mucin-containing lozenges in the treatment of intraoral problems associated with Sjögren's syndrome. A double-blind crossover study in 42 patients. *Oral Surgery, Oral Medicine, and Oral Pathology*, *75*(4), 466–471. doi:10.1016/0030-4220(93)90172-Z PMID:8464611

Ship, J. A., McCutcheon, J. A., Spivakovsky, S., & Kerr, A. R. (2007). Safety and effectiveness of topical dry mouth products containing olive oil, betaine, and xylitol in reducing xerostomia for polypharmacy-induced dry mouth. *Journal of Oral Rehabilitation*, *34*(10), 724–732. doi:10.1111/j.1365-2842.2006.01718.x PMID:17824884

Donatsky, O., Johnsen, T., Holmstrup, P., & Bertram, U. (1982). Effect of Saliment on parotid salivary gland secretion and on xerostomia caused by Sjögren's syndrome. *Scandinavian Journal of Dental Research*, *90*(2), 157–162. PMID:7041242

Jellema, A. P., Langendijk, H., Bergenhenegouwen, L., van der Reijden, W. A., Leemans, C. R., Smeele, L. E., & Slotman, B. J. (2001). The efficacy of Xialine in patients with xerostomia resulting from radiotherapy for head and neck cancer: A pilot-study. *Radiotherapy and Oncology: Journal of the European Society for Therapeutic Radiology and Oncology*, *59*(2), 157–160. doi:10.1016/S0167-8140(01)00336-X PMID:11325444

Persson, A., Lingström, P., Bergdahl, M., Claesson, R., & van Dijken, J. W. (2007). Buffering effect of a prophylactic gel on dental plaque in institutionalised elderly. *Gerodontology*, *24*(2), 98–104. doi:10.1111/j.1741-2358.2007.00151.x PMID:17518957

Stewart, C. M., Jones, A. C., Bates, R. E., Sandow, P., Pink, F., & Stillwell, J. (1998). Comparison between saliva stimulants and a saliva substitute in patients with xerostomia and hyposalivation. *Special Care in Dentistry*, *18*(4), 142–148. doi:10.1111/j.1754-4505.1998.tb01136.x PMID:10218061

Furumoto, E. K., Barker, G. J., Carter-Hanson, C., & Barker, B. F. (1998). Subjective and clinical evaluation of oral lubricants in xerostomic patients. *Special Care in Dentistry*, *18*(3), 113–118. doi:10.1111/j.1754-4505.1998.tb00915.x PMID:9680921

Fox, P. C., Cummins, M. J., & Cummins, J. M. (2001). Use of orally administered anhydrous crystalline maltose for relief of dry mouth. *Journal of Alternative and Complementary Medicine (New York, N.Y.)*, *7*(1), 33–43. doi:10.1089/107555301300004510 PMID:11246934

Khosravani, N., Birkhed, D., & Ekström, J. (2009). The cholinesterase inhibitor physostigmine for the local treatment of dry mouth: A randomized study. *European Journal of Oral Sciences*, *117*(3), 209–217. doi:10.1111/j.1600-0722.2009.00632.x PMID:19583746

Regelink, G., Vissink, A., Reintsema, H., & Nauta, J. M. (1998). Efficacy of a synthetic polymer saliva substitute in reducing oral complaints of patients suffering from irradiation-induced xerostomia. *Quintessence International*, *29*(6), 383–388. PMID:9728149

Jackiewicz-Barańska, D. (2007). Sztuczna ślina. *Polish Journal of Cosmetology*, *10*, 80–90.

Twycross, R., & Wilcock, A. (2012). Ear Nose and Oropharynx. In R. Twycross & A. Wilcock (Eds.), *PCF4-palliative care formulary* (pp. 569–573). Oxford: Radcliffe Press.

Sreebny, L. M., & Valdini, A. (1987). Xerostomia. A neglected symptom. *Archives of Internal Medicine*, *147*(7), 1333–1337. doi:10.1001/archinte.1987.00370070145022 PMID:3300589

Azodo, C. C., Ezeja, E. B., Omoaregba, J. O., & James, B. O. (2012). Oral health of psychiatric patients: The nurse's perspective. *International Journal of Dental Hygiene*, *10*(4), 245–249. doi:10.1111/j.1601-5037.2011.00537.x PMID:22192470

Trindade, E., Menon, D., Topfer, L. A., & Coloma, C. (1998). Adverse effects associated with selective serotonin reuptake inhibitors and tricyclic antidepressants: A meta-analysis. *Canadian Medical Association Journal*, *159*(10), 1245–1252. PMID:9861221

Strietzel, F. P., Martin-Granizo, R., Fedele, S., Lafaurie, G. I., Mendoza, G. R. B., Alajbeg, I., ... Kottinen, Y. T. (2011). Efficac.y and safety of an intraoral electrostimulation device for xerostomia relief: A multicenter, randomized trial. *Arthritis & Rheumatology (Hoboken, N.J.)*, *63*(1), 180–190. doi:10.1002/art.27766 PMID:20882668

Strietzel, F. P., Fedele, S., Lo Russo, L., Mignogna, M., Reichart, P. A., & Wolff, A. (2007). Electrostimulating device in the management of xerostomia. *Oral Diseases*, *13*(2), 206–213. doi:10.1111/j.1601-0825.2006.01268.x PMID:17305624

Alajbeg, I., Falcão, D. P., Tran, S. D., Martín-Granizo, R., Lafaurie, G. I., Matranga, D., ... Zunt, S. (2012). Intraor.al electrostimulator for xerostomia relief: A long-term, multicenter, open-label, uncontrolled, clinical trial. *Oral Surgery, Oral Medicine, Oral Pathology and Oral Radiology*, *113*(6), 773–781. doi:10.1016/j.oooo.2012.01.012 PMID:22668705

Simcock, R., Fallowfield, L., Monson, K., Solis-Trapala, I., Parlour, L., Langridge, C., & Jenkins, V. (2003). ARIX: A randomized trial of acupuncture vs. oral care sessions in patients with chronic xerostomia following treatment of head and neck cancer. *Annals of Oncology: Official Journal of the European Society for Medical Oncology*, *24*(3), 776–783. doi:10.1093/annonc/mds515 PMID:23104718

Blom, M., Dawidson, I., & Angmar-Månsson, B. (1992). The effect of acupuncture on salivary flow rates in patients with xerostomia. *Oral Surgery, Oral Medicine, and Oral Pathology*, *73*(3), 293–298. doi:10.1016/0030-4220(92)90124-9 PMID:1545961

O'Sullivan, E. M., & Higginson, I. J. (2010). Clinical effectiveness and safety of acupuncture in the treatment of irradiation-induced xerostomia in patients with head and neck cancer: A systematic review. *Acupuncture in Medicine*, *28*(4), 191–199. doi:10.1136/aim.2010.002733 PMID:21062848

Gu, J., Zhu, S., Li, X., Wu, H., Li, Y., & Hua, F. (2014). Effect of amifostine in head and neck cancer patients treated with radiotherapy: A systematic review and meta-analysis based on randomized controlled trials. *PLoS One*, *9*(5), e95968. doi:10.1371/journal.ponc.0095968 PMID:24788761

Pringle, S., van Os, R., & Coppes, R. P. (2013). Adult salivary gland stem cells and a potential therapy for xerostomia. *Stem Cells (Dayton, Ohio)*, *4*(4), 613–619. doi:10.1002tem.1327 PMID:23335219

Chapter 7
Parotid Injuries and Fistulae

ABSTRACT

Successful treatment of parotid injuries depends on early recognition and appropriate early intervention. Sequelae of inadequate diagnosis and treatment include parotid fistula and sialocele formation, which are inconvenient for the patient and more difficult to treat than the initial injury. A parotid fistula is a communication between the parotid gland (glandular fistula) or duct (ductal fistula) and the skin externally (external fistula) or to the oral cavity internally (internal fistula). A sialocele is a collection of saliva beneath the skin that occurs if the duct leaks but no fistula forms, or when the glandular substance, but not the duct, is disrupted. Management options include pressure dressings and use of anti-sialagogues, total parotidectomy, tympanic neurectomy, intra-oral transposition of the parotid duct, radiation therapy, the use of botulinum toxin A, and the use of fibrin glue.

ETIOLOGY

Causes of the parotid fistula include (1) trauma (Bergstrom & Hemenway, 1971), penetrating or blunt injury in the region of the parotid gland, or as a complication of facial fractures, (2) improper incision and drainage, or spontaneous rupture of a parotid abscess (or sialocele), (3) intra-operative iatrogenic injury of the gland or duct (following surgery in the maxillofacial region, or in the temporomandibular joint (TMJ) region, parotidectomy or secondary to drainage of facial/parotid abscess, mandibular osteotomy (Shapiro, 1978); Goldberg, 1973; Dierks, 1977; Ting, 2018), or the use

DOI: 10.4018/978-1-7998-5603-0.ch007

of external pin fixation (Laskin, 1978), (4) complication of parotid duct cannulation during sialography, and (5) malignant tumors invading to the surface (Ananthakrishnan & Parkash, 1982).

CLINICAL PRESENTATION

Males are twice as likely to experience parotid duct injury as females, and the mean age of individuals with parotid duct injury is approximately 30 years.

History

Important aspects of history of the wound include the circumstances surrounding the injury, precipitating cause, exact mechanism and site of injury, time of occurrence, and treatment initiated prior to presentation.Other important aspects of the history include tobacco, alcohol, or drug use; tetanus immune status; and co-morbid conditions that may place the patient at a higher risk for infection such as diabetes mellitus and immunosuppression.

Physical Examination

An internal fistula constitutes no consequences and requires *no treatment*. However, an external fistula connected with large ducts causes extreme discomfort every time the patient has a meal, smells or even thinks of food, due to excessive outpouring of saliva on the cheek causing skin excoriation (Figure 1). A sialogram will determine whether the fistula is ductal or glandular.

A thorough clinical examination is necessary for proper evaluation of the overall state of health, co-morbidities, nutritional status, and mental status of the patient. Important signs or symptoms related to the wound include pain, fever, edema, discharge, and/or odor. Important aspects of wound assessment include location, shape, size, type (blunt or penetrating), depth, drainage (quality, character, odor), presence of a foreign body (e.g. glass, tooth fragments), loss of tissue, tenderness, asymmetry, surrounding skin (erythema, edema, crepitus), and status of the facial nerve.

An injury classification system that divides the parotid duct into 3 regions has been devised for parotid duct injuries as follows:

Figure 1. Left external parotid fistula with out-pouring of saliva

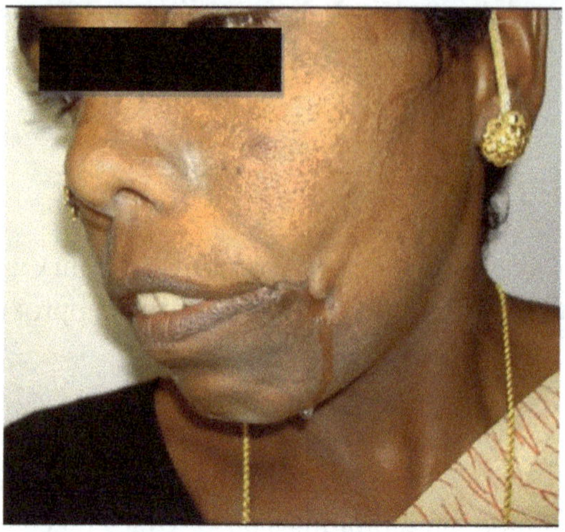

Site A: Posterior to the masseter muscle or intra-glandular (*glandular*).
Site B: Overlying the masseter muscle (*masseteric*).
Site C: Anterior to masseter muscle (*pre-masseteric*).

MANAGEMENT

Although there is consensus in the literature that acute parotid injury must be explored primarily and all injured structures be repaired accurately, the treatment of the chronic injury is controversial. Numerous methods of treatment, conservative as well as aggressive, have been described with varying success and morbidity. Management options include pressure dressings and use of anti-sialagogues (Parekh, Glezerson, Stewart, Esser, & Lawson, 1989), total parotidectomy, tympanic neurectomy (Davis, Holt, & Templer, 1977), intra-oral transposition of the parotid duct (Doctor, Rafii, Enepekides, & Tollefson, (2007), radiation therapy (Robinson, Khoury, & Robinson, 1989), the use of botulinum toxin A (Lim, 2008); Dessy, 2007; Arnaud, 2007), and the use of fibrin glue (Zwaveling, Steenvoorde, & da Costa, 2006).

Hu et al. (2018), retrospectively evaluated surgical treatment outcomes after delayed (1-3 months) parotid gland and duct injuries. Conservative treatment, microsurgical anastomosis, and diversion of salivary flow or ligation were chosen for delayed parotid gland and duct injuries concerning to their site of injury, time of repair and procedures. Assistant treatment as pressure dressing was adopted thereafter. All patients (n=9) experienced ultimately an uneventful recovery. Five patients received microsurgical anastomosis, two received Stensen's duct ligation, and two accepted salivary flow diversion. No recurrence was encountered.

Various treatment modalities to treat the parotid fistula have been advocated, if *conservative measures* fail. *Tympanic neurectomy* involves drilling into the temporal bone and disruption of the tympanic nerve, which carries parasympathetic secretory nerve fibers to the parotid gland (Chitre, 1997; Vasama, 2000). This technique aims at reducing salivary flow and causing spontaneous fistula resolution. Although popular in the past, this method tends to be *abandoned* due to short-term and poor results due to re-innervation of the gland with time (Mandour, El-Sheikh, & El-Garem, 1976).

Radiation has been used in the past to suppress the gland, but use of radiation for benign disease is now *avoided* because of its long-term ill-effects. Some authors advocate use of *anti-cholinergics* to suppress glandular function during healing, but this is *not* a frequently used modality.

Three operative techniques have been popularized over time. These include repair of the duct over a stent, ligation of the duct, and fistulization of the duct into the oral cavity. *Parotidectomy* has been discouraged as a treatment modality as postoperative facial palsy is seen in 75% of cases (Ananthakrishan & Prakash, 1982).

Non-Surgical Treatment

Wound Care

Wound care is the cornerstone of therapy. Prophylactic antibiotics should be administered and continued for 5-7 days but it should be noted that antibiotics cannot avert or cure infections in the setting of poor wound care. In rare cases, human saliva contains and occasionally transmits Clostridium tetani. Accordingly, all patients should be assessed for their tetanus immune status and immunization should be updated as appropriate.

Anti-Cholinergic Agents

Some authors choose to use *anti-cholinergic agents* to suppress glandular function during healing or in an attempt to close a fistula or resolve a sialocele spontaneously. A commonly used agent is propantheline bromide (Pro-

Banthine), which inhibits the action of acetylcholine at the postganglionic nerve endings of the parasympathetic nervous system (adult dose 15 mg PO qid half an hour prior to meals). Absence of reflex stimulation from mastication and chemical stimuli minimizes parotid secretions and allows healing of injured duct, but this method requires maximum patient compliance for prolonged time. Anti-cholinergic drugs are unlikely to be useful if used alone and are associated with numerous side effects like urinary retention, xerostomia, nausea, vomiting, vision disturbances, etc.

Pressure Dressings

Sialocele and salivary fistula can frequently be managed non-operatively with *antibiotics, pressure dressings, and serial aspiration.* Pressure dressings lead to atrophy of the gland as the lobules of the gland are contained in relatively inelastic capsule. The sustained rise in ductal pressure leads to compression of capillaries and veins, resulting in decrease in secretion and atrophy of gland (Parekh, Glezerson, Stewart, Esser, & Lawson, 1989). However, there is no adequate proof of their efficacy in literature.

Intermittent Serial Aspiration

Intermittent aspiration of sialoceles has led to resolution in many cases. Anti-cholinergics may be used to temporarily decrease salivary flow in order to effect wound healing.

Botulinum Toxin A

Botulinum toxin type A is one of eight distinct neurotoxins that are known, each with its own immunologic specificity (von Lindern, Niederhagen, Appel, Berge, & Reich, 2002). It leads to partial or complete muscle paralysis by inhibiting acetylcholine release at the neuromuscular synaptic end plate. Due to this paralytic function, it has become the mainstay of therapeutic non-surgical treatment for neuromuscular disorders such as hemifacial spasm, blepharospasm, spasmodic dysphonia, and dystonia (Christie, 1987). Because this toxin also blocks the release of acetylcholine at the cholinergic synapses of the autonomic nervous system, it also has effects on the cholinergic parasympathetic secretomotor fibers of the salivary gland. Hence, botulinum toxin has been tested in some autonomic disease, such as achalasia, hyperhiderosis and gustatory sweating (Frey's syndrome) (Laskawi, 1998; Tugnori, 1997).

Botulinum toxin A has been used nowadays, but it has a latency period and requires repeated injections for desired effects and the effects may not last long enough to bring about complete remission of disease. Moreover, it is a costly procedure (Gordin, Daniero, Krein, & Boon, 2010).

Fibrin Glue

Fibrin glue has also been used recently (Zwaveling, Steenvoorde, & da Costa, 2006); however, it is said that fibrin glue is rendered inactive by saliva leading to recurrence of fistula.

Hypertonic Saline Sclerotherapy

Hypertonic saline has been used in sclerotherapy in various concentrations. It has also been used for the treatment of varicose veins as an alternative to surgery (Parsons, 2004); and in the head and neck region for treatment of venous malformations with good results (Cabrera, Cabrera, Olmedo, & Redondo, 2003). Thermodynamic and physicochemical calculations suggest that these solutions work by causing conformational denaturation of the cell membrane proteins *in situ* and saline can be diluted to a point where there will be no cellular toxicity. The temperature of the saline can be raised above body temperature (60 degree) to enhance the fibrosing property of physiologic saline (Chhabra, Chhabra, & Kapila, 2009).

Hot hypertonic saline can be used for the purpose of fistula closure because it is cost effective, causes no foreign body reaction or hypersensitivity reaction to the patients, easily available, non-toxic and non-irritant to the surrounding structures. There are no chances of inadvertent injury to facial nerve and its branches and serves the purpose of causing fibrosis of gland parenchyma and spontaneous closure of fistula with no complications (Rao, Gehlot, Laxmy, & Vijay-Siwach, 2011).

Surgical Treatment

Copious irrigation of the wound with normal saline solution has been shown to decrease the incidence of wound infection. *Careful debridement* of devitalized tissue, particulate matter, and clot is necessary to reduce the infection risk and to improve the cosmetic result. Clean, surgically created wound margins allow for faster wound healing and better scarring.

Head and neck wounds, less than 12 hours old and not obviously infected, being in a cosmetically sensitive area, may be *closed directly* with a low incidence of infection. The low infection rate is probably related to the excellent regional blood supply and infrequency of edema in these areas. For a good cosmetic result, closure is performed in a simple interrupted fashion, using fine stitches and avoiding layered closure with buried sutures.

The most important initial step for proper surgical repair is the identification of key structures; namely, the buccal branches of the facial nerve (with the aid of a nerve stimulator intra-operatively if available) and the parotid duct itself. If the buccal branch was transected, repair it with fine sutures (8-0 to 10-0 monofilament is appropriate) under microscopic aid. The distal end of the parotid duct is identified by a silastic tube, placed via cannulation of the intra-oral papilla. The proximal parotid duct can usually be identified by the flow of saliva into the wound, with gentle pressure over the gland if necessary. Once all key structures are identified, a decision is made regarding which repair technique to employ.

Site C (Distal or Glandular)

Distal lacerations, occurring at site C, may be treated in several ways. If the *papilla is uninjured*, the proximal portion may be dissected free and re-implanted into the papilla. If the *papilla is injured* or if the proximal duct does not reach the papilla, the duct may be re-implanted (under magnification) into the oral mucosa posterior to the papilla, using fine interrupted absorbable sutures with meticulous approximation of duct epithelium to oral mucosa. If the distal injury is too short to be re-implanted into the oral mucosa without undue tension, then the best decision is to ligate the proximal duct.

Site B (Masseteric)

Injuries occurring over the masseter muscle, at site B, are the most common injuries to the parotid duct and may be treated by *repair or ligation*. If enough *length remains*, primary anastomosis over a silastic stent, using a single layer of interrupted fine sutures (8-0 to 10-0 monofilament) is performed under magnification. If a portion of the duct is *damaged* beyond repair or is missing, the proximal and distal duct should be ligated. Reports of attempts to use a vein graft (saphenous) in such cases have generally found such attempts unsuccessful. Sialoendoscopy-assisted repair of a transected Stensen duct in zone B has been reported (Koch, Iro, Bozzato, & Zenk, 2008).

Site A (Proximal or Pre-Masseteric)

Injuries of the proximal duct near the parotid substance, at ***site A***, are usually best treated by duct *ligation* as the amount of proximal duct remaining is usually insufficient to result in a useful repair. Laceration of the gland itself without disruption of the parotid duct may be repaired with fine absorbable sutures (5-0 or 6-0 Vicryl).

A drain in the wound bed is recommended to drain any residual salivary leak and prevent early sialocele formation. Drains are removed once drainage is minimal and the skin has become adherent to the operative site. *Post-operatively*, a compression dressing is placed over the operative field post-operatively for several days. If ductal injury required ligation of the proximal duct, marked temporary swelling of the gland followed by rapid glandular atrophy is expected. If leaking of saliva occurs as in the development of a fistula or sialocele, the pressure dressing should be continued or reinstituted.

In the case of a *chronic parotid duct fistula*, an *intra-oral diversion technique* to re-establish salivary flow in case of a non-functional parotid duct punctum has been described. The fistula tract and the surrounding ellipse of skin are passed in the oral cavity and sutured to the buccal mucosa with 4-0 chromic sutures without need for stenting. Alternatively, chronic fistula and sialocele have been medically managed with botulinum toxin (Arnaud, Batifol, Goudot, & Yachouh, 2008).

COMPLICATIONS

Persistent Salivary Fistula

If the fistula occurs in the oral cavity, it is of no consequence and requires no further therapy. If the fistula occurs to the overlying skin, the patient experiences saliva dripping down the cheek. Initial expectant management, with or without anti-cholinergic medications, has led to resolution in many cases. Other cases have required surgical excision of the fistula tract with repair of the duct or superficial parotidectomy.

Sialocele

Sialocele usually resolves with intermittent aspiration and compression and rarely requires drain placement. Anti-cholinergics may be beneficial in the treatment of sialoceles. Duct ligation may lead to early edema of the gland with accompanying pain from stretching of the capsule. This usually subsides spontaneously within 1-2 weeks as atrophy of the gland occurs. Infection of the remaining glandular substance may occur as a late complication of duct ligation.

Sialadenitis

Sialadenitis may result from manipulation of the intra-oral papilla or from sialography and may require drainage and antibiotics.

Nerve Injury

Facial nerve injury and sensory nerve injury may occur when surgery is conducted in the region of the parotid duct, particularly in cases where trauma and blood extravasation have discolored the tissues and disrupted tissue planes.

REFERENCES

Ananthakrishan, N., & Prakash, S. (1982). Parotid fistulas: A review. *British Journal of Surgery*, *69*(11), 641–643. doi:10.1002/bjs.1800691104 PMID:7127047

Ananthakrishnan, N., & Parkash, S. (1982). Parotid fistulas: A review. *British Journal of Surgery*, *69*(11), 641–643. doi:10.1002/bjs.1800691104 PMID:7127047

Arnaud, S., Batifol, D., Goudot, P., & Yachouh, J. (2008). Non-surgical management of parotid gland and duct injuries: Interest of botulinum toxin. *Annales de Chirurgie Plastique et Esthetique*, *53*, 36–40. doi:10.1016/j.anplas.2007.01.004 PMID:17382446

Bergstrom, L., & Hemenway, W. G. (1971). Parotid-antral fistula. Complication of facial fracture. *Archives of Otolaryngology*, *93*(5), 519–520. doi:10.1001/archotol.1971.00770060765016 PMID:5554889

Cabrera, J., Cabrera, J. Jr, Olmedo, A. G., & Redondo, P. (2003). Treatment of venous malformations with sclerosant in microfoam form. *Archives of Dermatology*, *139*(11), 1494–1496. doi:10.1001/archderm.139.11.1409 PMID:14623700

Chhabra, N., Chhabra, S., & Kapila, S. A. (2009). Use of hypertonic saline in the management of parotid fistulae and sialocele: A report of 2 cases. *Journal of Maxillofacial and Oral Surgery*, *8*(1), 64–67. doi:10.100712663-009-0016-9 PMID:23139474

Chitre, V. V., & Premchandra, D. J. (1997). Recurrent parotitis. *Archives of Disease in Childhood*, *77*(4), 359–363. doi:10.1136/adc.77.4.359 PMID:9389246

Christie, A. (1987). *Infectious Disease*. London: Churchill Livingstone.

Davis, W. E., Holt, G. R., & Templer, J. W. (1977). Parotid fistula and tympanic neurectomy. *American Journal of Surgery*, *133*(5), 587–589. doi:10.1016/0002-9610(77)90015-0 PMID:871188

Dessy, L. A., Mazzocchi, M., Monarca, C., Onesti, M. G., & Scuderi, N. (2007). Combined transdermal scopolamine and botulinum toxin A to treat a parotid fistula after a face-lift in a patient with siliconomas. *International Journal of Oral and Maxillofacial Surgery*, *36*(10), 949–952. doi:10.1016/j.ijom.2007.05.021 PMID:17662576

Dierks, E. J., & Granite, E. L. (1977). Parotid sialocele and fistula after mandibular osteotomy. *Journal of Oral Surgery*, *35*, 299–300. PMID:264948

Doctor, V. S., Rafii, A., Enepekides, D. J., & Tollefson, T. T. (2007). Intraoral transposition of traumatic parotid duct fistula. *Archives of Facial Plastic Surgery*, *9*(1), 44–47. doi:10.1001/archfaci.9.1.44 PMID:17224488

Goldberg, M. H., Marco, W., & Googel, F. (1973). Parotid fistula: A complication of mandibular osteotomy. *Journal of Oral Surgery*, *31*, 207–208. PMID:4509838

Gordin, E. A., Daniero, J. J., Krein, H., & Boon, M. S. (2010). Parotid gland trauma. *Facial Plastic Surgery*, *26*(6), 504–510. doi:10.1055-0030-1267725 PMID:21086237

Hu, C. Y., Shang, Z. J., Qin, X., & Shao, L. N. (2018). Application of Delayed Surgical Managements in Patients with Stensen's Duct Injury. *Current Medical Science*, *38*(3), 519–523. doi:10.100711596-018-1909-y PMID:30074221

Koch, M., Iro, H., Bozzato, A., & Zenk, J. (2008). Sialoendoscopy-assisted microsurgical repair of traumatic transection of Stensen's duct. *The Laryngoscope*, *123*(12), 3074–3477. doi:10.1002/lary.23412 PMID:24122915

Laskawi, R., Drobik, C., & Schonebeck, C. (1998). Up-to-date report of botulinum toxin type A treatment in patients with gustatory sweating (Frey's syndrome). *The Laryngoscope*, *108*(3), 381–384. doi:10.1097/00005537-199803000-00013 PMID:9504611

Laskin, J. L. (1978). Parotid fistula after the use of external pin fixation: Report of case. *Journal of Oral Surgery*, *36*, 621–622. PMID:277656

Lim, Y. C., & Choi, E. C. (2008). Treatment of an acute salivary fistula after parotid surgery: Botulinum toxin type A injection as primary treatment. *European Archives of Oto-Rhino-Laryngology*, *265*(2), 243–245. doi:10.100700405-007-0418-6 PMID:17704932

Mandour, M. A., El-Sheikh, M. M., & El-Garem, F. (1976). Tympanic neurectomy for parotid fistula. *Archives of Otolaryngology*, *102*(6), 327–329. doi:10.1001/archotol.1976.00780110039002 PMID:1275800

Parekh, D., Glezerson, G., Stewart, M., Esser, J., & Lawson, H. H. (1989). Post-traumatic parotid fistulae and sialoceles. A prospective study of conservative management in 51 cases. *Annals of Surgery*, *209*(1), 105–111. doi:10.1097/00000658-198901000-00015 PMID:2910210

Parsons, M. E. (2004). Sclerotherapy basics. *Dermatologist Clinic*, *22*(4), 501–508. doi:10.1016/j.det.2004.03.017 PMID:15450346

Rao, J. K. D., Gehlot, N., Laxmy, V., & Vijay-Siwach, V. (2011). Management of parotid fistula using hypertonic saline. *National Journal of Maxillofacial Surgery*, *2*(2), 177–180. doi:10.4103/0975-5950.94477 PMID:22639509

Robinson, A. C., Khoury, G. G., & Robinson, P. M. (1989). Role of irradiation in the suppression of parotid secretions. *The Journal of Laryngology and Otology*, *103*(6), 594–595. doi:10.1017/S0022215100109430 PMID:2769027

Shapiro, D. N., Gallo, J., & Moss, M. (1978). Subcutaneous parotid effusion after mandibular osteotomy. *Journal of Oral Surgery*, *36*, 397–398. PMID:273673

Ting, L., & Liew, Y. T. (2018). Parotid salivary fistula post-superficial parotidectomy. *Journal of Case Reports and Medical Images*, *1*(1), 1003. doi:10.33582/2639-9237/1003

Tugnoli, V., Eleopra, R., Montecucco, C., & DeGrandis, D. (1997). The therapeutic use of botulinum toxin. *Expert Opinion on Investigational Drugs*, *6*(10), 1383–1394. doi:10.1517/13543784.6.10.1383 PMID:15989508

Vasama, J. P. (2000). Tympanic neurectomy and chronic parotitis. *Acta Oto-Laryngologica*, *120*(8), 995–998. doi:10.1080/00016480050218762 PMID:11200598

von Lindern, J. J., Niederhagen, B., Appel, T., Berge, S., & Reich, R. H. (2002). New prospects in the treatment of traumatic and postoperative parotid fistulas with type A botulinum toxin. *Plastic and Reconstructive Surgery*, *109*(7), 2443–2445. doi:10.1097/00006534-200206000-00041 PMID:12045574

Zwaveling, S., Steenvoorde, P., & da Costa, S. A. (2006). Treatment of postparotidectomy fistulae with fibrin glue. *Acta Medica*, *49*, 67–69. PMID:16696446

Chapter 8
Calculi of the Parotid Gland

ABSTRACT

Sialolithiasis is the most common disorder of major salivary glands with approximately 80% to 95% occurring in the submandibular gland and 5% to 20% in the parotid gland. Parotid stones are composed of organic substances such as cellular debris, muco-polysaccharides and glycoproteins, and inorganic substances, mainly phosphates and calcium carbonates. Conventional x-ray sialography combined with US is the method of choice for visualization of salivary gland calculi. Sialography and US are also inevitable in patient's qualification for diagnostic and therapeutic sialoendoscopy, thus avoiding sialadenectomy. An alternative, non-invasive diagnostic method is magnetic resonance imaging (MRI), MR sialography (MRS), or unenhanced computed tomography (CT). Therapeutic options include parotidectomy, external lithtripsy, and interventional sialoendoscopy.

INCIDENCE

Sialolithiasis is the most common disorder of major salivary glands (Madani & Beale, 2006). The majority of salivary calculi (80% to 95%) occur in the submandibular gland, whereas 5% to 20% are found in the parotid gland (Madani, 2006; Drage, 2000; Rabinov, 2000; Yousem, 2000; Jager, 2000; Koischwitz, 2000; Alyas, 2005; Bialek, 2006; Erdem, 2018). The difference in incidence is attributed to a number of factors such as the difference in the composition of the saliva produced by each gland and the dependence of the submandibular (Wharton's) duct, which hinders easy drainage of its viscid

DOI: 10.4018/978-1-7998-5603-0.ch008

secretions. Sialothiasis rarely affects the sublingual gland and the minor salivary glands are rarely (1% to 2%) (Rabinov & Weber, 1985).

The majority of stones are single. In 25% of cases, the stones are multiple (Madani, 2006; Rabinov, 2000; Yousem, 2000; Alyas, 2005). The mean number of stones per one patient is 1.67 (range from 1 to 5), and the most symptomatic sialolithiasis can be observed in patients between 30 and 60 years old (Drage, Brown, Escudler, & McGurk, 2000).

COMPOSITION

Parotid stones are composed of *organic* substances such as cellular debris, muco-polysaccharides and glycoproteins, and *inorganic* substances, mainly phosphates and calcium carbonates (Langlais, 1995).

The organic substances are mainly found as the core of the stone, while the inorganic substances are in its periphery. *Hydroxyapatite* (calcium phosphate) is the most frequent component present throughout the calculus.

The annual growth rate of an established stone is about 1 mm per year and the average size is about 3.4 mm (range from 1.5 to 9 mm) (Drage, Brown, Escudler, & McGurk, 2000). Calculi within a major duct tend to be smooth and rounded, whereas those within the gland tend to be irregular in shape.

ETIOLOGY / PATHOGENESIS

According to one of the etiopathogenetic theories, the formation of the salivary gland calculi results from a deposition of calcium salts around a core made of desquamated epithelial cells, foreign bodies, bacteria, or mucus. Salivary gland calculi are of laminal structure.

Submandibular gland is the most common place for calculi formation because it produces a particularly viscous, mucous and more alkaline saliva, with a relatively high concentration of hydroxyapatites and phosphates. This predisposes to the precipitation of salts (Madani, 2006; Yousem, 2000). Moreover, the opening of the main salivary duct of the submandibular gland (Wharton's duct) is narrower than the diameter of the whole duct. What is more, the duct ascends towards its opening, which is also conducive to saliva retention (Yousem, 2000; Alyas, 2005; Langlais, 1995; Wong, 2003).

CLINICAL PRESENTATION

Parotid calculi can occur in the gland or Stensen's duct (Figure 1) Sialolithiasis can occur at any *age* - however most cases occur in patients in their third to sixth decade. Sialothiasis rarely occurs in children. Males and females are equally affected.

Figure 1. Parotid calculi in Stensen's duct, which is dilated behind the stone

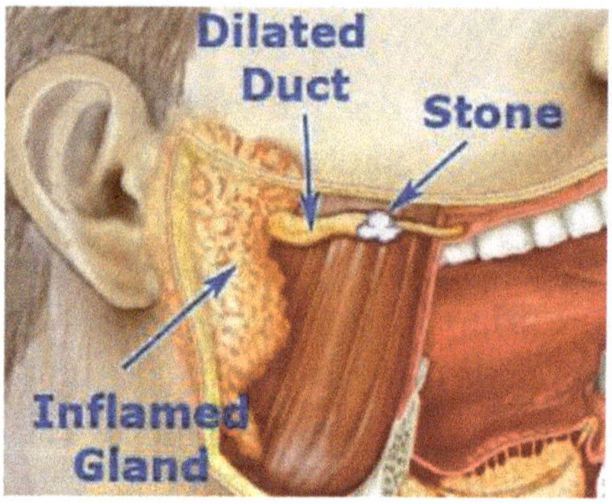

Clinical presentations of a parotid stone vary from being *asymptomatic*, to intermittent obstructive parotitis (sialolithiasis is the cause of 42-77% of cases of salivary duct obstruction) (Nahlieli, 2001; Yuasa, 1997), to an acute abscess. The patient usually presents with swelling and pain, aggravated by eating, but subsiding within the next hour or so after the meal. A decreased production of the saliva may be observed as well (Madani, 2006; Yousem, 2000; Loischwitz, 2000; Bialek, 2006; Hasson, 2007). Palpation of the gland confirms that it is enlarged and should be done on both sides for comparison. *Complications* of sialolithiasis include acute suppurative sialadenitis, ductal ulceration and stricture (Madani, 2006; Drage, 2009).

INVESTIGATIONS

Calculi must be differentiated from *stenosis* of the duct caused by repeated trauma and fibrosis. The basic imaging methods of sialolithiasis are: plain X-ray images, X-ray sialography, ultrasonography (US), computed tomography

(CT), magnetic resonance imaging (MRI). Sialoendoscopy, which is also a therapeutic method, is becoming increasingly common.

Plain X-rays may reveal larger stones but the soft tissue image of the cheek makes this method less suited for the detection of smaller ones. Sialograms (contrast radiology of the duct system) are more likely to be able to reveal the stones but still may be difficult to interpret. Other investigative options include US, CT scanning and MRI, all of which are particularly useful in evaluating masses in the salivary glands.

In the USA, a major role in sialolithiasis diagnostics is played by unenhanced CT, while in Europe this is US and digital subtraction sialography (Madani & Beale, 2006). MR sialography is also gaining on popularity.

Plain X-Ray

Occlusal and lateral-oblique views demonstrate radio-opaque calculi. Radiolucent calculi are undetectable by plain radiography. It was reported that stones of the submandibular gland produce opacity in 80–90% of cases, while stones of the parotid gland only in 60% (Figure 2) (Madani, 2006; Rabinov, 2000; Jager, 2000).

A single X-ray is normally performed before contrast administration for sialography.

Sialography

Sialography allows examination of the architecture of the salivary gland and duct. Parotid stones are usually imaged through sialography being mostly radiolucent. The sensitivity of conventional sialography in calculi detection ranges from 64 to 100%, while its specificity from 88 to 100%. Digitalization of that examination, with the use of subtraction (digital subtraction sialography - DSS), increased its sensitivity of stone detection up to 96-100%, and its specificity to 88-91.1% (Jager et al, 2000).

Ultrasonography (US)

Ultrasonography can be used to differentiate between solid and cystic lesions of the gland. It can be used to differentiate intrinsic from extrinsic disease and is helpful in identification of abscess formation.

Figure 2. Plain X-ray showing a round radio-opaque shadow (stone) in the parotid (black arrow)

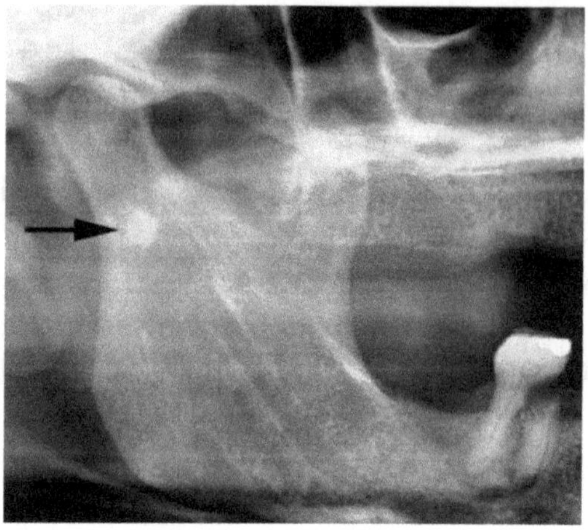

Ultrasonography is regarded by some authors as a method of choice in salivary stone diagnostics. In calculi detection, it has a sensitivity of 94%, specificity of 100% and accuracy of 96% (Madani, 2006, Yousem, 2000; Wong, 2003). Ultrasonography has been reported to allow for *non-opaque* calculi detection with a sensitivity of 80-96% (Koischwitz, 2000; Alyas, 2005). A typical US image of a stone involves: an echogenic, round or oval structure, producing an acoustic shadow (Figure 3) (Madani, 2006; Koischwitz, 2000; Bialek, 2006). Stones in salivary ducts may lead to the distension of the duct above the obstacle, which may be shown on US.[7] Stones smaller than 2 mm may not produce any acoustic shadow (Madani, 2006; Jager, 2000; Koischwitz, 2000; Alyas, 2005). Diagnostic mistakes may concern very small stones in intra-parenchymal ducts, with no duct distension (Madani, 2006; Koischwitz, 2000). Moreover, hyperechogenic air-bubbles mixed with the saliva and simulating stones, may also be misleading (Białek, Jakubowski, Zajkowski, Szopinski, & Osmolski, 2006).

The detection of fine stones may be helped by sialogogue injection, which causes salivary duct dilatation and thus facilitates calculi visualization (Madani, 2006; Koischwitz, 2000). In about 50% of the sialolithiasis cases, US images show features of inflammation.

Despite many advantages of US, it turns out to be less precise in differentiating a cluster of stones from a single, large stone (Yousem, Kraut, & Chalian, 2000).

Figure 3. Ultrasound showing a stone (white arrow) with an acoustic shadow behind the calculus

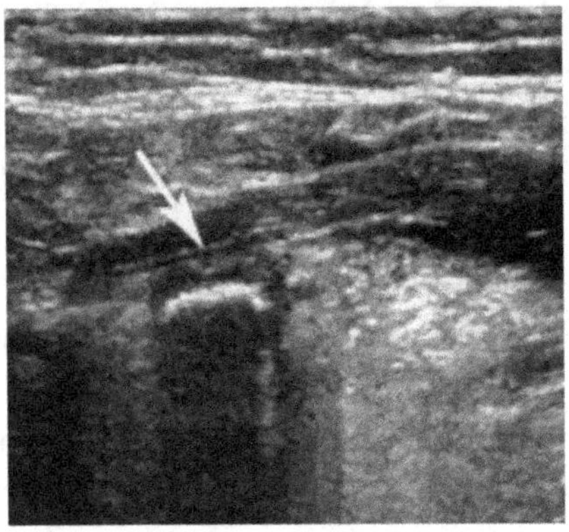

Computed Tomography (CT) Scanning

CT scan is useful in differentiating intrinsic from extrinsic glandular disease (Figure 4). It can be used in defining abscess formation versus phlegmon, but has limited usefulness in evaluation of ductal system unless combined with simultaneous sialography in addition to patient exposure to ionizing radiation and a relatively high cost of the examination (Drage, Brown, Escudler, & McGurk, 2000).

Figure 4. CT scan showing parotid gland calculus (arrow)

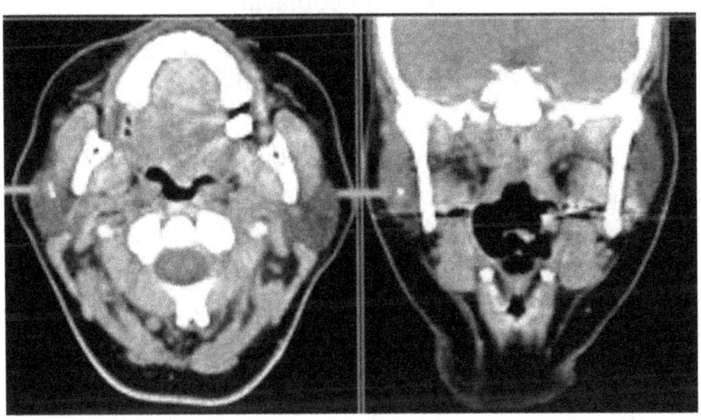

CT sialography, similarly to the conventional sialography, requires cannulation of the duct opening. Moreover, it exposes patients to a higher dose of radiation, as compared with the conventional sialography. This method allows for simultaneous visualization of the glandular tissue and the salivary ducts. The salivary glands may be shown in 3D reconstruction. However, CT sialography cannot visualize the secondary and the tertiary branches (Jäger et al, 2000).

According to some authors, unenhanced CT scan is the best method in detection of sialolithiasis, especially in case of painful salivary glands and suspicion of a few, very tiny calculi (Madani, 2006; Yousem, 2000). A cluster of fine stones is hard to differentiate from one, large stone. That is when CT is recommended (Madani & Beale, 2006). The phenomenon of the post-contrast enhancement in CT should be used in suspicion of an abscess that cannot be detected with US.

Recently, some authors reported encouraging results on the use of the volumetric tomography (alternatively called Cone Beam Computed Tomography – CBCT) in sialolithiasis diagnostics (Drage & Brown, 2009). This method produces high-resolution, 3D images of bony structures of the head and neck, with the use of up to 15 times lower ionizing radiation dose, and being much cheaper (Ludlow, 2008; Scarfe, 2006).

Magnetic Resonance Imaging (MRI)

MRI does *not* allow evaluation of the ductal system, and it is *not* helpful in defining calcifications. It is an excellent tool for soft tissue definition (invaluable in instances of suspected neoplasia).

Magnetic Resonance Sialography (MRS)

Being a non-invasive method, it does *not* require cannulation of the salivary duct opening, and it *does* not expose patients to ionizing radiation or iodine contrast administration. MR sialography allows for a precise morphological evaluation of the salivary ducts, enabling the visualization of their tertiary branches (Capaccio et al, 2008). Moreover, the examination may be carried out in acute inflammation of the salivary gland. It is considered an alternative to digital subtraction sialography, especially in cases of acute sialoadenitis or failure of salivary opening cannulation (Obaid, 2006; Kalinowski, 2002; McGahan, 1984; Becker, 2000).

Capaccio et al. (2008) compared the results of MRS versus US. Examinations were performed before and after stimulation with lemon juice. MRS showed secondary branches of the salivary ducts within submandibular salivary glands, and tertiary branches within the parotid glands. MRS allowed visualization of very tiny stones that could not be found with US.

According to Becker et al. (20000), MRS is a better method for salivary gland evaluation than conventional X-ray sialography or US, as it allows visualization of distal salivary ducts. Moreover, by adding extra MRI sequences for parenchymal imaging, it is possible to detect some lesions located outside the system of the salivary ducts (e.g. Warthin's tumor) (Rabinov, 2000).

Becker et al. (2000) compared MRS precision in detection of calculi as compared to conventional sialography, US, and sialoendoscopy. MRS showed a sensitivity of 91%, a specificity of 94-97%, a positive predictive value of 93-97%, and a negative predictive value of 91%. False negative results were obtained in calculi measuring 2-3 mm, located in undilated salivary ducts. MRS did not distinguish a stone from a dense mucosal plug. Moreover, amalgam fillings veiled tiny calculi and stenoses of the salivary ducts. Results also revealed that the peripheral salivary ducts could be better visualized with the conventional X-ray sialography than with MRS. Limitation of MRS is also connected with its lower spatial resolution enabling the differentiation of partial and of complete occlusions of the salivary ducts (Kalinowski, Heverhagen, Rehberg, Klose, & Wagner, 2002). In conclusion, MRS is considered as a highly effective, non-invasive diagnostic method of visualization of salivary ducts of large salivary glands, especially in cases of acute sialoadenitis.

Sialendoscopy

The causes of salivary duct stenosis remain unknown by imaging modalities in 5-10% of cases. The diagnostic gap is filled by sialoendoscopy that allows direct visualization of the salivary duct lumen, i.e. visualization of calculi (Figure 5B), mucosal plugs, foreign bodies and polyps.

Sialoendoscopy enabled the surgeons to examine the salivary ducts from the inside (Figure 5A). Combination of sialoendoscopy with therapeutic procedures increases the frequency of sialography (Yu, Zheng, Yang, & Shen, 2008). Yu et al. (2008) recommended dilatation of the ductal openings before performing sialoendoscopy. Others recommend papillotomy. During sialoendoscopy, the operators use very small tools and a camcorder, to reach the proximal parts of the salivary ducts. Sialoendoscopy includes performance of the following procedures: calculi removal with the use of the Dormia basket (Figure 5C), dilatation of the stenosed salivary ducts with the use of balloons (Figure 5D), as well as stenosis correction (Nahlieli, Shacham, Yoffe, & Eliav, 2001). At the end of the sialoendoscopic procedure, a stent, 2–3 cm long, is left in the salivary duct for 7-10 days to facilitate healing and drainage.

Figure 5. Sialoendoscopy. (A) Sialoendoscopic view of intra-glandular branches of Stensen's duct; (B) View of the calculus inside the Wharton's duct; (C) Dormia basket, in the left lower corner the retrieved calculus; (D) Balloon-tipped catheter

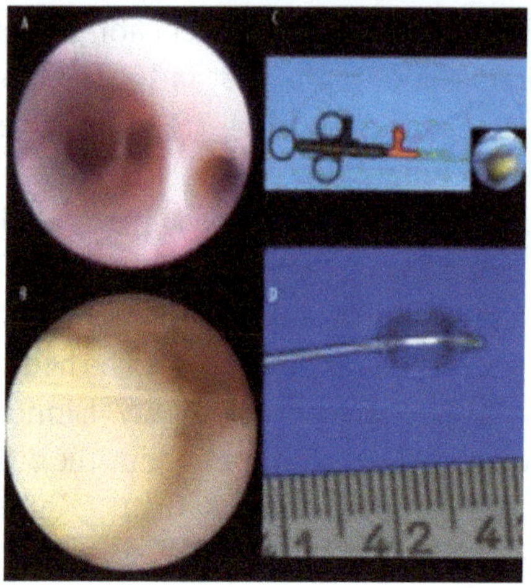

Conclusion

Conventional X-ray sialography (especially DSS) combined with US is the method of choice in visualization of salivary gland calculi. Sialography precisely shows the location and number of stones. Interventional sialography is less invasive than surgical treatment. Moreover, sialography and US are inevitable in patient's qualification for diagnostic and therapeutic sialoendoscopy; thus, avoiding sialadenectomy. An alternative, non-invasive diagnostic method of salivary gland calculi and salivary duct stenosis detection is MRI or MRS. These methods neither require cannulation of the salivary duct openings, nor the administration of the contrast medium or exposure to ionizing radiation either. MRS may also be carried out in acute sialoadenitis. As the last resort, in search for very fine and multiple calculi, it is possible to apply the unenhanced computed tomography of the salivary glands.

TREATMENT

Surgical Treatment

Glandular or ductal stones can be treated with *parotidectomy*, while those close to the duct orifice are removed by ductal dilation and massage or by longitudinal slitting of the duct and releasing the stone.

External Lithotripsy

New therapeutic modalities use extracorporeal or intracorporeal crushing of the salivary gland calculi. The crushed stones can be flushed out with saliva, through natural salivary duct openings (Drage, Brown, Escudler, & McGurk, 2000). The advent of *external lithotripsy* in the early 1990s paved the way for conservative treatment of all calculi, with a success rate of 40% in the submandibular gland and 75% in the parotid. Unfortunately, results were discouraging, specifically in patients with large calculi (Aidan, 1996; Capaccio, 2004; Iro, 1998; Gutmann, 1995).

Interventional Sialoendoscopy

Interventional Sialendoscopy, first described in the 1990s, offered much less invasive therapeutic options and became popular later with technological improvements (Marchal, 2003; Marchal 2000; Marchal, 1999; Marchal, 2001; Marchal, 2002; Nahlieli, 1999).

Interventional sialoendoscopy can be used to retrieve *stones* from the ducts as shown in Figure 6 as well as dilating ductal *strictures*. When the diameter of the stone is 5 mm or less, it can be removed purely by an endoscopic technique, particularly when the stone is located above the muscles that comprise the floor of the mouth.

Kopec et al. (2016) presented the results of treatment of sialolithiasis of the submandibular and parotid glands using sialendoscopy and sialendoscopy-assisted surgery. During the period from 2009-2013, 239 consecutive patients were treated for sialolithiasis of the major salivary glands. Sixty-four patients had 71 stones removed from the parotid gland by endoscopic retrieval or surgical release and 43 (67%) were free of stones (by sialendoscopy alone (n=25), and sialendoscopy-assisted surgery (n=18). Twenty patients (31%) had residual stones and one (2%) required removal of the gland. They thus

Figure 6. Sialoendoscopy showing interior of parotid (Stensen's) duct (A); and intra-ductal stones (B)

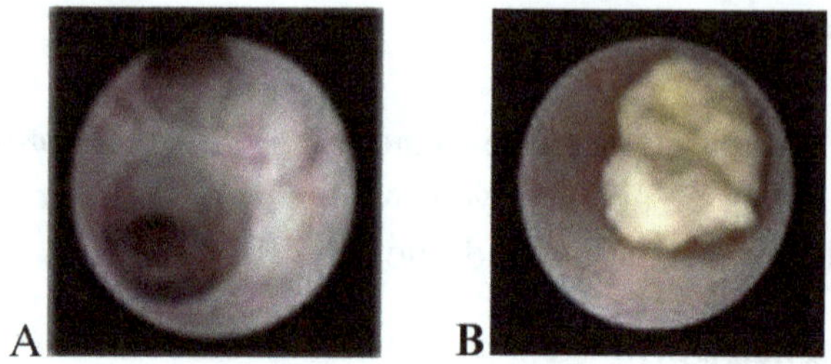

confirmed that sialendoscopy and sialendoscopy-assisted removal is the current treatment of choice for stones in the major salivary glands. The indications for excision of the gland are becoming less common as first-line treatment, although it is still indispensable in some cases.

The 4 common techniques used to remove the salivary gland stones are (1) the grasping technique, (2) using a small wire basket retrieval system, (3) mechanical fragmentation, and (4) laser fragmentation (Nahlieli, Nakar, Nazarian, & Turner, 2006). Nevertheless, success rates of interventional sialoendoscopy with intra-ductal laser fragmentation and basket extraction of calculi remained possible in only 80% of patients (Marchal & Dulguerov, 2003). Unsuccessful treatment was attributed to large-sized calculi (6 mm and larger) and to associated ductal stenosis (Marchal, 2007). In such cases, the only solution was to remove the gland, with its associated significant morbidity (Aidan, 1996; Capaccio, 2004; Iro, 1998).

When the diameter is larger than 5 mm, a twofold (endoscopic-assisted) approach can also be utilized. The endoscope is introduced and the stone localized, and then dissected and removed through an intra-oral approach. After a sialolith is removed from an affected gland, a silastic *stent* is inserted into the duct for 2-4 weeks for the duration of the healing process of the oral region and until normal function of the gland is restored. This prevents *scar* formation, which can develop over the ductal opening into the mouth.

In presence of *strictures* or *adhesions*, the diagnosis and exact location of obstruction are established using a *sialogram*. The surgeon can use the endoscopic method. The first step is anesthetizing and lavaging the duct with 2% lidocaine and saline solution. If there is no improvement, the surgeon then can insert a *dilation balloon*, which can be inflated up to 3 mm. The pressure created by the inflation can be sufficient to dilate most strictures.

Another technique for dilating strictures is to expand the stricture region with *grasping forceps* used as a dilator.

PROGNOSIS/RECURRENCE

In cases in which only the calculus is removed, the recurrence rate may be as high as 18% because the underlying cause, which is unknown, has not been corrected.

REFERENCES

Aidan, P., De Kerviler, E., LeDuc, A., & Monteil, J. P. (1996). Treatment of salivary stones by extracorporeal lithotripsy. *American Journal of Otolaryngology*, *17*(4), 246–250. doi:10.1016/S0196-0709(96)90089-7 PMID:8827289

Alyas, F., Lewis, K., Williams, M., Moody, A. B., Wong, K. T., Ahuja, A. T., & Howlett, D. C. (2005). Diseases of the submandibular gland as demonstrating using high resolution ultrasound. *The British Journal of Radiology*, *78*(928), 362–369. doi:10.1259/bjr/93120352 PMID:15774602

Becker, M., Marchal, F., Becker, C. D., Dulguerov, P., Georgakopoulos, G., Lehmann, W., & Terrier, F. (2000). Sialolithiasis and Salivary Ductal Stenosis: Diagnostic Accuracy of MR Sialography with a Three-dimensional Extended-Phase Conjugate-Symmetry Rapid Spin-Echo Sequence. *Radiology*, *217*(2), 347–358. doi:10.1148/radiology.217.2.r00oc02347 PMID:11058627

Białek, E. J., Jakubowski, W., Zajkowski, P., Szopinski, K. T., & Osmolski, A. (2006). US of the major salivary glands: Anatomy and spatial relationships, pathologic conditions, and pitfalls. *Radiographics*, *26*(3), 745–763. doi:10.1148/rg.263055024 PMID:16702452

Capaccio, P., Cuccarini, V., Ottaviani, F., Minorati, D., Sambataro, G., Cornalba, P., & Pignataro, L. (2008). Comparative Ultrasonographic, Magnetic Resonance Sialographic and Video-endoscopic Assessment of Salivary Duct Disorders. *The Annals of Otology, Rhinology, and Laryngology*, *117*(4), 245–252. doi:10.1177/000348940811700402 PMID:18478832

Capaccio, P., Ottaviani, F., Manzo, R., Schindler, A., & Cesana, B. (2004). Extracorporeal lithotripsy for salivary calculi: A long-term clinical experience. *The Laryngoscope*, *114*(6), 1069–1073. doi:10.1097/00005537-200406000-00021 PMID:15179215

Drage, N. A., & Brown, J. E. (2009). Cone beam computed sialography of sialoliths. *Dento Maxillo Facial Radiology*, *38*(5), 301–305. doi:10.1259/dmfr/90784441 PMID:19474259

Drage, N. A., Brown, J. E., Escudler, M. P., & McGurk, M. (2000). Interventional radiology in the removal of salivary calcluli. *Radiology*, *214*(1), 139–142. doi:10.1148/radiology.214.1.r00ja02139 PMID:10644113

Erdem, S., Abilov, A., Erdem, S., Zengin, A. Z., & Sumer, M. (2018). An unusual parotid sialolith diagnosis and treatment: A case report. *Journal of Dental Research and Reports*, *1*(1), 1–4. doi:10.15761/JDRR.1000104

Gutmann, R., Ziegler, G., Leunig, A., Jacob, K., & Feyh, J. (1995). Endoscopic and extracorporeal shock wave lithotripsy of salivary calculi. *Laryngo- Rhino- Otologie*, *74*(4), 249–253. doi:10.1055-2007-997732 PMID:7772227

Hasson, O. (2007). Sialoendoscopy and Sialography: Strategies for Assessment and Treatment of Salivary Gland Obstructions. *Journal of Oral and Maxillofacial Surgery*, *65*(2), 300–304. doi:10.1016/j.joms.2005.12.052 PMID:17236938

Iro, H., Zenk, J., Waldfahrer, F., Benzel, W., Schneider, T., & Ell, C. (1998). Extracorporeal shock wave lithotripsy of parotid stones. Results of a prospective clinical trial. *The Annals of Otology, Rhinology, and Laryngology*, *107*(10 Pt 1), 860–864. doi:10.1177/000348949810701009 PMID:9794616

Jäger, L., Menauer, F., Holzknecht, N., Scholz, V., Grevers, G., & Resier, M. (2000). Sialolithiasis: MR Sialography of the Submandibular Duct – An Alternative to Conventional Sialography and US? *Radiology*, *216*(3), 665–671. doi:10.1148/radiology.216.3.r00se12665 PMID:10966693

Kalinowski, M., Heverhagen, J. T., Rehberg, E., Klose, K. J., & Wagner, H.-J. (2002). Comparative Study of MR Sialography and Digital Subtraction Sialography for Benign Salivary Gland Disorders. *AJNR. American Journal of Neuroradiology*, *23*(9), 1485–1492. PMID:12372736

Koischwitz, D., & Gritzmann, N. (2000). Ultrasound of the neck. *Radiologic Clinics of North America, 38*(5), 1029–1045. doi:10.1016/S0033-8389(05)70219-0 PMID:11054967

Kopec, T., Wierzbicka, M., Kałużny, J., Młodkowska, A., & Szyfter, W. (2016). Sialendoscopy and sialendoscopically-assisted operations in the treatment of lithiasis of the submandibular and parotid glands: Our experience of 239 cases. *British Journal of Oral & Maxillofacial Surgery, 54*(7), 767–771. doi:10.1016/j.bjoms.2016.04.026 PMID:27185233

Langlais, R. P. (1995). *Diagnostic Imaging of the Jaws*. Williams and Wilkins.

Ludlow, J. B., & Ivanovic, M. (2008). Comparative dosimetry of dental CBCT devices and 64-slice CT for oral and maxillofacial radiology. *Oral Surgery, Oral Medicine, Oral Pathology, Oral Radiology, and Endodontics, 106*(1), 106–114. doi:10.1016/j.tripleo.2008.03.018 PMID:18504152

Madani, G., & Beale, T. (2006). Inflammatory Conditions of the Salivary Glands. *Seminars in Ultrasound. CT and MRI, 27*(6), 440–451. PMID:17233227

Marchal, F. (2007). A combined endoscopic and external approach for extraction of large stones with preservation of parotid and submandibular glands. *The Laryngoscope, 117*(2), 373–377. doi:10.1097/mlg.0b013e31802c06e9 PMID:17204984

Marchal, F., Becker, M., Dulguerov, P., & Lehmann, W. (2000). Interventional sialoendoscopy. *The Laryngoscope, 110*(2 Pt 1), 318–320. doi:10.1097/00005537-200002010-00026 PMID:10680937

Marchal, F., & Dulguerov, P. (2003). Sialolithiasis management: The state of the art. *Archives of Otolaryngology--Head & Neck Surgery, 129*(9), 951–956. doi:10.1001/archotol.129.9.951 PMID:12975267

Marchal, F., Dulguerov, P., Becker, M., Barki, G., Disant, F., & Lehmann, W. (2001). Specificity of parotid sialendoscopy. *The Laryngoscope, 111*(2), 264–271. doi:10.1097/00005537-200102000-00015 PMID:11210873

Marchal, F., Dulguerov, P., Becker, M., Barki, G., Disant, F., & Lehmann, W. (2002). Submandibular diagnostic and interventional sialendoscopy: New procedure for ductal disorders. *The Annals of Otology, Rhinology, and Laryngology, 111*(1), 27–35. doi:10.1177/000348940211100105 PMID:11800367

Marchal, F., Dulguerov, P., & Lehmann, W. (1999). Interventional sialoendoscopy. *The New England Journal of Medicine*, *341*(16), 1242–1243. doi:10.1056/NEJM199910143411620 PMID:10523164

McGahan, J. P., Walter, J. P., & Bernstein, L. (1984). Evaluation of the Parotid Gland. Comparison of Sialography, Non-contrast Computed Tomography and CT Sialography. *Radiology*, *152*(2), 453–458. doi:10.1148/radiology.152.2.6739814 PMID:6739814

Nahlieli, O., & Baruchin, A. M. (1999). Endoscopic technique for the diagnosis and treatment of obstructive salivary gland diseases. *Journal of Oral and Maxillofacial Surgery*, *57*(12), 1394–1401. doi:10.1016/S0278-2391(99)90716-4 PMID:10596658

Nahlieli, O., Nakar, L. H., Nazarian, Y., & Turner, M. D. (2006). Sialoendoscopy: A new approach to salivary gland obstructive pathology. *The Journal of the American Dental Association*, *137*(10), 1394–1400. doi:10.14219/jada.archive.2006.0051 PMID:17012718

Nahlieli, O., Shacham, R., Yoffe, B., & Eliav, E. (2001). Diagnosis and treatment of strictures and kinks in salivary gland ducts. *Journal of Oral and Maxillofacial Surgery*, *59*(5), 484–490. doi:10.1053/joms.2001.22667 PMID:11326365

Obaid, H., Sinha, R., & Robinson, L. (2006). Submandibular sialogram performed through a Wharton's duct fistula: Technical adaptation of conventional technique. *European Journal of Radiology*, *60*(1), 56–57. doi:10.1016/j.ejrad.2006.05.015 PMID:16815660

Rabinov, J. D. (2000). Imaging of salivary gland pathology. *Radiologic Clinics of North America*, *38*(5), 1047–1057. doi:10.1016/S0033-8389(05)70220-7 PMID:11054968

Rabinov, K., & Weber, A. L. (1985). *Radiology of the Salivary Glands*. Boston: G.K. Hall Medical Publishers.

Scarfe, W. C., Farman, A. G., & Sukovic, P. (2006). Clinical applications of cone-beam computed tomography in dental practice. *Journal - Canadian Dental Association*, *72*(1), 75–80. PMID:16480609

Wong, K. T., Ahuja, A. T., & Yuen, H. Y. (2003). Ultrasound of salivary glands. *Australasian Society for Ultrasound in Medicine Ultrasound Bulletin*, *6*(3), 18–22.

Yousem, D. M., Kraut, M. A., & Chalian, A. A. (2000). Major Salivary Gland Imaging. *Radiology, 216*(1), 19–29. doi:10.1148/radiology.216.1.r00jl4519 PMID:10887223

Yu, C., Zheng, L., Yang, C., & Shen, N. (2008). Causes of chronic obstructive parotitis and management by sialoendoscopy. *Oral Surgery, Oral Medicine, Oral Pathology, Oral Radiology, and Endodontics, 105*(3), 365–370. doi:10.1016/j.tripleo.2007.08.008 PMID:18280969

Yuasa, K., Nakhayama, E., Ban, S., Kawazu, T., Chikui, T., Shimizu, M., & Kanda, S. (1997). Submandibular gland duct endoscopy. Diagnostic value for salivary duct disorders in comparison to conventional radiography, sialography, and ultrasonography. *Oral Surgery, Oral Medicine, Oral Pathology, Oral Radiology, and Endodontics, 84*(5), 578–581. doi:10.1016/S1079-2104(97)90276-6 PMID:9394392

Chapter 9
Sialadenitis and Sialadenosis

ABSTRACT

In this chapter, the etiology and management of salivary gland inflammation (sialadenitis) and sialadenosis (sioalosis) are discussed. Causes of inflammatory disorders of the parotid gland include viral infections; bacterial infections; recurrent parotitis of childhood; papillary obstructive parotitis; granulomatous sialadenitis; autoimmune sialadenitis including Mickulicz disease, Sjogren's syndrome; and other autoimmune sialadenitis such as Wegener's granulomatosis, Kimura's disease, and chronic sclerosing sialadenitis. Sialadenosis is a chronic, diffuse, non-inflammatory, non-neoplastic disorder causing diffuse enlargement of salivary glands, usually the parotid glands. Grossly, there is only diffuse enlargement of the affected gland, and histologically, the condition is characterized by acinar hypertrophy and fatty infiltration. Patients present with painless, soft, and diffuse enlargement of both parotid glands. Treatment in the form of controlling the underlying disorder or withdrawing the incriminated drug helps sialosis to resolve.

SIALADENITIS

Inflammatory disorders (sialadenitis) of the parotid gland may be caused by viral infections, bacterial infections, recurrent parotitis of childhood, papillary obstructive parotitis, granulomatous sialadenitis, autoimmune sialadenitis, and post-radiation sialadenitis.

DOI: 10.4018/978-1-7998-5603-0.ch009

Viral Infections

Mumps

In the United States, aggressive vaccination has significantly decreased the prevalence of mumps sialadenitis, with approximately 300 cases reported annually (Barskey, et al, 2013).

Mumps is a specific acute viral infection due to a paramyxovirus, an RNA virus that belongs to the influenza and para-influenza family. In 85% of cases, it affects the school-age children under the age of 15 years, with an incubation period of 2 to 3 weeks. The illness starts by 1 to 2 days of prodromal influenza-like syndrome (discomfort, loss of appetite, nausea, chills, fever, sore throat, and headache), followed by the appearance of the characteristic face swelling. The patient is infectious from 3 days before the onset of salivary swellings to 7 days after, through airborne droplets of infected saliva. A single episode of infection confers lifelong immunity. Fortunately, this condition has been mostly eradicated as a result of vaccination (McQuone, 1999).

The swelling, which that usually starts unilateral and in a few days becomes bilateral, lasts from a couple of days to one week (Figure 1). The virus causes fever and is considered the commonest cause of acute painful profuse swelling of the parotid gland.

The gland is soft and tender, but never suppurates. Impingement on the auriculotemporal and great auricular nerves causes much pain as the gland is pressured during mastication. Symptoms usually resolve within 5 to 10 days.

Mumps may be complicated by pancreatitis, orchitis, and oophoritis. It might be a cause of abortion during the first trimester of pregnancy because of fetal endocardial fibroelastosis. Sensorineural deafness (1/20,000) and meningo-encephalitis are rare, but are more likely to occur in adults.

Laboratory findings include leukocytopenia with relative lymphocytosis. Serum amylase peaks in the 1st week and normalizes by the 2nd or 3rd week. Soluble antibodies directed against the nucleoprotein core of the virus appear within the final week of infection, and disappear within 8 months. Antibodies directed against the outer surface appear several weeks after soluble antibodies, and persist for 5 years. Mumps is a self-limited disease that requires rest and symptomatic treatment only, which includes antibiotics, sialagogues and rehydration (McQuone, 1999).

Figure 1. Mumps in a 10-month child with a smooth enlargement of the right parotid gland

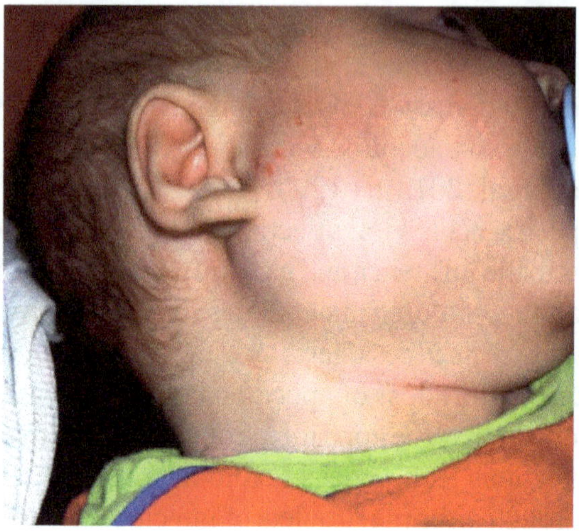

Non-Mumps Viral Parotitis

Parotitis with the same clinical picture as that described for mumps can be caused by other viral agents; namely, Coxsackie A and B, para-influenza types 1 and 3, echovirus and lymphocytic choriomeningitis virus.

Human Immunodeficiency Virus (HIV)-Associated Sialadenitis

The presentation of HIV-associated sialadenitis is in the form of chronic, bilateral enlargement of parotid glands where the glands are painless, hard and nodular. The disease is more common among children than among adults. The condition may be associated with xerostomia and xerophthalmia, being so similar to the classical Sjogren's syndrome in adulthood. Although, both conditions share similar histological characteristics, yet, HIV-associated sialadenitis is usually associated with a negative autoantibody screen. Multiple glandular cysts causing gross parotid swelling and facial disfigurement is another pattern of presentation. Thirty percent of HIV-infected children have been reported to have enlargement of their parotid glands. In addition, patients with HIV are more susceptible to infection with cytomegalovirus (CMV) and adenoviruses as causative agents for non-mumps parotitis (Huang, 1991; Schoidt, 1989).

Useful imaging tools include ultrasound (US), computed tomography (CT) scan and magnetic resonance imaging (MRI). The latter two demonstrate the characteristic 'Swiss cheese' appearance of multiple large cystic lesions (Figure 2). These tools can also guide fine-needle aspiration (FNA), which reveals serous fluid with the presence of lymphocytes and macrophages. As the parotid gland contains many lymph nodes (LNs) at different levels, they might be enlarged as the HIV virus mainly affects the lymphoid tissue. The sole indication of surgery in such cases might be to improve the esthetic appearance (Huang, 1991; Schoidt, 1989).

Bacterial Infections

Acute Suppurative Parotitis (Brook, 2003)

The infective organism can be any of the following bacteria; staphylococcus aureus, streptococcus viridans, Penicillin-resistant coagulase positive staphylococcus, streptococcus pneumonia, beta-hemolytic streptococcus, Methicillin-resistant Staphylococcus aureus (MRSA), or gram-negative germs, such as coli. Studies have shown the presence of 30-40% of anaerobic bacteria; bacteroides, peptostreptococcus, fusobacteria. In South-East Asia, Pseudomonas pseudomallei have been reported. In many cases the infection is a mixed one.

Ascending retrograde infection spreads from an infected dry mouth through the duct into the gland, or it may be blood-borne. One or more of the following factors that cause dehydration and/or electrolyte imbalance are usually evident, septicemia, obstruction of Stensen's duct by a stone, after major surgery or bad oral hygiene. However, sometimes the condition is totally idiopathic. Parotids are affected more frequently than submandibular glands. One of the possible reasons is that the bacteriostatic activity of the saliva secreted by the parotid gland is inferior to that secreted by the submandibular gland as the former is predominantly serous and thus lacks the protective constituents (IgA, sialic acid and lysozomes) seen in mucinous secretions of the other salivary glands.

Acute suppurative parotitis is more commonly seen in elderly, debilitated, diabetic, or immunocompromised, patients (Chi, 2014; Ganesh, 2005; Ozkan, 2015). The patient generally complains of anorexia, fever, tachycardia and malaise. Over several hours, the local condition starts with a swelling which is very tender, hot and with throbbing pain that is exacerbated by mastication.

Figure 2. MRI showing the characteristic Swiss-cheese appearance of multiple large cystic lesions

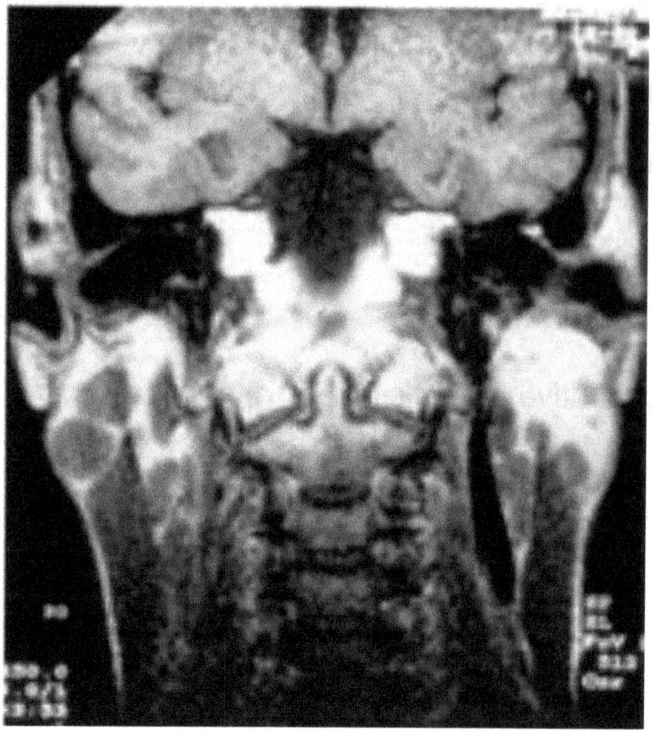

The gland size may reach 3 to 4 times larger than that of the normal gland, which is usually diffuse but may localize to the lower pole. The skin overlying the gland is red, edematous and tethered (Figure 3). Movements of the ipsilateral temporo-mandibular joint (TMJ) are restricted and painful. Upper deep cervical LNs are enlarged and tender.

The parotid gland, being enclosed in a dense capsule, is liable to fulminating inflammation and necrosis due to increased tension within this tightly closed fascial compartment. Fluctuation is difficult to elicit and is never waited for. Pus may exude from the duct orifice on massage of the gland, which is in spite of being painful at the moment; it relieves the pressure inside the ductal system and thence the pain. Diseases of the parotid gland cause pain to be referred to the ear, the TMJ, and the external auditory meatus. This is due to the overlapping of sensory branches of various nerves serving the regions of the parotid bed, ear, and TMJ. Infections of the parotid gland may be confused with toothache as a result of trigeminal nerve (CN V) involvement.

Figure 3. Large left parotid abscess with erythematous edematous and tethered overlying skin

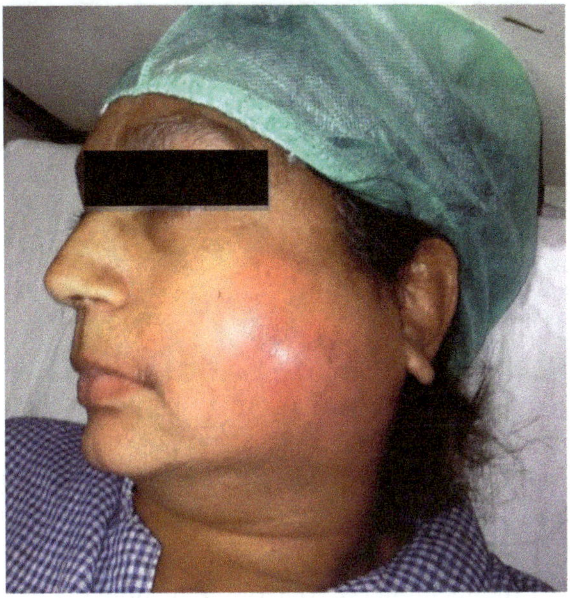

An inflamed parotid papilla (parotid duct orifice in the oral cavity) provides clue to diagnosis.

A parotid abscess may be *complicated* by local spread in the form of cellulitis, chronicity due to inadequate management, development of a fistula, septicemia, and rupture into the external auditory meatus (EAM) or along the carotid sheath. The patient shows increased white blood cell count and culture and sensitivity should be done from the pus. Sialography is *contraindicated* during acute infection and ultrasonography (US) or computed tomography (CT) scan (Figure 4) may be needed, however, the diagnosis is mostly done on clinical grounds.

Prophylaxis against the development of such suppuration is considered much safer through adopting good oral hygiene, preventing dehydration and early adequate correction of electrolyte imbalance. As an early treatment of any inflammatory condition affecting the parotid gland, one should use warm local fomentations, intravenous antibiotics, anti-inflammatory agents and analgesics. When suppuration ensues (known by throbbing pain, hectic fever, aspirated pus or US identified abscess formation), formal drainage under general anesthesia becomes necessary.

Figure 4. CT scan showing enlarged right parotid gland with increased density and streaking opacities in the overlying fat

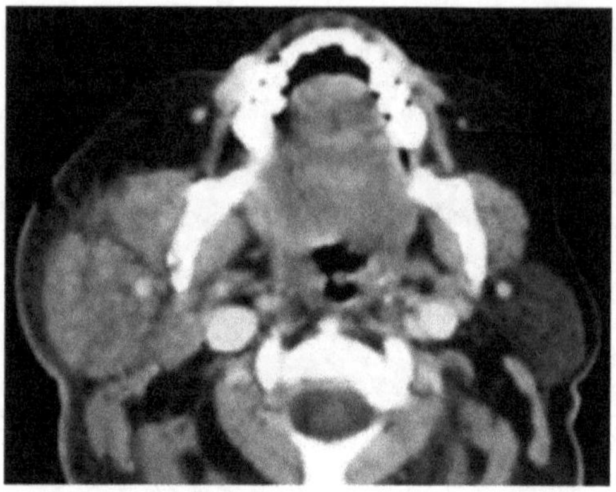

Decompression of the parotid (Hilton's method): Do not wait for fluctuation. Under general anesthesia, a *vertical* incision is done in the skin down to the parotid capsule. The capsule in then incised *transversely* along the course of the branches of the facial nerve to avoid their injury. Pus is evacuated, a drain is put in the lower part of the incision for 24 to 72 hours then closure is achieved. Complications of this procedure include parotid fistula and facial nerve injury. Alternatively, the skin incision may be made low to avoid damage to the lower branch of the facial nerve. Lee et al. (2018) reported the results of management of 13 patients with acute suppurative parotitis. Patients were treated with empirical intravenous broad-spectrum antibiotics and seven patients underwent surgical incision and drainage. There was no recurrence or death associated with parotid abscess; however, one patient developed facial nerve palsy that persisted at three-years follow-up, despite adequate treatment.

Chronic Pyogenic Parotitis

Chronic bacterial sialadenitis is rare in the parotid gland. It may result from improper treatment of acute parotitis, presence of stones in the duct, or stenosis of the Stensen's duct (Arriaga & Myers, 1990).

Actinomycosis

Actinomycosis affects LNs adjacent to salivary glands, mimicking a salivary gland infection. The pathogen is Actinomyces israelii, A. proprionica, A. viscosus, or A. odontolyticus. Infection may be acute, subacute or chronic. The *acute* form is associated with suppuration, the *subacute* with a slightly tender and tumor-like mass attached to the mandible, and the *chronic* with marked induration that may be misdiagnosed as a neoplasm. The finding of pollen grain like "sulfur granules" on clinical examination or "sulfur grounds" on pathological evaluation are pathognomonic of this condition. Treatment of the acute phase is surgical, with eventual drainage of the exudates and administration of broad-spectrum antibiotics (Belmont, Behar, & Wax, 1999).

Cat Scratch Disease

It is caused a gram negative bacillus; called *Bartonella Henslae*. The disease originally involves LNs adjacent to salivary glands, which may be secondarily involved by continuous spread. It results from contact with cats, and children or young adults are the most often involved. Laboratory tests include specific PCR or serology. Antibiotics do not seem to shorten the course of the disease, but may be given as prophylaxis against secondary bacterial infection. The affected LNs disappear spontaneously within a few months (Ben-Salma, 2008; Malakskey, 2000).

RECURRENT PAROTITIS OF CHILDHOOD

This is a distinct clinical entity of unknown etiology and unsure prognosis. It is the most frequent non-viral disorder of salivary glands in children (Wooley, 1996). Suggested etiologies include congenital malformation of the parotid ducts, primary or secondary infections and local manifestations of systemic immunological disease.

The clinical picture comprises fever, malaise, rapid swelling of one or both parotid glands and pain which is made worse by mastication. This usually lasts from 3 to 7 days followed by a quiescent period of weeks to several months. The condition may rarely start as early as 4 months of age, but usually children present between the ages of 3 and 6 years and usually resolve around puberty. The diagnosis is made by obtaining typical history, and findings of the clinical examination. Sialography may be confirmatory. It shows a characteristic punctate sialectasis likened to a 'snowstorm' (Figure 5) which persists until adult life. Sialendoscopy may show diffuse reduction of the caliber of Stensen's duct, associated sometimes with multiple localized stenoses and may be salivary calculi. Endoscopy may also show sialectasia (dilated ductules and acini). Sialendoscopy has proven recently to be effective therapeutically through injection of antiseptic solutions in some cases (Woolley, 1996).

No specific treatment is available; however therapeutic options include good oral hygiene, prophylactic low-dose antibiotics for several months or even years especially if recurrence is frequent, anti-inflammatory agents, sialendoscopy and total conservative parotidectomy (Baurmash, 2004).

Figure 5. Sialography showing a characteristic punctate sialectasis (snow-storm appearance)

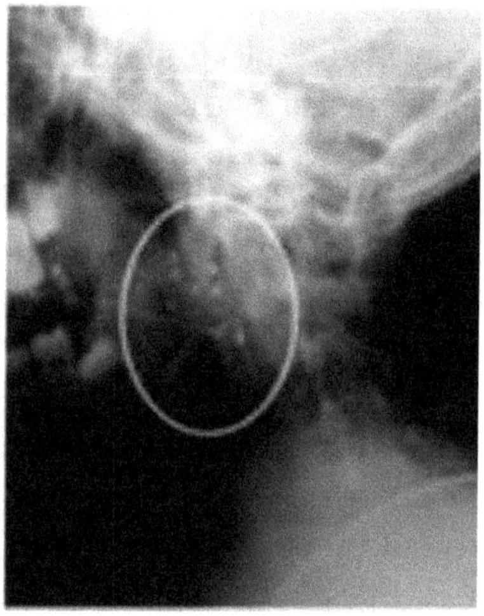

PAPILLARY OBSTRUCTIVE PAROTITIS

Although there are many recognized causes of obstructive parotitis, however, papillary obstruction due to trauma to the parotid papilla through either an overextended upper denture flange or a fractured upper molar tooth is merely the commonest of all. Subsequent edema then fibrosis of the papilla obstructs salivary flow, especially at mealtimes, in intermittent then chronic forms, respectively. Thus, the patient suffers from an intermittent painful swelling of the parotid, accumulating over minutes after the start of his meal. If stenosis ensues, the symptoms will not resolve except by a papillotomy. Obstructive parotitis is less common than obstructive submandibular sialadenitis.

GRANULOMATOUS SIALADENITIS

Granulomatous sialadenitis can result from tuberculosis, mycosis, sarcoidosis, or duct obstruction from calculi or malignant tumors. In the latter instance, granulomas result from rupture of ducts and may contain small pools of mucin.

Tuberculosis (TB)

Mycobacterium tuberculosis and atypical mycobacterium both affect LNs adjacent to salivary glands or intra-glandular LNs. The patient may suffer from one or more of the systemic manifestations of TB such as low grade fever, night sweating and anemia. The gland is firm and nodular but may become cystic with sinuses and little pain. Polymerase chain reaction is the best pre-operative laboratory diagnostic tool, but diagnosis is only confirmed with histopathology after parotidectomy, if needed. Specific treatment includes multi-drug therapy for an average of one year together with exposure to direct sunlight, good aeration and well-balanced nutrition to enhance general health and immunity (Thakur, 2011; Ozcan, 2008).

Sarcoidosis

Sarcoidosis is a systemic disease involving multiple organs. Its etiology remains unclear, but several hypotheses have been made, including auto-antigens and infectious organisms. It resembles TB but with no caseation. Salivary glands are usually affected, and specifically the parotid glands. Symptoms include swellings and xerostomia. Sometimes, the disease my present as a mass and the diagnosis is only made after surgical excision of the presumed tumor; the *sarcoid pseudotumor*. Laboratory diagnosis is made through amylase, kallikrein and the ACE test. Radiological and histological evidence of non-caseous epithelial granulomas are confirmatory. Corticosteroids are the best therapeutic option.

Heerfordt's syndrome is a rare form of sarcoidosis that involves parotid swelling, anterior uveitis, facial palsy and fever (uveoparotid fever). It affects young patients in their third decade (Mandel & Surattanont, 2002).

AUTOIMMUNE SIALADENITIS

Mickulicz Disease (MD)

It is an autoimmune disease, which is characterized by chronic, symmetrical, bilateral enlargement of all salivary and lacrimal glands. It is named after *Johann von Mickulicz Radecki* (1888) (Figure 6) and is also called *benign lympho-epithelial lesion* or *myoepithelial sialadenitis.*

Figure 6. Johann von Mickulicz Radecki (1888)

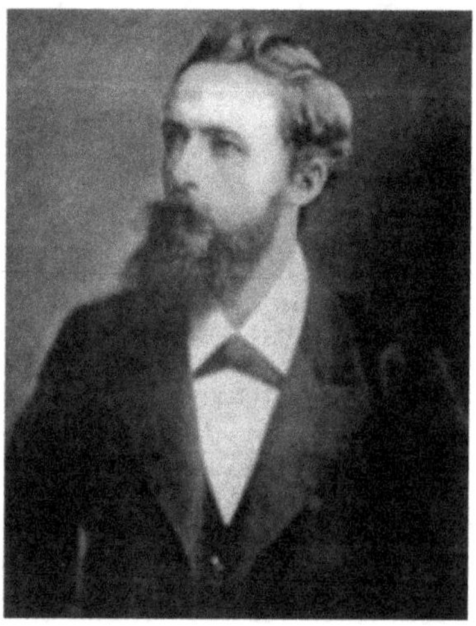

The disease almost always occurs in association with another underlying disease such as TB, leukemia, syphilis or systemic lupus erythematosis. Patients may experience recurring fever. There is lymphocytic infiltration, parenchymal atrophy and myoepithelial islands.

It affects the parotid glands in 85% and the submandibular glands in 15% of cases, occurring more among women (60-80%) with a mean age of 50 years and causing firm, diffuse enlargement of the affected gland. Patients are usually asymptomatic but may complain of mild pain and are at a higher risk of developing lymphomas. Some authors believe that it should be considered a form of Sjogren's syndrome. Actually, the main clinical difference between MD and SS is the preservation of the lacrimation and salivation in MD due to much less gland cell apoptosis than that found in SS (Fox, 2005).

Sjogren's Syndrome (SS)

This disease is an autoimmune one involving the parotid glands more frequently than the submandibular glands. It is named after *Henrik Samuel Conrad Sjogrin* (1933), a Swedish ophthalmologist (Figure 7).

Figure 7. Henrik Samuel Conrad Sjogrin (1933)

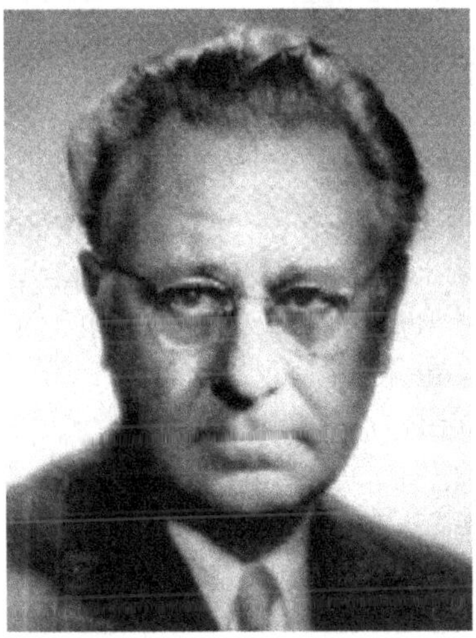

Females are affected more than males (10:1). It leads to *xerostomia* and *kerato conjunctivitis* sicca due to progressive destruction of both salivary and lacrimal glands. The diseased gland is occasionally enlarged and is occasionally painful. Secondary bacterial ascending infection may occur as a result of dry mouth.

Computed tomography (CT) scan and magnetic resonance imaging (MRI) show bilateral parotid enlargement with heterogeneously enhancing parenchyma. The CT scan may show a honey-comb appearance with low-density foci in a generally enhancing gland (Figure 8).

Histologically, SS is characterized by massive progressive lymphocytic infiltration, acinar cell destruction and ductal epithelial cell proliferation

Figure 8. CT scan showing honey-comb appearance in a bilaterally enlarged parotid gland (Sjogrin syndrome)

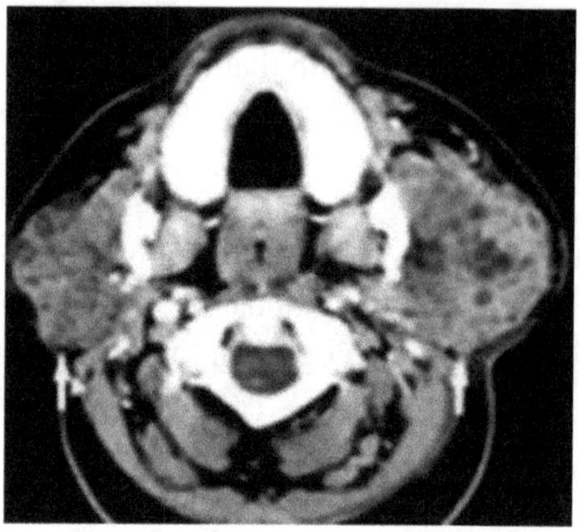

affecting all salivary and lacrimal glands. This is the *primary* SS (pSS). *Secondary* SS differs in that it is associated with a connective tissue disorder, symptoms are less severe and the incidence of lymphomatous transformation (most commonly monocytoid B-cell lymphoma) is also less (Fox, 2005).

To date, there is no known specific treatment available to stop Sjogren's syndrome and thus management is considered to be *symptomatic* (Table 1). Artificial tears and periodic ophthalmological examination is mandatory to avoid corneal ulcerations. Artificial salivary substitutes are available and their importance increases in the dentate patient where fluoride should be added as well. Usually the patient consumes a large amount of water daily carrying a bottle of water with him all the time (Petrone et al, 2002).

Table 1. Symptomatic treatment of Sjogren's Syndrome

Dry Eyes	Dry Mouth	Dry Nasal Mucosa
- Lubricants: Artificial tears, ointments - Punctal plugs - Lateral tarsorrhaphy	- Saliva substitutes: sprays, rinses. - Salivary Stimulation: hard candy, pilocarpine. - Cholinergic agents: cevimeline hydrochloride - Special toothpaste, oral gel - Active dental care	- Saline nasal sprays - Lavage

The pathological hallmark of pSS is the mucosa-associated lymphoid tissue (MALT) arising in chronically inflamed tissues, mainly in salivary glands, where inflammation, autoimmunity and lymphoproliferation coexist.

The B-lymphocyte activating factor (BAFF or BLys) is one of the main factors contributing to B-cell survival and hyperactivity in pSS. Due to such a lymphoproliferative background, targeting B-lymphocytes represents a promising new treatment approach for pSS and other immune-mediated diseases, but is only investigational at present. Immunobiological evidences support a sequential scheme of administration with belimumab preceding rituximab, aiming to firstly target the micro-environmental BAFF to improve the success of the subsequent depleting treatment in the MALT pathological tissue with rituximab. Hopefully, further trials will assess if improvement in B-cell targeting will lead to the decrease in salivary gland lymphoid infiltrate as well as to a possible reduction of lymphoma development in pSS (Gandolfo & De Vita, 2019).

Benign Lymphoepithelial Lesion (Myoepithelial Sialadenitis, MESA)

This disease mostly affects females over 50 years of age. Patients present with a diffusely enlarged, firm and often painful parotid gland, which is bilateral in 20% of cases. Sialography shows sialectasia, which ranges from punctuate to cavitary. Management is usually parotidectomy to establish a final diagnosis.

Histopathological examination of the excised gland carries the very same previously described histopathological features of Sjogren's syndrome and so the differentiation between both is only done on clinical grounds. Prolonged follow-up of such patients is mandatory as 20% of them will develop lymphoma at a certain time (Peel, 2001).

Other Autoimmune Sialadenitis

Wegener's granulomatosis is an autoimmune disease characterized by upper and lower respiratory and renal disease. The most common salivary gland to be involved is the parotid gland (Mandel & Surattanont, 2002); however, this occurs in less than 1% of the cases (Fauci, Haynes, Katz, & Wolff, 1983).

Kimura's disease occurs typically in young Asian males and is characterized clinically by painless lymphadenopathy of the head and neck region, including peri-parotid and intra-parotid LNs (Mandel, 2002; Peel, 2001; Som, 1992).

Chronic sclerosing sialadenitis presents as a firm localized swelling of the salivary gland mimicking a neoplasm, most commonly involving the submandibular gland. It may be associated with autoimmune extra-salivary disease such as primary sclerosing cholangitis, and idiopathic retro-peritoneal fibrosis (Peel, 2001).

POST-RADIATION SIALADENITIS

Radiation-induced sialadenitis is frequently seen in patients who receive radiation for treatment of oropharyngeal cancer. The first clinical sign is reduced saliva flow and has been reported to occur with radiation dose thresholds as low as 15 Gy (Cheng, Wu, Kwong, & Ying, 2011). The classical imaging findings of radiation-induced sialadenitis include hyper-enhancement of the salivary glands that progresses to atrophy over time. This hyperenhancement occurs with doses >45 Gy and is thought to represent contrast expanding the extracellular space that was once occupied by acinar cells lost from radiation (Bronstein, Nyberg, Schwartz, Shuman, & Griffin, 1987). Over time, chronic scarring/fibrosis leads to volume loss and magnetic resonance imaging typically demonstrates low-to-intermediate signal intensity on all sequences (Houweling, van den Berg, Roesink, Terhaard, & Raaijmakers, 2010).

SIALADENOSIS

Sialadenosis (sialosis) is a chronic, diffuse, non-inflammatory, non-neoplastic disorder that causes diffuse enlargement of salivary glands, usually the parotid glands, and less commonly the submandibular (Peel, 2001; Chilla, 1981; Donath, 1976) and minor salivary glands (Mignogna, Fedele, Lo, & Russo, 2004).

Etiology

Causes of sialadenosis can be categorized as: (1) *nutritional* (alcoholism, cirrhosis, cystic fibrosis, bulimia, anorexia nervosa, kwashiorkor, and pellagra). Any disorder that affects digestion of food over a prolonged period can result in sialosis. (2) *endocrinal* (diabetes mellitus, thyroid disorders such as acromegaly, pregnancy, gonadal dysfunction, following oophorectomy), and (3) *neurochemical / drugs* (vegetative state, lead and mercury poisoning, iodine, Thiouracil [anti-thyroid], isoproterenol [sympatho-mimetic], and phenothiazines) (Peel, 2001; Chilla, 1981; Donath, 1976). Among the many drugs that may induce sialosis, anti-hypertensive agents are prominent. However, in many cases *no underlying disorder* can be detected.

Pathogenesis

The proposed pathogeneses include prolonged *malnutrition* with resultant glandular atrophy and fatty replacement. Sialadenosis is also thought to be a *neuro-secretory* disorder. Diabetic neuropathy may be the clue causing acinar cell atrophy, in some cases.

Ultra-structural and animal experimental studies point to a disturbance in the autonomic innervation of salivary glands (*autonomic neuropathy*). This is considered to be the initiating factor for sialadenosis (Chilla, 1981; Donath, 1976; Donath, 1975; Donath, 1974).

Multiple emetic episodes (bulimia) cause autonomic neuropathy. With *sympathetic nerve impairment*, individual acinar cells enlarge because of zymogen granule engorgement. One explanation is that the sympathetic nerve supply to the secreting acinar cell is concerned with the production and secretion of zymogen, the precursor of amylase. Because of sympathetic nerve dysfunction, there may be an increase in zymogen storage in the cell, owing to increased production, decreased secretion of the granules or both. The ensuing cellular enlargement, which is evidenced by fine needle aspiration biopsy (FNAB), leads to the clinically visible bilateral parotid gland enlargement (Chilla, 1981; Donath, 1976; Donath, 1975; Donath, 1974).

Pathology

Grossly, there is only diffuse enlargement of the affected gland. *Histologically*, the condition is characterized by acinar hypertrophy and fatty infiltration (Figure 9) (Gupta & Sodhani, 1998). Zymogen granules are increased in size and number by light and electron microscopy. No inflammation or fibrosis can be detected, which differentiates sialadenosis from sialadenitis. While amyloidosis may also present with diffuse enlargement of the salivary glands, histologically, there will be interstitial fibrosis as well as the characteristic pale amyloid deposition that can be demonstrated with a Congo red stain (Eversole, 2001).

Figure 9. Microscopy showing atrophy of parotid parenchymal tissue and increased intraglandular fat. Inflammatory infiltrates are absent.

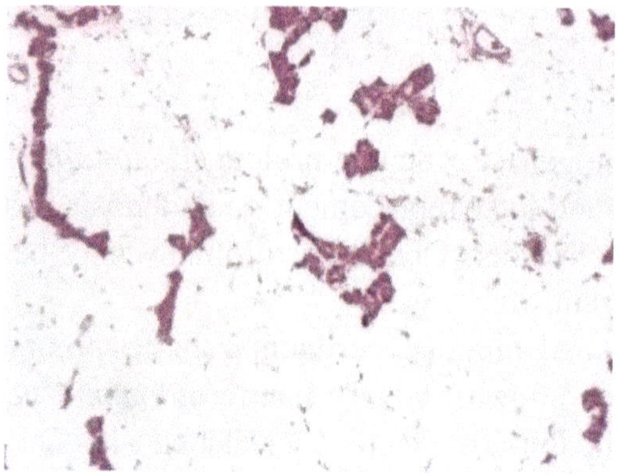

Clinical Presentation

Sialadenosis is usually *bilateral* and has an equal sex distribution. Most of the patients are between 40 and 70 years of age. There is painless, soft, and diffuse enlargement of both parotid glands (Figure 10, A and B) giving the patient a striking facial feature, known as the "*hamster-like appearance*".

Figure 10. Bilateral diffuse enlargement of the parotid glands (sialadenosis) due to alcoholism in two middle-aged male patients

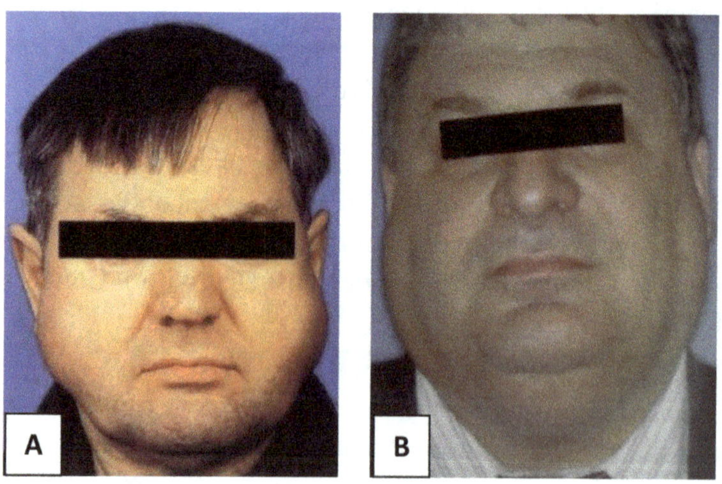

Investigations / Diagnosis

- *Blood tests* may reveal hyperglycemia (diabetes mellitus), and abnormal liver function tests (cirrhosis, alcoholism);
- *Sialochemistry* may show increased serum potassium and calcium levels;
- *Imaging* (ultrasound, magnetic resonance imaging or sialography) helps differentiate space occupying lesions in the parotid glands;
- *Biopsy* is rarely indicated, and may show enlarged acinar cells to almost twice the normal diameter and packed cytoplasm with enzyme granules.

Treatment

Usually, no specific treatment is necessary. Treatment in the form of controlling the underlying disorder or withdrawing the incriminated drug helps sialosis to resolve. There is usually little morbidity associated with the condition itself, and surgery (superficial parotidectomy) is resorted to only in case of significant disfigurement and cosmetic complaint.

In some instances, anorexic or bulimic patients may seek advice about removal of the glands. Anorexia or bulimia would need to be treated first before any such surgery could be contemplated.

REFERENCES

Arriaga, M. A., & Myers, E. N. (1990). The surgical management of chronic parotitis. *The Laryngoscope*, *100*(12), 1270–1275. doi:10.1288/00005537-199012000-00004 PMID:2243516

Barskey, A. E., Juieng, P., Whitaker, B. L., Erdman, D. D., Oberste, M. S., Chern, S. W., ... Rota, P. A. (2013). Viruses. detected among sporadic cases of parotitis, United States, 2009-2011. *The Journal of Infectious Diseases*, *208*(12), 1979–1986. doi:10.1093/infdis/jit408 PMID:23935203

Baurmash, H. D. (2004). Chronic recurrent parotitis: A closer look at its origin, diagnosis, and management. *Journal of Oral and Maxillofacial Surgery*, *62*(8), 1010–1018. doi:10.1016/j.joms.2003.08.041 PMID:15278868

Belmont, M. J., Behar, P. M., & Wax, M. K. (1999). Atypical presentations of actinomycosis. *Head & Neck, 21*(3), 264–268. doi:10.1002/(SICI)1097-0347(199905)21:3<264::AID-HED12>3.0.CO;2-Y PMID:10208670

Ben-Slama, L., Hasni, W., & Royer, B. (2008). Cat-scratch disease localisation in the parotid gland. *Revue de Stomatologie et de Chirurgie Maxillo-Faciale, 109*(3), 183–186. PMID:18533210

Bronstein, A. D., Nyberg, D. A., Schwartz, A. N., Shuman, W. P., & Griffin, B. R. (1987). Increased salivary gland density on contrast-enhanced CT after head and neck radiation. *AJR. American Journal of Roentgenology, 149*(6), 1259–1263. doi:10.2214/ajr.149.6.1259 PMID:3500619

Brook, I. (2003). Acute bacterial suppurative parotitis: Microbiology and management. *The Journal of Craniofacial Surgery, 14*(1), 37–40. doi:10.1097/00001665-200301000-00006 PMID:12544218

Cheng, S. C., Wu, V. W., Kwong, D. L., & Ying, M. T. (2011). Assessment of post-radiotherapy salivary glands. *The British Journal of Radiology, 84*(1001), 393–402. doi:10.1259/bjr/66754762 PMID:21511748

Chi, T. H., Yuan, C. H., & Chen, H. S. (2014). Parotid abscess: A retrospective study of 14 cases at a regional hospital in Taiwan. *B-ENT, 10*, 315–318. PMID:25654957

Chilla, R. (1981). Sialadenosis of the salivary glands of the head. Studies on the physiology and pathophysiology of parotid secretion. *Advances in Oto-Rhino-Laryngology, 26*, 1–38. doi:10.1159/000395287 PMID:7020371

Chilla, R., Witzemann, V., Opaitz, M., & Arglebe, C. (1981). Possible involvement of parotid beta-adrenergic receptors in the etiology of sialadenosis. *Archives of Oto-Rhino-Laryngology, 230*(2), 113–120. doi:10.1007/BF00456140 PMID:6271110

Donath, K. (1976). Sialadenosis of the parotid gland. Ultrastructural, clinical and experimental findings in disturbances of secretion (author's transl). *Veröffentlichungen aus der Pathologie, 103*, 1–122. PMID:1007613

Donath, K., & Seifert, G. (1975). Ultrastructural studies of the parotid glands in sialadenosis. *Virchows Archiv. A, Pathological Anatomy and Histology, 365*(2), 119–135. doi:10.1007/BF00432384 PMID:804743

Donath, K., Spillner, M., & Seifert, G. (1974). The influence of the autonomic nervous system on the ultrastructure of the parotid acinar cells. Experimental contribution to the neurohormonal sialadenosis. *Virchows Archiv. A, Pathological Anatomy and Histology, 364*(1), 15–33. doi:10.1007/BF01230855 PMID:4217027

Eversole, L. (2001). Salivary Gland Pathology. In Y. Fu, B. M. Wenig, E. Abemayor, & B. L. Wenig (Eds.), *Head and Neck Pathology: with Clinical Correlations* (pp. 242–291). Philadelphia, PA: Churchill-Livingstone.

Fauci, A. S., Haynes, B. F., Katz, P., & Wolff, S. M. (1983). Wegener's granulomatosis: Prospective clinical and therapeutic experience with 85 patients for 21 years. *Annals of Internal Medicine, 98*(1), 76–85. doi:10.7326/0003-4819-98-1-76 PMID:6336643

Fox, R. I. (2005). Sjogren's syndrome. *Lancet, 366*(9482), 321–331. doi:10.1016/S0140-6736(05)66990-5 PMID:16039337

Gandolfo, S., & De Vita, S. (2019). Double anti-B cell and anti-BAFF targeting for the treatment of primary Sjögren's syndrome. *Clinical and Experimental Rheumatology, 37*(3), 199-208.

Ganesh, R., & Leese, T. (2005). Parotid abscess in Singapore. *Singapore Medical Journal, 46*, 553–556. PMID:16172776

Gupta, S., & Sodhani, P. (1998). Sialadenosis of parotid gland: A cytomorphologic and morphometric study of four cases. *Analytical and Quantitative Cytology and Histology, 20*(3), 225–228. PMID:9642451

Houweling, A. C., van den Berg, C. A., Roesink, J. M., Terhaard, C. H., & Raaijmakers, C. P. (2010). Magnetic resonance imaging at 3.0T for submandibular gland sparing radiotherapy. *Radiotherapy and Oncology: Journal of the European Society for Therapeutic Radiology and Oncology, 97*(2), 239–243. doi:10.1016/j.radonc.2010.08.014 PMID:20846735

Huang, R. D., Pearlman, S., Friedman, W. H., & Loree, T. (1991). Benign cystic vs. solid lesions of the parotid gland in HIV patients. *Head & Neck, 13*(6), 522–527. doi:10.1002/hed.2880130608 PMID:1724235

Kim, Y. Y., Lee, D. H., Yoon, T. M., Lee, J. K., & Lim, S. C. (2018). Parotid abscess at a single institute in Korea. *Medicine, 97*(30), e11700. doi:10.1097/MD.0000000000011700 PMID:30045329

Malatskey, S., Fradis, M., Ben-David, J., & Podoshin, L. (2000). Cat-scratch disease of the parotid gland: An often-misdiagnosed entity. *The Annals of Otology, Rhinology, and Laryngology, 109*(7), 679–682. doi:10.1177/000348940010900712 PMID:10903051

Mandel, L., & Surattanont, F. (2002). Bilateral parotid swelling: A review. *Oral Surgery, Oral Medicine, Oral Pathology, Oral Radiology, and Endodontics, 93*(3), 221–237. doi:10.1067/moe.2002.121163 PMID:11925529

McQuone, S. J. (1999). Acute viral and bacterial infections of the salivary glands. *Otolaryngologic Clinics of North America, 32*(5), 793–811. doi:10.1016/S0030-6665(05)70173-0 PMID:10477787

Mignogna, M. D., Fedele, S., & Lo Russo, L. (2004). Anorexia/bulimia-related sialadenosis of palatal minor salivary glands. *Journal of Oral Pathology & Medicine, 33*(7), 441–442. doi:10.1111/j.1600-0714.2004.00208.x PMID:15250838

Ozcan, C., Apa, D. D., Aslan, G., Gulhan, S., & Gorur, K. (2008). Mycobacterium tuberculosis infection within parotid gland Warthin's tumor. *The Journal of Craniofacial Surgery, 19*(6), 1561–1565. doi:10.1097/SCS.0b013e31818ac146 PMID:19098552

Ozkan, A., Ors, C. H., Kosar, S., & Karaman, H. I. (2015). Parotid abscess with involvement of facial nerve branches. *Journal of the College of Physicians and Surgeons--Pakistan, 25*, 613–614. PMID:26305311

Peel, R. (2001). Diseases of the salivary gland. In L. Barnes (Ed.), *Surgical Pathology of the Head and Neck* (pp. 634–757). New York, NY: Marcel-Dekker.

Petrone, D., Condemi, J. J., Fife, R., Gluck, O., Cohen, S., & Dalgin, P. (2002). A double-blind, randomized, placebo-controlled study of cevimeline in Sjogren's syndrome patients with xerostomia and kerato-conjunctivitis sicca. *Arthritis & Rheumatology (Hoboken, N.J.), 46*(3), 748–754. doi:10.1002/art.510 PMID:11920411

Schiodt, M., Greenspan, D., Levy, J. A., Nelson, J. A., Chernoff, D., Hollander, H., & Greenspan, J. S. (1989). Does HIV cause salivary gland disease? *AIDS (London, England), 3*(12), 819–822. doi:10.1097/00002030-198912000-00006 PMID:2517203

Som, P. M., & Biller, H. F. (1992). Kimura disease involving parotid gland and cervical nodes: CT and MR findings. *Journal of Computer Assisted Tomography*, *16*(2), 320–322. doi:10.1097/00004728-199203000-00028 PMID:1545036

Thakur, J., Thakur, A., Mohindroo, N., Mohindroo, S., & Sharma, D. (2011). Bilateral parotid tuberculosis. *Journal of Global Infectious Diseases*, *3*(3), 296–299. doi:10.4103/0974-777X.83543 PMID:21887065

Woolley, A. L. (1996). Salivary gland diseases in children. *Current Opinion in Otolaryngology & Head & Neck Surgery*, *4*(6), 385–391. doi:10.1097/00020840-199612000-00004

Chapter 10
Cystic Parotid Lesions and Classification of Parotid Tumors

ABSTRACT

The causes of cystic parotid lesions may be congenital or acquired and may cause bilateral or unilateral cysts. Bilateral cystic lesions include Warthin's tumor, benign lymphepithelial lesions of human immunodeficiency virus, Sjorgrin's syndrome, and sialocele. Unilateral cystic lesions include Warthin's tumor, sialocele, first-branchial cleft cyst, parotid lymphoepithelial cyst, parotid lymphangioma, necrotic and infected lymph node. This chapter describes in more detail the etiology, clinical presentation, evaluation, and treatment of "sialocele" and "dermoid cyst of the parotid gland." It also summarizes parotid gland tumors based on the World Health Organization histological classification, which categorizes parotid tumors into benign epithelial tumors (most commonly pleomorphic adenoma), soft tissue tumors (hemangioma), hematolymphoid tumors (lymphoma), and secondary tumors (represent less than 2% of all head and neck neoplasms).

DOI: 10.4018/978-1-7998-5603-0.ch010

Table 1. Cystic parotid lesions

Bilateral	Unilateral
- Warthin's tumor - Benign lymphoepithelial lesions of HIV - Sjogren's syndrome - Sialocele	- Warthin's tumor - Sialocele - First branchial cleft cyst: parotid lymphoepithelial cyst. - Parotid lymphangioma - Necrotic LN(s), especially SCC. - Infected LN(s)

CYSTIC LESIONS OF THE PAROTID GLAND

Cysts of the parotid gland represent a clinical dilemma. They may be congenital or acquired caused by neoplasms, benign lymphoepithelial lesion of human immunodeficiency virus (HIV), trauma, parotitis, calculi, duct obstruction or mucus extravasation.

ETIOLOGY / CLASSIFICATION

Unilateral or Bilateral?

Cystic parotid lesions may be *bilateral* or *unilateral*; their causes are summarized in Table 1. Apart from the cystic forms of benign and malignant neoplasms, cysts of the parotid gland may be the presentation of a variety of diseases. Such non-neoplastic cysts are uncommon and represent 2-5% of all salivary gland lesions (Williams, Bulstrode, & O'Connell, 2008). A *first branchial arch anomaly* must be considered when one encounters a case of parotid cyst (Tripti-Maithani & Seema, 2014).

Sialoceles result from trauma to the parotid gland or duct. *Dermoid cysts* (Yigit, Karslioglu, Yildizoglu, & Karakoc, 2014) and *hydatid* cysts Kara T, et al, 2014) have also been reported in the parotid, though exceptionally rare.

Parotid duct cysts, also known as *sialocysts*, *simple cysts*, and *retention cysts*, result from duct *obstruction* due to various causes (Yigit, 2014; Eversole, 2001; Batsakis, 1989). They are true cysts lined by epithelium, unlike *mucocele*, which is lined by granulation tissue (Batsakis & Raymond 1989). Parotid duct cysts should not be confused with duct ectasia (Figure 1).

Figure 1. Left parotid duct ectasia, simulating a parotid cyst, in a 41-year-old gentleman

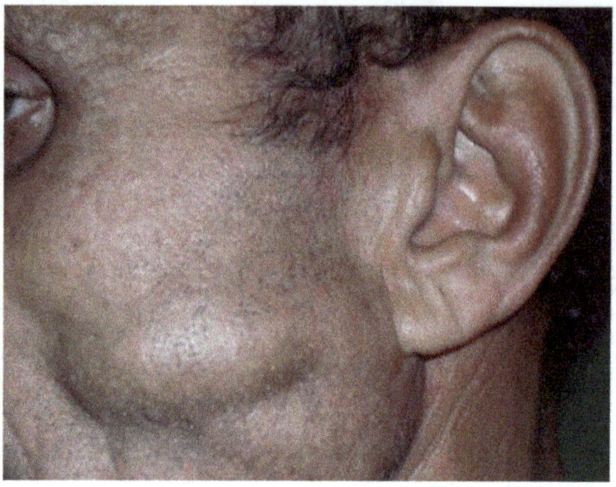

Congenital or Acquired?

Parotid cystic lesions may be *congenital* or *acquired.*

Congenital Cysts

Congenital cysts of the parotid gland are of three types as follows:

1. **Dermoid cyst:** It consists of keratinizing squamous epithelium with associated skin appendages and is treated by complete removal with preservation of the facial nerve;
2. **Congenital ductal cyst:** It is generally seen in infancy. No therapy is required unless repeated infections occur (Work, 1977);
3. **Cysts of the first branchial groove (Figure 2):** These account for less than 1% of all branchial arch anomalies. There are two types: *Type I* is ectodermal and is a duplication anomaly of the membranous external auditory canal. It typically occurs posterior, inferior or anterior to the ear and is related to the facial nerve. Complete excision during a quiescent period, with preservation of the facial nerve, is curative. *Type II* is both, ectodermal and mesodermal, and is a duplication anomaly of the membranous and cartilaginous external auditory canal. It may occur from the pre-auricular area to the hyoid bone. Regardless of the location, the tract is intimately associated with the facial nerve. As with

Type I, treatment entails complete excision during a quiescent period, with preservation of the facial nerve.

Figure 2. Branchial cleft cyst. Axial CT image showing a large hypodense lesion in right parotid gland (arrow) with calcific content in the dependent portion.

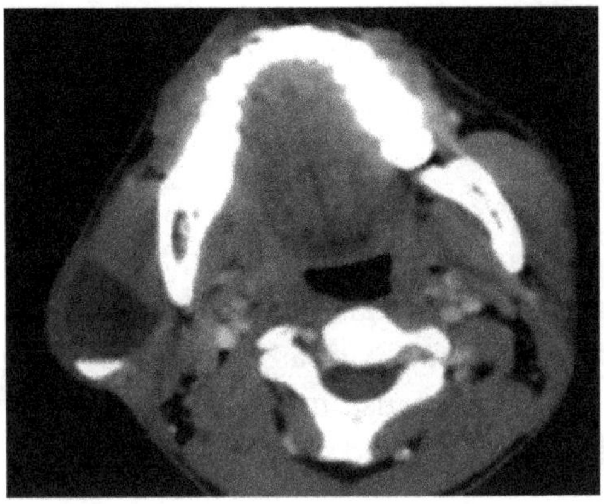

Acquired Cysts

Acquired cysts may be due to *neoplasms*, a benign *lymphoepithelial lesion of HIV, trauma, parotitis, calculi, duct obstruction or mucus extravasation* (Work & Hecht, 1968; Ogasawara, 2017). Aquired parotid cysts due to lymphoepithelial lesion of HIV are rather rare. Ogasawara et al. (2017), reported two patients who were treated with medical treatment (anti-viral and anti-histaminc drugs). Computed tomography scan revealed a complete response 4 weeks after treatment. These findings suggested that the parotid gland swelling associated with HIV was due to various factors including immune reconstitution inflammatory syndromc (IRIS). In case such a parotid gland cystic swelling, invasive treatments can be avoided.

The presence of a cyst does not preclude the possibility of a neoplasm, especially a pleomorphic adenoma, an adenoid cystic carcinoma, a mucoepidermoid carcinoma or Warthin's tumor. These are the most common parotid tumors and most commonly cystic. For an acquired cyst with an identifiable underlying cause, the latter should be treated first. If that fails, the cyst should be excised.

Mucoceles and mucus-retention cysts usually involve minor salivary glands and not the parotid gland, occurring mostly in the lips, buccal mucosa and ventral tongue. Mucus-retention cysts are true cysts with an epithelial lining and result from partial duct obstruction. Complete duct obstruction leads to glandular atrophy (Sela & Ulmansky, 1969). Mucoceles do not possess an epithelial lining (i.e. pseudocysts). They represent mucus extravasation into the soft tissue.

SIALOCELE

Etiology

Disruption of the parotid duct or parenchyma results in extravasation of saliva into the glandular or peri-glandular tissues. When the rate of saliva accumulation within these areas surpasses the body's capacity to reabsorb it, a *sialocele* can form. The cause might be facial trauma (assault, traffic accident, sport injury, etc) or parotid surgery especially when surgicel is used.

Pathology

Duct cysts are unilocular and may grossly contain mucoid material, or sialoliths in long-standing cases. *Histologically*, they are lined by a cuboidal, columnar, or squamous epithelium, though oncocytic metaplasia may be seen in older patients. However, these cysts are not associated with lymphoid elements.[(10)]

Clinical Presentation

Sialoceles / parotid cysts are relatively benign and may present with no symptoms apart from a *swelling* (lump) in the parotid region (Figure 3), but they can be associated with the following *complications*:

- Pain due to accumulation of saliva and stretching/compression of surrounding tissues;
- Infection due to stagnation of salivary flow rate;
- Interference with speech or chewing;
- Undesirable cosmetic change;
- Recurrence (rare) due to incomplete excision (Peel, 2001).

Figure 3. Parotid cyst presenting as a lump (cyst) in front of the tragus of the right ear (arrow) of a 38-year gentleman

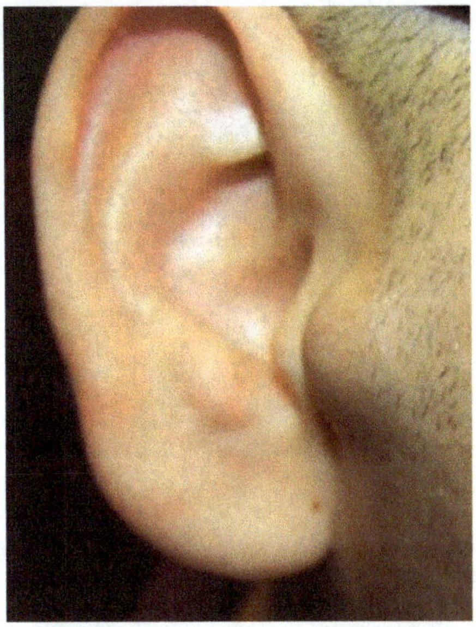

Evaluation

Imaging with ultrasound will clearly demonstrate the cystic nature of the parotid lesion and accurately measures its size (Figure 4).

Computed tomography (CT) scan can also delineate the parotid lesion and provide anatomical relations to surrounding structures (Figure 5).

Treatment

Adequate management of a parotid cyst entails (1) precise removal of the affected parotid gland pathology, (2) proper management of the remaining glandular tissue and associated ductal structures, and (3) close post-operative management and care to prevent complications.

The parotid cyst should be meticulously dissected (Figures 6 and 7) and resected thereby preventing potentially serious complications such as facial paralysis, taste distortion, and disfigurement. Once resection of the cyst or affected salivary gland has been completed, proper management of the remaining glandular tissues is crucial to avoid sialocele formation.

Figure 4. Ultrasound of the parotid gland showing a simple parotid cystic lesion (arrow)

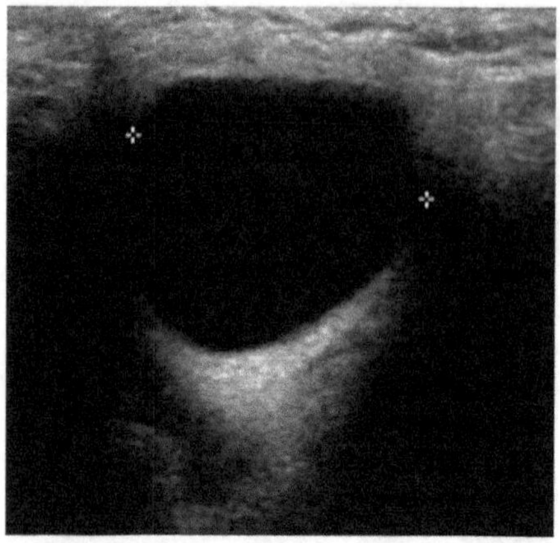

Figure 5. CT scan showing a parotid cystic lesion and its dimensions

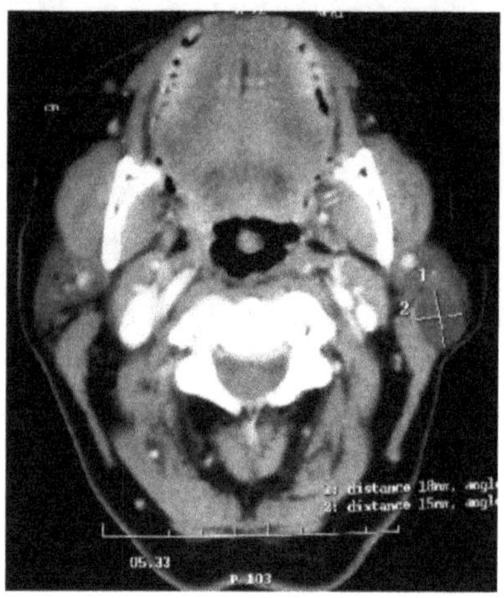

Proper post-operative care is comprised of close follow-up and dietary modifications. The surgical site is closely followed-up for proper drain management, wound healing, quality of scar formation, and for infection prevention.

Special compressive dressings and small drains are placed at the surgical site to promote proper fluid drainage as well as to close off any potential areas where saliva can accumulate. In addition to suppressing sialocele formation,

Figure 6. Intra-operative dissection of a left parotid cyst

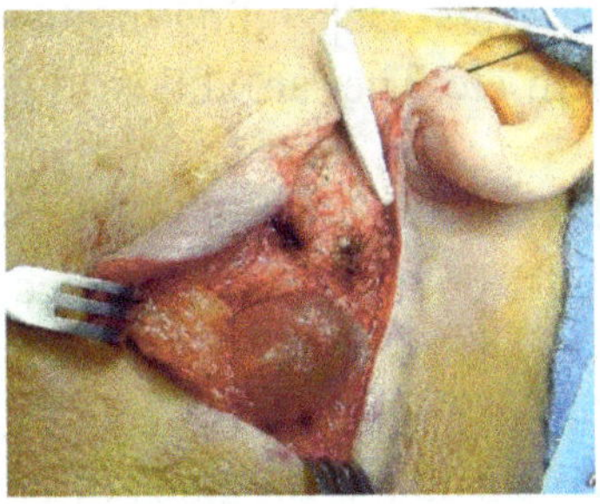

this deters bacterial accumulation and infection. Dietary modifications are also prescribed to prevent the production of excess saliva during the healing phase.

It should be remembered that sialoceles that are treated by *drainage* or *aspiration* are associated with a high rate of *recurrence* because the mechanism which initially led to the formation of the sialocele has not been treated.

DERMOID CYST OF THE PAROTID GLAND

Classification of Dermoid Cysts

New and Erich (1937), on the basis of hypothesized pathogenesis and histopathological appearance, classified dermoid cysts into the following three categories:

Figure 7. Intra-operative dissection of a right parotid cyst

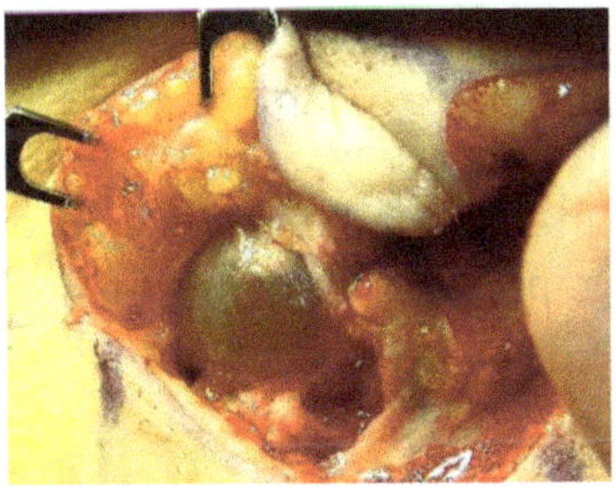

1. **Congenital dermoid cysts of teratoma type:** These arise from the embryonic germinal layers. Depending on the dormant layer, they can contain skin, hair, teeth, etc. They are almost always limited to the ovaries and testes;
2. **Acquired dermoid cysts:** These are inclusion cysts due to traumatically implanted skin in the deeper tissues. They occur on the hands and the other exposed parts of the body;
3. **Congenital inclusion dermoid cysts:** These develop from inclusions of displaced dermal cells along the lines of embryologic fusion. This category is further subdivided into four subgroups: (a) cysts around the eyes and orbits, originating along the naso-optic groove, (b) those around the nose, resulting from intrusion of the fronto-nasal plate, (c) those around the floor of the mouth, and in submental and submaxillary regions, originating from the first and second branchial arches, (d) those around the suprasternal, suboccipital, thyroidal, lower lip and palate, most of which occur along the mid-ventral or mid-dorsal lines of the body.

Incidence

Dermoid cysts of the head and neck are rare benign lesions that usually present as a midline neck mass and rarely appear in lateral region. Approximately, 7% of all dermoid cysts are seen in head and neck region (Moody, Avery, & Harrison, 1998) and 80% of them predominantly occur in the orbit, floor of mouth and nose (New, 1937; Tylor, 1967; Smirniopoulas, 1995). These locations are the fusion sites of many embryonic structures and hence prone for dermoid cyst formation (Islam & Hoffman, 2009).

Dermoid cyst in parotid gland is rare and only few case reports are available in literature. Cystic lesions account for 2-5% of all parotid gland lesions (Choi et al, 1988).

Etiology

Dermoid cystic lesions are either congenital or acquired (Naujoks et al, 2007). *Congenital* lesions are most often ectodermal in origin and they include branchial cleft cysts / lymphoepithelial cysts. *Acquired* cysts can be due to obstructions, neoplasms, calculi and traumatic implantation of epithelium in deeper layers (Pryor, Lewis, Weaver, & Orvidas, 2005).

Pathology

Dermoid cysts can be congenital or acquired. Congenital cysts arise from a rest of embryonic epithelium whereas acquired cysts are a result of traumatic implanted skin in deeper layers.

Histologically, dermoid cysts are composed of tissues originating from ectoderm and mesoderm. These are lined by stratified squamous epithelium with variable amount of pilosebaceous units and sweat glands supported by a fibrous connective tissue wall.

Clinical Presentation

More than 50% of dermoid cysts in the head and neck region are usually detected by the age of six, though approximately one-third are present at birth (Pryor, Lewis, Weaver, & Orvidas, 2005). Dermoid cysts generally are painless swellings (Figure 8) without infiltration into surrounding important structures such as the facial nerve or skin or fixation to the deeper structures.

Figure 8. A mass in the right parotid gland in a 37-year-old lady (arrow). It proved to be a dermoid cyst (Dwivedi et al, 2018).

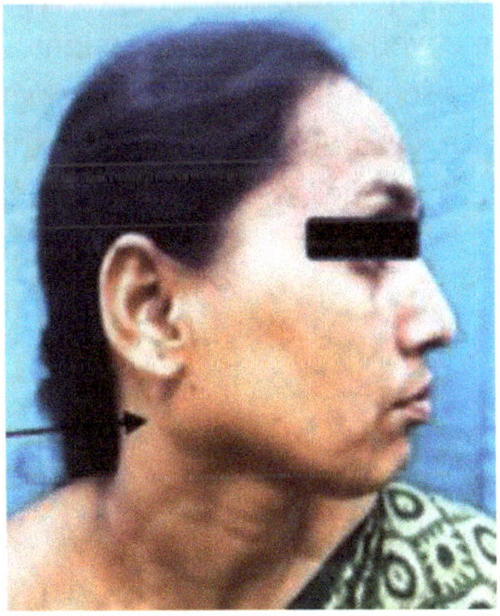

Diagnosis

Clinico-radiological evaluation is often ambiguous which makes pre-operative diagnosis difficult. *Differential diagnosis* includes mucous retention cyst, unilateral obstruction of the parotid duct, benign mesenchymal tumors (e.g. lipoma, fibroma, hemangioma or neurofibroma), branchial cleft cyst, benign parotid gland tumors (e.g. pleomorphic adenoma or Warthin's tumor), and malignant parotid gland tumors (e.g. muco-epidermoid tumor) (Islam, 2009; Choi, 1988).

Ultrasonography (US), computed tomography (CT), magnetic resonance imaging (MRI), and fine-needle aspiration cytology (FNAC) can be performed. *Ultrasound* is able to differentiate between solid, vascular and cystic lesions. Both, *MRI* and *CT* scan may give an idea about the location and relations of the mass with the surrounding tissue, but cannot give a final pre-operative diagnosis.

MRI of a dermoid cyst typically depicts a cystic mass, hypointense on T1-weighted images and hyperintense on T2-weighted ones with peripheral enhancement on contrast (Figure 9). Some dermoid cysts have variable signal intensity on T1 weighted images, which may be hyperintense because of the presence of sebaceous lipid (Mukunyadzi, 2002).

Fine needle aspiration cytology may provide reliable information on cystic lesions if there are supporting radiological findings, but can also be misleading because some well-differentiated squamous cell carcinomas and malignant lesions showing squamous metaplasia may share the benign-looking cytological features with dermoid cysts. Hence, the definitive diagnosis should always be made by histopathological examination (Naujoks, 2007; Baschinsky, 1999).

Treatment

Superficial parotidectomy is generally performed for the treatment of parotid dermoid cyst. Dwivedi et al (2018); however, performed enucleation of the cyst and not superficial parotidectomy as it was easily dissected in-toto without sacrificing the superficial lobe (Figure 10). In all kinds of surgical intervention, careful dissection of the facial nerve from the cyst wall is paramount to prevent damage which may potentially cause neurologic deficits (Damar, Erdem, Dinç, Bişkin, & Bahadır, 2015).

Figure 9. MRI showing: (A) Hypointense mass on T1 image; and (B) Hyperintense on T2. Fat planes are preserved.

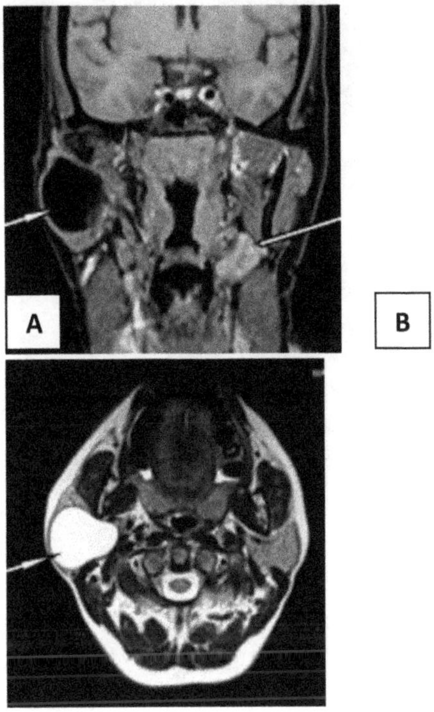

CLASSIFICATION OF PAROTID GLAND TUMORS

Salivary gland tumors calssified according to their pathological entities have a wide morphologic spectrum, and there may be considerable overlap between non-neoplastic, benign, and malignant entities.

WHO Hiostological Classification (Seifert, 1992; Everson, 2005)

Benign Epithelieal Tumors

- Pleomorphic Adenoma (PA) (Mixed salivary tumor)
- Myoepithelioma
- Basal cell adenoma
- Warthin's Tumor (Adenolymphoma, Papillary Cystadenoma Lymphomatosum)

Figure 10. The excised (enucleated) parotid dermoid cyst (Dwivedi et al, 2018)

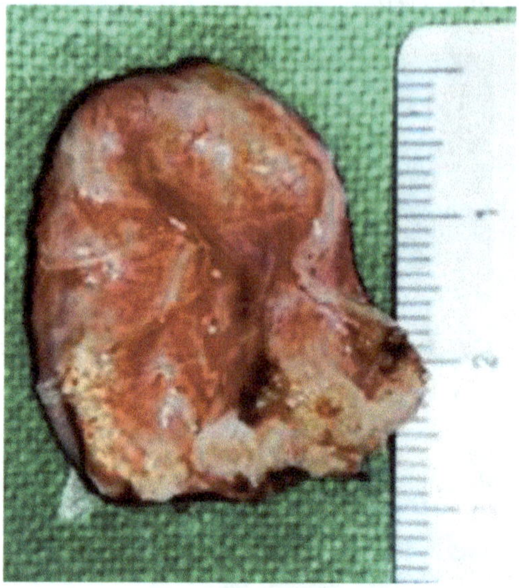

- Oncocytoma
- Canalicular adenoma
- Sebaceous adenoma
- Lymphadenoma:
    - Sebaceous
    - Non-sebaceous
- Duct papilloma:
    - Inverted duct papilloma
    - Intraductal papilloma
    - Sialadenoma papilliferum
- Cystadenoma

Malignant Epithelieal Tumors

- Acinic cell carcinoma
- Mucoepidermoid carcinoma (MEP)
- Adenoid cystic Carcinoma (ACC)
- Polymorphous low-grade adenocarcinoma (PLGA)
- Epithelial-myoepithelial carcinoma
- Clear cell carcinoma, not otherwise specified
- Basal cell adenocarcinoma

- Sebaceous carcinoma
- Sebaceous lymphadenocarcinoma
- Cystadenocarcinoma
- Low grade cribriform cystadenocarcinoma
- Mucinous adenocarcinoma
- Oncocytic carcinoma
- Salivary duct carcinoma
- Adenocarcinoma, not otherwise specified
- Myoepithelial carcinoma
- Carcinoma ex-pleomorphic adenoma (CEPA)
- Carcinosarcoma (Malignant mixed salivary tumor)
- Metastasizing pleomorphic adenoma
- Squamous cell carcinoma
- Small cell carcinoma (SCC)
- Large cell carcinoma
- Lymphoepithelial carcinoma
- Sialoblastoma

Soft Tissue Tumors

- Hemangioma

Hematolymphoid Tumors

- Hodgkin's lymphoma
- Diffuse large B-cell lymphoma
- Extra-nodal marginal zone B-cell lymphoma

Secondary Tumors

Secondary tumors of the salivary glands are relatively uncommon and represent less than 2 percent of all head and neck neoplasms.

Tumor-Like Lesions

- Ranula
- Venous malformation
- Lymphatic malformation
- Arterio-venous malformation

REFERENCES

Baschinsky, D., Hameed, A., & Keyhani-Rofagha, S. (1999). Fine-needle aspiration cytological features of dermoid cyst of the parotid gland: A report of two cases. *Diagnostic Cytopathology*, *20*(6), 387–388. doi:10.1002/(SICI)1097-0339(199906)20:6<387::AID-DC13>3.0.CO;2-0 PMID:10352915

Batsakis, J. G., & Raymond, A. K. (1989). Sialocysts of the parotid glands. *The Annals of Otology, Rhinology, and Laryngology*, *98*(6), 487–489. doi:10.1177/000348948909800618 PMID:2729835

Choi, E. C., Jin, J. B., Kim, J. Y., Hong, W. P., Kim, M. J., & Park, Y. K. (1988). Dermoid cyst of the parotid gland. *Yonsei Medical Journal*, *29*(2), 199–203. doi:10.3349/ymj.1988.29.2.199 PMID:3064438

Damar, M., Erdem, D., Dinç, A. E., Bişkin, S., & Bahadır, B. (2015). Dermoid cyst of the parotid gland. *ENT Cases*, *1*(3), 191–194.

Dwivedi, G., Gupta, V., Patnaik, U., Kumar, M., Amit-Sood, A, & Upadhyay, M. (2018). Dermoid Cyst of the Parotid Gland: A Rare Entity. *Indian Journal of Otolaryngology and Head & Neck Surgery*, 1-4.

Eversole, L. (2001). Salivary gland pathology. In Y. Fu, B. M. Wenig, E. Abemayor, & B. L. Wenig (Eds.), *Head and Neck Pathology: with Clinical Correlations* (pp. 242–291). Philadelphia, PA: Churchill-Livingstone.

Everson, J. W., Auclair, P., Gnepp, D. R., & El-Naggar, A. K. (2005). Tumors of the salivary glands. In L. Barnes, J. W. Eveson, P. Reichart, & D. Sidransky (Eds.), *World Health Organization Classification of Tumors. Pathology and Genetics of Head and Neck Tumors* (pp. 212–215). Lyon: IARC Press.

Islam, S., & Hoffman, G. R. (2009). Parotid dermoid cyst: A rare entity. *The Journal of Laryngology and Otology*, *123*(2), 1–4. doi:10.1017/S0022215109004447 PMID:19152721

Kara, T., Arpaci, R. B., Vayisoglu, Y., Serinsoz, E., Gursoy, D., & Ozgur, A. (2014). … Ozcan. (2014). Hydatid Cyst of Parotid Gland: An Unusual Case Diagnosed by Fine Needle Aspiration Biopsy. *Turkish Journal of Pathology*, *4*, 1–4.

Moody, A. B., Avery, C. M., & Harrison, J. D. (1998). Dermoid cyst of the parotid gland. *International Journal of Oral and Maxillofacial Surgery*, *27*(6), 461–462. doi:10.1016/S0901-5027(98)80038-6 PMID:9869288

Mukunyadzi, P. (2002). Review of fine-needle aspiration cytology of salivary gland neoplasms, with emphasis on differential diagnosis. *Pathology Patterns Reviews*, *118*(1suppl_1), S100–S115. doi:10.1309/WVVR-30E4-13TW-494D PMID:14569817

Naujoks, C., Handschel, J., Braunstein, S., Emaetig, F., Depprich, R., Meyer, U., & Kübler, N. (2007). Dermoid cyst of the parotid gland-a case report and brief review of the literature. *International Journal of Oral and Maxillofacial Surgery*, *36*(9), 861–863. doi:10.1016/j.ijom.2007.03.011 PMID:17498925

New, G. B. (1937). Dermoid cysts of the head and neck. *Surgery, Gynecology & Obstetrics*, *65*, 48–55.

Ogasawara, N., Takano, K. I., Kobayashi, H., Kikuchi, K., Matsumiya, H., Yoshioka, I., & Himi, T. (2017). HIV-associated cystic lesions of the parotid gland. *Auris, Nasus, Larynx*, *44*(1), 126–130. doi:10.1016/j.anl.2016.05.011 PMID:27264875

Peel, R. (2001). Diseases of the salivary gland. In L. Barnes (Ed.), *Surgical Pathology of the Head and Neck* (pp. 634–757). New York, NY: Marcel-Dekker.

Pryor, S. G., Lewis, J. E., Weaver, A. L., & Orvidas, L. J. (2005). Pediatric dermoid cysts of the head and neck. *Otolaryngology - Head and Neck Surgery*, *132*(6), 938–942. doi:10.1016/j.otohns.2005.03.005 PMID:15944568

Seifert, G., & Sobin, L. H. (1992). The World Health Organization's classification of salivary gland tumors. A commentary on the second edition. Cancer, 70(2), 379-385.

Sela, J., & Ulmansky, M. (1969). Mucous retention cyst of salivary glands. *Journal of Oral Surgery*, *27*, 619–623. PMID:5265202

Smirniotopoulos, J. G., & Chiechi, M. V. (1995). Teratomas, dermoids, and epidermoids of the head and neck. *Radiographics*, *15*(6), 1437–1455. doi:10.1148/radiographics.15.6.8577967 PMID:8577967

Taylor, B. W., & Erich, J. B. (1967). Dermoid cysts of nose. *Mayo Clinic Proceedings*, *42*(8), 488.

Tripti-Maithani, A. P., & Seema, A. (2014). Congenital agenesis of unilateral parotid gland with ipsilateral type I first branchial cleft anomaly: A rare presentation. *Egyptian Journal of Ear, Nose. Throat and Allied Sciences, 15*, 53–56.

Williams, N. S., Bulstrode, C., & O'Connell, P. R. (2008). *Bailey & Love's Short Practice of Surgery* (25th ed.). London: Hodder Arnold. doi:10.1201/b13454

Work, W. P. (1977). Cysts and congenital lesions of the parotid gland. *Otolaryngologic Clinics of North America, 10*, 339–343. PMID:896198

Work, W. P., & Hecht, D. W. (1968). Non-neoplastic lesions of the parotid gland. *The Annals of Otology, Rhinology, and Laryngology, 77*(3), 462–467. doi:10.1177/000348946807700308 PMID:5667940

Yigit, N., Karslioglu, Y., Yildizoglu, U., & Karakoc, O. (2014). Dermoid Cyst of the Parotid Gland: Report of a Rare Entity with Literature Review. *Head and Neck Pathology, 9*(2), 286–292. doi:10.100712105-014-0563-3 PMID:25113038

Chapter 11
Benign Tumors of the Parotid Gland

ABSTRACT

Benign tumors of the salivary glands are varied and named after their cell type. They occur most commonly in the parotid gland, and the majority (approximately 80%) are pleomorphic adenoma. This benign tumor arises from the superficial lobe of the gland in approximately 80% of cases. Less commonly, the mass presents as a cheek mass overlying the masseter muscle, arising from the accessory parotid lobe. If the tumor arises from the deep lobe, it presents as a para-pharyngeal mass with a completely different clinical presentation. In this instance, the patient will complain of snoring and difficultly in swallowing. Physical examination will reveal a soft palate and tonsillar, diffuse bulge, which is firm in consistency. Malignant transformation is extremely rare. Ultrasonography, computed tomography scan and magnetic resonance imaging are the best imaging tools. Treatment is usually through superficial or total conservative parotidectomy, with preservation of the facial nerve.

PLEOMORPHIC ADENOMA (PA)

Incidence

Pleomorphic adenoma, the most common salivary gland tumor, is also known as benign mixed tumor because of its dual origin from epithelial

DOI: 10.4018/978-1-7998-5603-0.ch011

and myoepithelial elements. It constitutes up 75-80% of all benign parotid tumors (McLoughlin, 2019; Lee, 2019; Meshram, 2018). It may affect as well the submandibular and minor salivary glands. Its incidence is slightly higher in females, and affects most commonly patients between 30 to 50 years of age (Bueting, 1998; Honda, 2005; Kici, 2001). Though uncommon, it has been reported in the first two decades of life. It is uncommon to be bilateral (Eveson, Kusafuka, & Stenman, 2005). It is usually a solitary lesion, although synchronous or metachronous involvement of two or more salivary glands can occur. It may also occur in combination with other tumors, mostly Warthin's tumor.

Etiology

The etiology of pleomorphic adenoma is unknown, but the incidence of this tumor has been increasing in the last two decades in relation to the exposure of radiation. One study suggested that oncogenic simian virus (SV40) may play a role in the onset or progression of pleomorphic adenoma. Prior head and neck irradiation is also a risk factor for the development of these tumors (Gündüz, Yeşiltaş, & Shields, 2018).

Pathology

It is a well-defined tumor, but with small extensions into the adjacent normal tissue through an incomplete capsule, which explains recurrence after enucleation. It has a pleomorphic matrix, with a non-cystic cut-section that may show some islets of cartilage. *Microscopically*, it is formed of epithelial cells intermingled with a pleomorphic stroma; fibrous, myxomatous and pseudo-cartilaginous (Figure 1). It is categorized into 4 types as follows (Chaplin, Darke, & Patel, 1983): (1) principally myxoid, (2) mixed myxoid and cellular components in equal proportions, (3) predominantly cellular, and (4) extremely cellular.

The tumor carries a malignant potential of 5-10%. The presence of hyalinized stroma is the most predictive histological parameter of malignant transformation. It may rarely metastasize without having the histological features of malignancy, but this almost always occurs after inadequate surgical excision, possibly due to altered anatomy secondary to surgery, which gave access to vascular and lymphatic channels.

Figure 1. Pleomorphic adenoma: Biphasic population of epithelial and mesenchymal cells. Epithelial cells assume tubular profiles, cords or nests. Stroma is myxoid (H&E, x100).

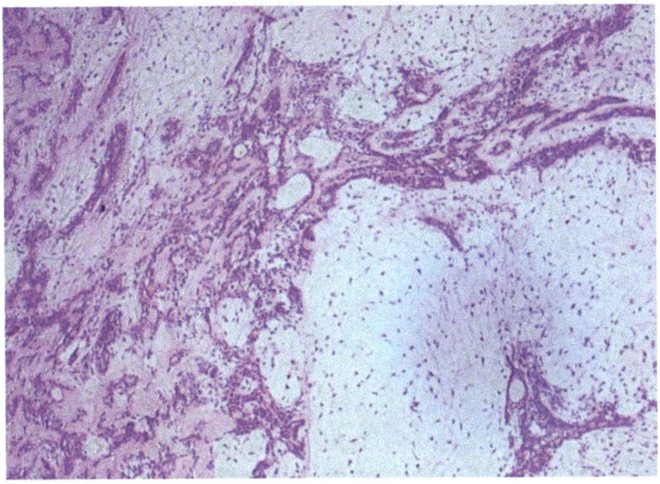

Roughly 70% of PAs have cytogenetic alterations that likely play a major role in *tumorigenesis*, and can be categorized into 4 groups: (1) tumors with 8q12 rearrangements, (2) those with 12q13-15 rearrangements, (3) those with miscellaneous clonal changes, and (4) those that are karyotypically normal (Kas, 1997; Voz, 1998).

Clinical Presentation

The patient presents with a painless, slowly growing, spherical mass, of variable size ranging from pea-size to a large mass, 20-50 cm across (Lee, 1992; Seifert, 1999; Skalova, 2001), as shown in Figure 2. The mass usually lies over the angle of the mandible and below the lobule of the ear (Figure 3). However, a swelling of the lower pole of the parotid gland may present in the lateral side of the neck, below and behind the angle of the mandible, giving rise to clinical diagnostic difficulty (Figure 4). The patient's complaint is usually disfigurement. The mass is of heterogonous consistency and mobile, being neither attached to the skin nor to the deep structures. Bosselation of the tumor is demonstrable if it is bigger than 3 cm. A fibrous capsule may not be apparent, but the tumor is clearly demarcated from surrounding tissues.

While most PAs occur in the superficial lobe of the parotid gland (80%) (Seifert, 1996; Yu, 1996; Everson, 1985), the deep lobe can be involved (20%)

Figure 2. A large left-sided pleomorphic adenoma (PA) of the parotid gland in a 56-year-old male patient. Note displacement of the left ear lobule.

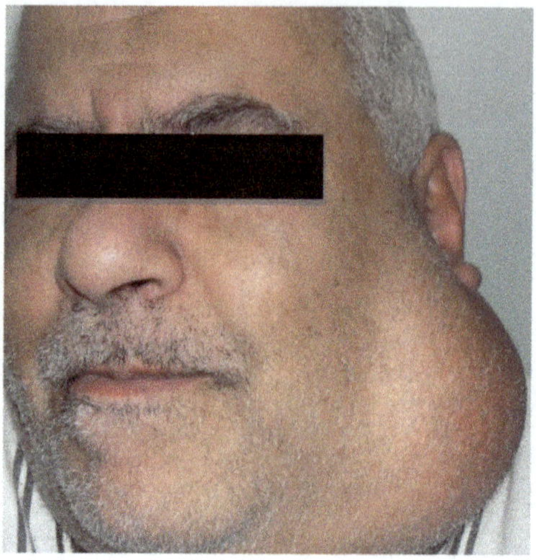

Figure 3. Pleomorphic adenoma in its typical position over the angle of the mandible and below the lobule of the ear

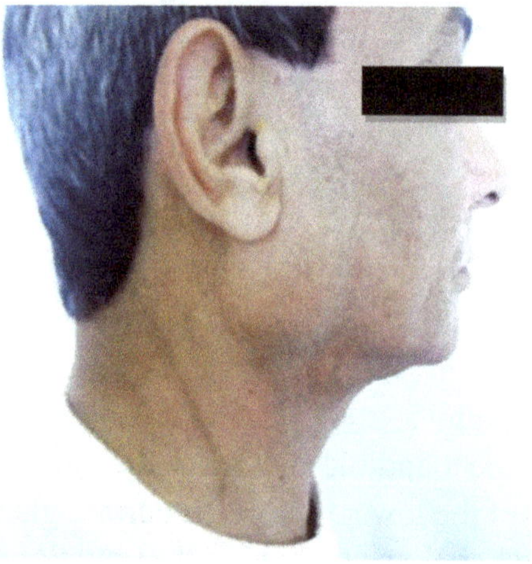

and is clearly demonstrable by computed tomography (CT) scan (Figure 5). Extensions of deep lobe PAs are the most common tumors of the para-pharyngeal space constituting 40% of tumors in this region (Everson, 2005; Everson, 1985). The draining lymph nodes (LNs) are not enlarged and the facial nerve is always intact.

Figure 4. Pleo-morphic adenoma in its typical position over the angle of the mandible and below the lobule of the ear

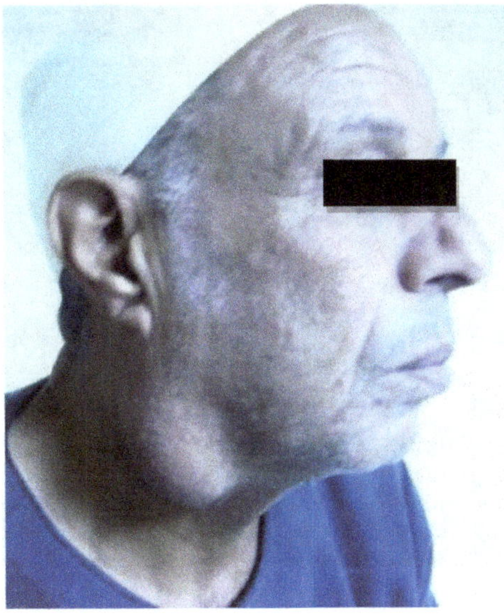

Investigations

The diagnosis of PA is based both on tissue sampling and radiographical studies. Tissue sampling procedures including fine needle aspiration (FNA) and core-needle biopsy can be done in an outpatient setting. These procedures are associated with very low tumor seeding rates (Kato, 2018; Shalley, 2018).

As for any parotid mass, ultrasonography (US), CT and magnetic resonance imaging (MRI) (preferably with diffusion-weighted and perfusion sequences) are the best imaging tools. *Ultrasound* PAs characteristically appear hypoechoic in texture. They usually show a lobulated distinct border with or without posterior acoustic enhancement. CT scan usually appears as smoothly marginated or lobulated homogeneous soft tissue density globular mass. Necrosis can be seen in larger masses. Few foci of calcification are common. Smaller tumors show early homogenous prominent enhancement while in the case of larger tumors enhancement is less marked and delayed. MRI is similar to CT; smaller masses appear well-circumscribed and homogeneous whereas larger tumors appear heterogeneous (Kato et al., 2018). Zaghi et al. (2014) suggested that if a parotid mass demonstrates bright T2 signal, sharp margins, heterogeneous nodular enhancement, lobulated contours, and a dark T2 rim, this combination of features carries 95% specificity for PA.

Figure 5. CT scan showing extension of the PA to involve the deep lobe of the parotid gland (red arrow)

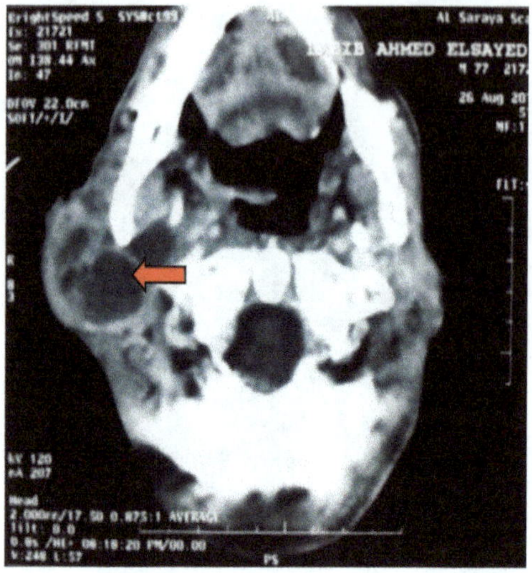

Fine needle aspiration cytology (FNAC) is a recognized method for obtaining pre-operative diagnosis and is advised to be done after imaging for the fear of hemorrhage. FNAC can determine whether the tumor is malignant in nature with an approximate sensitivity of 90%. Core needle biopsy is more invasive but provides more accurate histological typing of the tumor with a diagnostic accuracy of around 97%. Immuno-histochemistry (IHC) may prove to be supportive in delineating the different cell components. Many studies showed that the use of flow cytometry as a biological parameter for the prediction of recurrence in PAs should be considered. Tumors of a larger size showed a higher percentage of cells in the S-phase fraction and probably a greater tendency for recurrence (Junquera et al, 1999).

Treatment

Treatment of PA is through superficial or total conservative parotidectomy, with preservation of the facial nerve. Partial superficial parotidectomy and extra-capsular dissection are other recognized options of resection (Zbaren, 2013; Bradley, 2005; Fukushima, 2011). Partial superficial parotidectomy entails dissection of the main trunk of the facial nerve and only one division with its terminal branches (Figure 6). *Enucleation* is *never done* for its high

Figure 6. Dissection of the main trunk and only one division, related to the parotid mass arrow

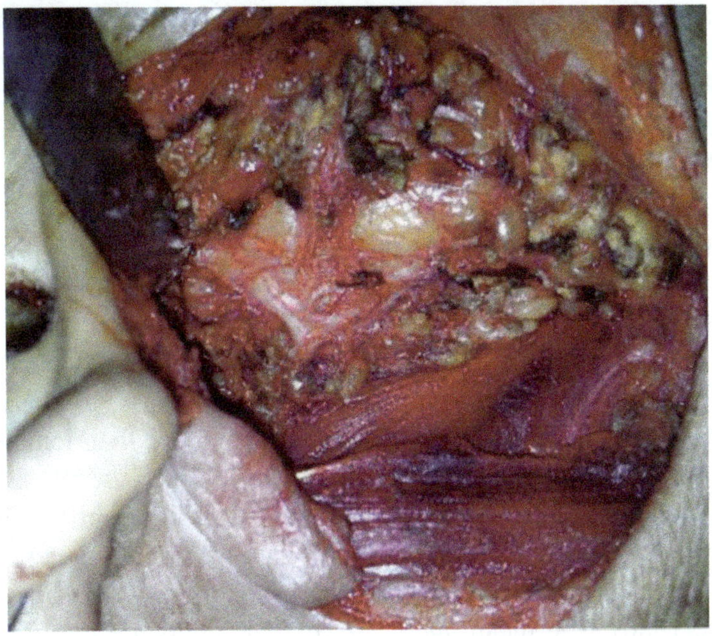

recurrence rate. The skin incision can be the classical lazy-S incision or recently one can resort to the cosmetically better face lift incision.

Flaps are raised and the facial nerve trunk is exposed at the stylomastoid foramen and all its five terminal branches are followed to the muscles to avoid their injury. If the facial nerve is injured, the patient must be taught an eye care program and how to use lubricating drops to prevent keratopathy. A referral to an ophthalmologist in this case is highly recommended. Depending on the severity of nerve injury, it may take months or years to fully recover eyelid function (Infante-Cossio et al, 2018).

The incidence of *recurrence* following surgery varies depending on the surgical technique used, surgeon's experience and duration of patient's follow-up (Ayoub, Bhatia, & Mal, 2002). In general, a recurrence rate of less than 1% is considered acceptable. Recurrent PAs have a higher likelihood for a second recurrence of about 6%-15% (Henriksson, Westrin, Carlsoo, & Silfversward, 1998). Uninodular recurrences have a better outcome than multinodular recurrences (Klinworth, 2010; Orita, 2010).

WARTHIN'S TUMOR (ADENOLYMPHOMA)

Warthin's tumor, also known as *papillary cystadenoma Lymphomatosum* and *adenolymphoma* is a benign cystic tumor of the parotid gland containing abundant lymphocytes and germinal centers (lymph node-like stroma). It is named for pathologist *Aldred Scott Warthin*, who described two cases in 1929. *It should not be confused with Wharton's duct of the submandibular gland.*

Incidence

Warthin's tumor represents about 5% of all benign parotid tumors, and is *bilateral* in 5%-10% of cases (Figure 7), but the two masses usually are at different times. It is the most common *parotid tail* mass. It occurs almost exclusively in the parotid gland, affecting males more than females (8:1); however, the ratio has decreased drastically during the past 50 years to 2:1 (Fascicle, 1996; Simpson, 2005). This gender predilection shift is referred to that it is highly linked to *smoking*. Smokers have an 8 times higher incidence of developing Warthin's tumors than non-smokers (Snyderman, Johnson, & Barnes, 1986). The mean *age* is 62 years. Patients are rarely below 40 years (Kotwall, 1992; Pinkston, 1996). Autoimmune disease or exposure to radiation increases the *risk* of Warthin's tumor progression.

Pathogenesis

The exact pathogenesis of Warthin's tumors is unknown (Cope, 2014; Teymoortash, 2013; Orabona, 2015). The predominant hypothesis suggests that this lesion arises from the salivary gland tissue entrapped within parotid lymph nodes (LNs) during embryogenesis. Carcinogens in smoke seem to be an important risk factor for the occurrence of Warthin's tumors. Several studies have also shown the role of progesterone receptors in the etiology of Warthin tumors. There are few studies assessing the role of viruses in the pathogenesis of this tumor (Lee, Yoon, Lee, & Lim, 2019).

Pathology

Macroscopically, it is a reddish brown mass with a true capsule. Its cut section has many cystic spaces and the fluid content is characteristically granular brown resembling "motor oil".

Figure 7. CT scan showing bilateral parotid tail masses (yellow arrows)

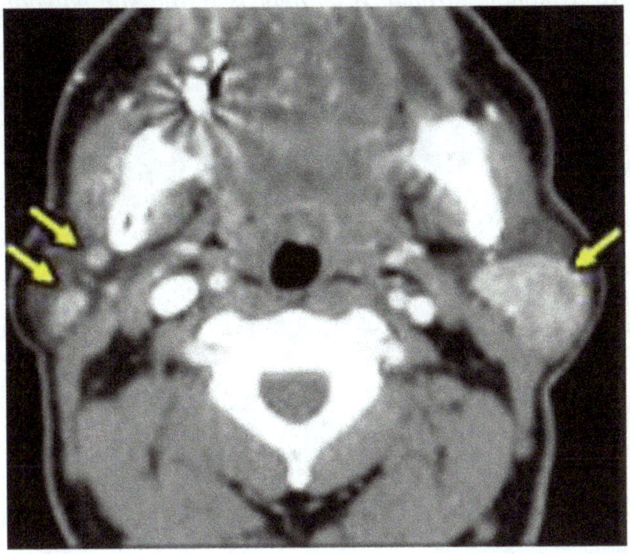

Microscopically, it is comprised of a papillary proliferation lined by a double layer composed of surface columnar oncocytic epithelium and a smaller basal layer of small cuboidal cells with myoepithelial characteristics. The surrounding stroma contains a highly ordered lymphoid architecture similar to an actual LN (Figure 8). When Warthin's tumor arises in a cervical LN, it may be mistaken for metastatic carcinoma, particularly from a papillary thyroid carcinoma. Malignant transformation is extremely rare (< 1%). The lymphoid component may lead to lymphoma.

Diagnosis

Clinically, the mass is painless, slowly-growing, soft in consistency, freely mobile, and usually 1 to 3 cm in diameter. It rarely attains a large size (Figure 9). It has a smooth surface, homogenous consistency and is sometimes cystic (30%). It is often multifocal (20%) and may be fixed to the overlying skin (van der Wal, Davids, & van der Waal, 1993). Rarely, infarcted Warthin's tumors may cause pain and heaviness in the mouth (Simpson, & Eveson, 2005).

As for any parotid swelling, US, CT scan and MRI are the best imaging tools. Adenolymphoma (Warthin's tumor) is characteristically the only parotid tumor that can give a *hot spot in* ^{99Tm}*Tc scan*. Ultrasound-guided FNAC is a recognized method for obtaining pre-operative diagnosis.

Figure 8. Warthin's Tumor: Cystic spaces lined by double layer of epithelial cells resting on dense lymphoid stroma. Inset depicts intracystic polypoid projections with lymphoid stroma (H&E, x100).

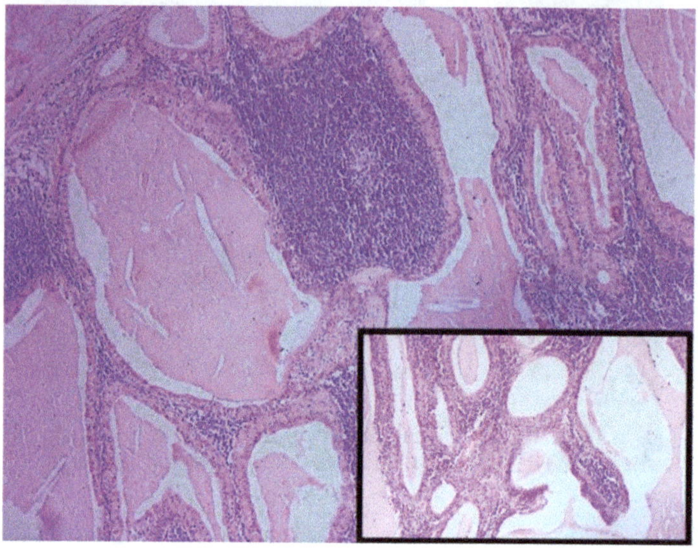

Treatment

The type and extent of surgery is dependent on the location of tumors by CT scan and the result of FNAC. Recently, Lee et al. (2019), reported the results of 118 operations performed for 110 patients (8 patients had bilateral tumors) from December 2006 to December 2016. All patients underwent a macroscopically complete oncologic resection. *Partial parotidectomy*, including *enucleation* or removal of the inferior half of the superficial lobe, was performed if the Warthin's tumor was located in the tail (inferior) portion of the parotid gland (n=77). *Superficial parotidectomy* was performed if the tumor was located in the superficial lobe (n=34). *Total parotidectomy* was performed if the tumor was located in the deep lobe (n=7). Partial facial dysfunction after the operation was detected in 12 pateints and recovered spontaneously within 3 months. Only one patient experienced a recurrence, and was disease-free after re-operation.

Figure 9. Right adeno-lymphoma presenting as a small (3 cm), smooth, mass in a 61-year-old gentleman

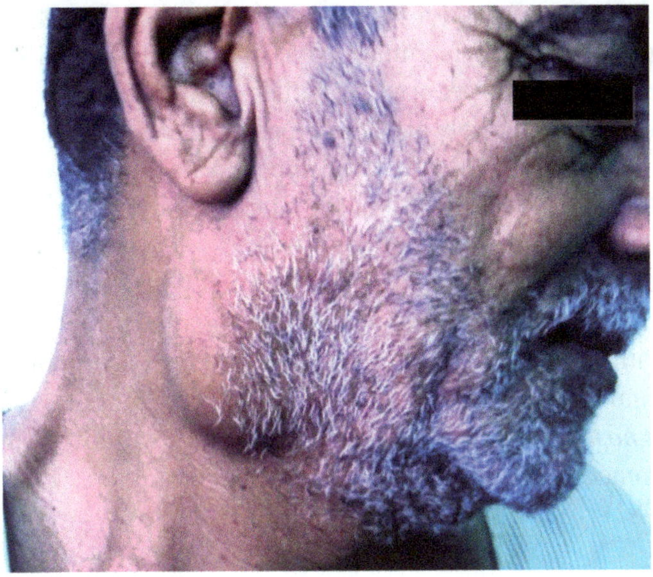

BASAL CELL ADENOMA (BCA)

Basal cell adenoma tends to occur over the *age* of 50 years with a *female-to-male* ratio of 2:1. (Eveson & Cawson, 1985). It usually occurs in the parotid gland (75%), much less commonly in the submandibular gland (5%) (Zarbo, 2002), and rarely in the minor salivary glands with the exclusion of canalicular adenomas, which were previously categorized with BCA (Yu, 1996; Yu, 1998). It typically *presents* as a slowly growing solitary painless mass. A special variant of BCA, the membranous type (dermal analog tumor) has a propensity for multifocality, and can be associated with multiple tricho-epitheliomas and cylindromas (*Brooke-Spiegler syndrome*) (Nagao et al, 1982).

Prognosis of BCA is generally excellent. Recurrence rate is low, except for the membranous subtype, which may recur in about 25% of cases. Malignant transformation is rare, again favoring the membranous subtype (Fascicle, 1996; Daley, 1984; Ferriero, 2005).

CANALICULAR ADENOMA

Canalicular adenoma, previously categorized with BCA, is a rare tumor comprising <1% of all salivary tumors (Fascicle, 1996; Daley, 1984; Ferriero, 2005). The mean age is 65 years with a female-to-male ratio of 1.8:1 (Fascicle, 1996; Suarez, 1998). It rarely affects the parotid glands (Fascicle, & Auclair, 1996). The minor salivary glands of the upper lip are the ones most commonly involved (80%) followed by the buccal mucosa (Ferreiro, 2005) and palate (Rousseau, Mock, Dover, & Jordan, 1999).

It typically *presents* as painless, slowly growing submucosal nodule. Rarely, multiple/multifocal canalicular adenomas may occur and present clinically with multiple discrete masses, typically occurring in the upper lip and buccal mucosa.

The *prognosis* is excellent and recurrences are extremely rare. Some of these recurrences may be considered as separate tumors (Fascicle, 1996; Sciubba, 1982).

MYOEPITHELIOMA

Myoepitheliomas account for about 1.5% of all salivary tumors. This tumor primarily affects adults with a peak incidence in the third to fourth decades (range 8–82 years) (Begin, 1993; Begin, 1991). The parotid gland is the most common site affected (40%-50%), followed by the minor salivary glands in the palate. It usually presents as a slow-growing painless mass.

Prognosis is generally favorable; recurrences are relatively rare and are usually the result of incomplete excision (Savera, Sloman, Huvos, & Klimstra, 2000). Malignant transformation is uncommon (Rosai, 1996).

CYSTADENOMA

Cystadenoma is a rare benign cystic salivary tumor that resembles Warthin's tumor, though with different clinico-pathological features. Unlike Warthin's tumor, there is a slight female predilection, there is no association with smoking (Fascicle, 1996; Waldron, 1988), and is not exclusive for the parotid gland, though it is affected in nearly half of the cases.

Other sites include the lip and buccal mucosa (Skalova & Michal, 2005), and rarely the supra-glottic larynx (Gilcrease, Nelson, & Guzman-Paz, 1998). It affects adults with a mean age of 57 years (Brandwein & Huvos, 1995).

Prognosis of cystadenoma is excellent; complete excision is curative.

LIPOMA

Lipomas are benign neoplasms composed of mature adipose tissue surrounded by a fibrous capsule. Salivary gland lipomas are very rare and most commonly involve the parotid gland. They may be located with the gland itself or extra-capsular within the adjacent parotid space (Paparo, Massarelli, & Giuliani, 2016).

On imaging, lipomas appear as well-circumscribed lesions with imaging appearance similar to fat. On CT, they demonstrate attenuation of approximately -60 to -120 HU. On MRI, they demonstrate T1 and T2 hyper-intensity and will become hypo-intense with fat-suppression techniques. In the rare variant, *sialolipoma*, a lipoma undergoes secondary entrapment of normal salivary gland tissue, which alters the appearance of the lesion on imaging, producing a fatty lesion with heterogeneous internal composition owing to incorporation of salivary tissue (Pandey, Vats, Akhtar, & Pathania, 2015). Although this may be confusing at first, any well encapsulated heterogeneous lesion with clear fatty components should raise the suspicion for sialolipoma.

HEMANGIOMA

Hemangiomas (hemangioendotheliomas) are vascular lesions that result from abnormal proliferation of endothelial cells. It is the most common parotid tumor of childhood and tends to have a female predominance (3:1). Clinically, these patients usually present at 4 months of age with a rapidly growing mass that may have an overlying red/blue cutaneous lesion. MRI is extremely accurate in diagnosing these lesions as they classically appear as lobulated masses with T2 hyperintensity and homogeneous enhancement. The vascular nature of these lesions renders them at greater risk of hemorrhage during biopsy. Therefore, many authors recommend that biopsy should not be performed when the MRI demonstrates features suggestive of a hemangioma (Lara-Sánchez, Peral-Cagigal, Madrigal-Rubiales, & Verrier-Hernández,

2014). Spontaneous regression of this tumor is often seen after 18 months, although if large enough, surgery or sclerotherapy may be needed.

REFERENCES

Mc Loughlin, L., Gillanders, S. L., Smith, S., & Young, O. (2019). The role of adjuvant radiotherapy in management of recurrent pleomorphic adenoma of the parotid gland: A systematic review. *European Archives of Oto-Rhino-Laryngology, 276*(2), 283–295. doi:10.100700405-018-5205-z PMID:30426229

Lee, J. H., Kang, H. J., Yoo, C. W., Park, W. S., Ryu, J. S., Jung, Y. S., ... Han, N. (2019). PLAG1, SOX10, and Myb Expression in Benign and Malignant Salivary Gland Neoplasms. *Journal of Pathology and Translational Medicine, 53*(1), 23–30. doi:10.4132/jptm.2018.10.12 PMID:30424592

Meshram, G.G., Kaur, N., & Hura, K.S. (2018). Pediatric Pleomorphic Adenoma of the Parotid: Case Report, Review of Literature and Novel Therapeutic Targets. *Children (Basel), 18*(9), 127-131.

Gündüz, A. K., Yeşiltaş, Y. S., & Shields, C. L. (2018). Overview of benign and malignant lacrimal gland tumors. *Current Opinion in Ophthalmology, 29*(5), 458–468. doi:10.1097/ICU.0000000000000515 PMID:30028745

Buenting, J. E., Smith, T. L., & Holmes, D. K. (1998). Giant pleomorphic adenoma of the parotid gland: Case report and review of the literature. *Ear, Nose, and Throat Journal, 77*(8), 634–640. doi:10.1177/014556139807700812 PMID:9745180

Honda, T., Yamamoto, Y., Isago, T., Nakazawa, H., Nozaki, M., & Hirayama, T. (2005). Giant pleomorphic adenoma of the parotid gland with malignant transformation. *Annals of Plastic Surgery, 5*(5), 524–527. doi:10.1097/01.sap.0000176023.94693.b7 PMID:16258307

Kici, S., & Peytral, C. (2001). *Giant pleomorphic adenoma of the parotid gland: a case report and review of the literature*. Academic Press.

Eveson, J. W., Kusafuka, K., & Stenman, G. (2005). Pleomorphic adenoma. In E. L. Barnes, J. W. Eveson, P. Reichart, & D. Sidransky (Eds.), *Pathology and Classification of Head and Neck Tumours*. Lyon: IARC.

Chaplin, A. J., Darke, P., & Patel, S. (1983). Tyrosine-rich crystals in pleomorphic adenomas of parotid glands. *Journal of Oral Pathology*, *12*(5), 342–346. doi:10.1111/j.1600-0714.1983.tb00346.x PMID:6195320

Kas, K., Voz, M. L., Roijer, E., Astrom, A. K., Meyen, E., Stenman, G., & Van de Ven, W. J. M. (1997). Promoter swapping between the genes for a novel zinc finger protein and beta-catenin in pleiomorphic adenomas with t(3;8)(p21;q12) translocations. *Nature Genetics*, *15*(2), 170–174. doi:10.1038/ng0297-170 PMID:9020842

Voz, M. L., Astrom, A. K., Kas, K., Mark, J., Stenman, G., & Van de Ven, W. J. (1998). The recurrent translocation t(5;8)(p13;q12) in pleomorphic adenomas results in upregulation of PLAG1 gene expression under control of the LIFR promoter. *Oncogene*, *16*(11), 1409–1416. doi:10.1038j.onc.1201660 PMID:9525740

Lee, K. C., Chan, J. K., & Chong, Y. W. (1992). Ossifying pleomorphic adenoma of the maxillary antrum. *The Journal of Laryngology and Otology*, *106*(1), 50–52. doi:10.1017/S0022215100118596 PMID:1311743

Seifert, G., Donath, K., & Schafer, R. (1999). Lipomatous pleomorphic adenoma of the parotid gland. Classification of lipomatous tissue in salivary glands. *Pathology, Research and Practice*, *195*(4), 247–252. doi:10.1016/S0344-0338(99)80042-9 PMID:10337663

Skalova, A., Starek, I., Simpson, R. H., Kucerova, V., Dvorackova, J., Curik, R., & Dusková, M. (2001). Spindle cell myoepithelial tumours of the parotid gland with extensive lipomatous metaplasia. A report of four cases with immunohistochemical and ultrastructural findings. *Virchows Archiv*, *439*(6), 762–767. doi:10.1007004280100469 PMID:11787848

Seifert, G., & Donath, K. (1996). Multiple tumours of the salivary glands--terminology and nomenclature. *European Journal of Cancer Part B Oral Oncology*, *32B*(1), 3-7.

Yu, G. Y., Ma, D. Q., Zhang, Y., Peng, X., Cai, Z. G., Gao, Y., & Chen, Y. (2004). Multiple primary tumours of the parotid gland. *International Journal of Oral and Maxillofacial Surgery*, *33*(6), 531–534. doi:10.1016/j.ijom.2004.03.010 PMID:15308250

Eveson, J. W., & Cawson, R. A. (1985). Salivary gland tumours. A review of 2410 cases with particular reference to histological types, site, age and sex distribution. *The Journal of Pathology*, *146*(1), 51–58. doi:10.1002/path.1711460106 PMID:4009321

Kato, H., Kawaguchi, M., Ando, T., Mizuta, K., Aoki, M., & Matsuo, M. (2018). Pleomorphic adenoma of salivary glands: Common and uncommon CT and MR imaging features. *Japanese Journal of Radiology*, *36*(8), 463–471. doi:10.100711604-018-0747-y PMID:29845358

Zaghi, S., Hendizadeh, L., Hung, T., Farahvar, S., Abemayor, E., & Sepahdari, A. R. (2014). MRI criteria for the diagnosis of pleomorphic adenoma: A validation study. *American Journal of Otolaryngology*, *35*(6), 713–718. doi:10.1016/j.amjoto.2014.07.013 PMID:25128908

Shalley, S., Chand, N., Aggarwal, A., Garg, L. N., Yadav, V., & Yadav, A. (2018). Diagnostic Accuracy of Fine Needle Aspiration Cytology in Lesions of Oral Cavity and Salivary Glands: A Clinico-Pathological Study. *The Open Dentistry Journal*, *12*(1), 782–790. doi:10.2174/1745017901814010782 PMID:30369988

Junquera, L., Alonso, D., Sampedro, A., Fresno, F., Albertos, J. M., & Lopez-Arranz, J. S. (1999). Pleomorphic adenoma of the salivary glands: Prospective clinicopathologic and flow cytometric study. *Head & Neck*, *21*(7), 652–656. doi:10.1002/(SICI)1097-0347(199910)21:7<652::AID-HED10>3.0.CO;2-E PMID:10487953

Zbaren, P., Poorten, V., Witt, R. L., Woolgar, J. A., Shaha, A. R., Triantafyllou, A., ... Ferlito, A. (2013). Pleomorphic adenoma of the parotid: Formal parotidectomy or limited surgery? *American Journal of Surgery*, *205*(1), 109–118. doi:10.1016/j.amjsurg.2012.05.026 PMID:23062782

Bradley, P. J. (2005). Metastasizing pleomorphic salivary adenoma' should now be considered a low-grade malignancy with a lethal potential. *Current Opinion in Otolaryngology & Head & Neck Surgery*, *13*(2), 123–126. doi:10.1097/01.moo.0000153450.87288.2a PMID:15761289

Fukushima, M., Miyaguchi, M., & Kitahara, T. (2011). Extracapsular dissection: Minimally invasive surgery applied to patients with parotid pleomorphic adenoma. *Acta Oto-Laryngologica*, *131*(6), 653–659. doi:10.3109/00016489.2010.543148 PMID:21254958

Infante-Cossio, P., Gonzalez-Cardero, E., Garcia-Perla-Garcia, A., Montes-Latorre, E., Gutierrez-Perez, J. L., & Prats-Golczer, V. E. (2018). Complications after superficial parotidectomy for pleomorphic adenoma. *Medicina Oral, Patologia Oral y Cirugia Bucal*, *23*(4), e485–e492. doi:10.4317/medoral.22386 PMID:29924764

Ayoub, O. M., Bhatia, K., & Mal, R. K. (2002). Pleomorphic adenoma of the parotid gland: Is long-term follow-up needed? *Auris, Nasus, Larynx*, *29*(3), 283–285. doi:10.1016/S0385-8146(02)00013-5 PMID:12167452

Henriksson, G., Westrin, K.M., Carlsoo, B., & Silfversward, C. (1998). Recurrent primary pleomorphic adenomas of salivary gland origin: intrasurgical rupture, histopathologic features, and pseudopodia. *Cancer*, *82*(4), 617-620.

Klintworth, N., Zenk, J., Koch, M., & Iro, H. (2010). Postoperative complications after extracapsular dissection of benign parotid lesions with particular reference to facial nerve function. *The Laryngoscope*, *120*(3), 484–490. doi:10.1002/lary.20801 PMID:20112414

Orita, Y., Hamaya, K., Miki, K., Sugaya, A., Hirai, M., Nakai, K., ... Yoshino, T. (2010). Satelli.te tumors surrounding primary pleomorphic adenomas of the parotid gland Europea.n. *Archives of Oto-Rhino-Laryngology*, *267*(5), 801 806. doi:10.100700405 009 1149 7 PMID:19898859

Fascicle, G. L., & Auclair, P. L. (1996). *Tumors of the Salivary Glands, Atlas of Tumor Pathology*. Washington, DC: Armed Forces Institute of Pathology.

Simpson, R. H. W., & Eveson, J. W. (2005). Warthin tumor. In E. L. Barnes, J. W. Eveson, & D. Sidransky (Eds.), *Pathology and Classification of Head and Neck Tumours* (pp. 263–265). Lyon: IARC.

Snyderman, C., Johnson, J. T., & Barnes, E. L. (1986). Extraparotid Warthin's tumor. *Otolaryngology - Head and Neck Surgery*, *94*(2), 169–175. doi:10.1177/019459988609400207 PMID:3083330

Kotwall, C. A. (1992). Smoking as an etiologic factor in the development of Warthin's tumor of the parotid gland. *American Journal of Surgery*, *164*(6), 646–647. doi:10.1016/S0002-9610(05)80725-1 PMID:1334381

Pinkston, J. A., & Cole, P. (1996). Cigarette smoking and Warthin's tumor. *American Journal of Epidemiology*, *144*(2), 183–187. doi:10.1093/oxfordjournals.aje.a008906 PMID:8678050

Cope, W., Naugler, C., Taylor, S. M., Trites, J., Hart, R. D., & Bullock, M. J. (2014). The association of Warthin tumor with salivary ductal inclusions in intra- and peri-parotid lymph nodes. *Head and Neck Pathology*, *8*(1), 73–76. doi:10.100712105-013-0477-5 PMID:23868565

Teymoortash, A., Bohne, F., Jonsdottir, T., Hoch, S., Eivasi, B., & Roessler, M. (2013). Human papilloma virus (HPV) is not implicated in the etiology of Warthin's tumor of the parotid gland. *Acta Oto-Laryngologica*, *133*(9), 972–976. doi:10.3109/00016489.2013.797603 PMID:23944949

Orabona, G., Abbate, V., Piombino, P., Romano, A., Schonauer, F., Iaconetta, G., ... Califano, L. (2015). Warthin's tumour: Aetiopathogenesis dilemma, ten years of our experience. *Journal of Cranio-Maxillo-Facial Surgery*, *43*(4), 427–431. doi:10.1016/j.jcms.2014.11.019 PMID:25814196

Lee, D. H., Yoon, T. M., Lee, J. K., & Lim, S. C. (2019). Surgical treatment strategy in Warthin's tumor of the parotid gland. *Revista Brasileira de Otorrinolaringologia (English Ed.)*, *85*(5), 546–550. doi:10.1016/j.bjorl.2018.04.004 PMID:29807810

van der Wal, J. E., Davids, J. J., & van der Waal, I. (1993). Extraparotid Warthin's tumours--report of 10 cases. *British Journal of Oral & Maxillofacial Surgery*, *31*(1), 43–44. doi:10.1016/0266-4356(93)90098-H PMID:8431414

Eveson, J. W., & Cawson, R. A. (1985). Tumours of the minor (oropharyngeal) salivary glands: A demographic study of 336 cases. *Journal of Oral Pathology*, *14*(6), 500–509. doi:10.1111/j.1600-0714.1985.tb00522.x PMID:2991488

Zarbo, R. J. (2002). Salivary gland neoplasia: A review for the practicing pathologist. *Modern Pathology*, *15*(3), 298–323. doi:10.1038/modpathol.3880525 PMID:11904344

Yu, G., Ussmueller, J., & Donath, K. (1996). Histogenesis and development of membranous basal cell adenoma of the salivary gland. *Zhonghua Kou Qiang Yi Xue Za Zhi*, *35*(1), 31–33. PMID:11831959

Yu, G. Y., Ubmuller, J., & Donath, K. (1998). Membranous basal cell adenoma of the salivary gland: A clinicopathologic study of 12 cases. *Acta Oto-Laryngologica*, *118*(4), 588–593. doi:10.1080/00016489850154775 PMID:9726688

Nagao, K., Matsuzaki, O., Saiga, H., Sugano, I., Shigematsu, H., Kaneko, T., ... Kitamur.a, T. (1982). Histopa.thologic studies of basal cell adenoma of the parotid gland. *Cancer*, *50*(4), 736–745. doi:10.1002/1097-0142(19820815)50:4<736::AID-CNCR2820500419>3.0.CO;2-M PMID:6284339

Daley, T. D., Gardner, D. G., & Smout, M. S. (1984). Canalicular adenoma: Not a basal cell adenoma. *Oral Surgery, Oral Medicine, and Oral Pathology*, *57*(2), 181–188. doi:10.1016/0030-4220(84)90209-3 PMID:6366687

Ferreiro, J. A. (2005). Canalicular adenoma. In E. L. Barnes, J. W. Eveson, P. Reichart, & D. Sidransky (Eds.), *Pathology and Classification of Head and Neck Tumours* (p. 267). Lyon: IARC.

Suarez, P., Hammond, H. L., Luna, M. A., & Stimson, P. G. (1998). Palatal canalicular adenoma: Report of 12 cases and review of the literature. *Annals of Diagnostic Pathology*, *2*(4), 224–228. doi:10.1016/S1092-9134(98)80011-7 PMID:9845742

Rousseau, A., Mock, D., Dover, D. G., & Jordan, R. C. (1999). Multiple canalicular adenomas: A case report and review of the literature. *Oral Surgery, Oral Medicine, Oral Pathology, Oral Radiology, and Endodontics*, *87*(3), 346–350. doi:10.1016/S1079-2104(99)70221-0 PMID:10102598

Sciubba, J. J., & Brannon, R. B. (1982). Myoepithelioma of salivary glands: Report of 23 cases. *Cancer*, *49*(3), 562–572. doi:10.1002/1097-0142(19820201)49:3<562::AID-CNCR2820490328>3.0.CO;2-6 PMID:6277451

Begin, L. R., & Black, M. J. (1993). Salivary-type myxoid myoepithelioma of the sinonasal tract: A potential diagnostic pitfall. *Histopathology*, *23*(3), 283–285. doi:10.1111/j.1365-2559.1993.tb01204.x PMID:8225249

Begin, L. R., Rochon, L., & Frenkiel, S. (1991). Spindle cell myoepithelioma of thc nasal cavity. *The American Journal of Surgical Pathology*, *15*(2), 184–190. doi:10.1097/00000478-199102000-00012 PMID:1846508

Savera, A. T., Sloman, A., Huvos, A. G., & Klimstra, D. S. (2000). Myoepithelial carcinoma of the salivary glands: A clinicopathologic study of 25 patients. *The American Journal of Surgical Pathology*, *24*(6), 761–774. doi:10.1097/00000478-200006000-00001 PMID:10843278

Rosai, J. (1996). Major and minor salivary glands. In J. Rosai (Ed.), *Ackerman's Surgical Pathology* (pp. 834–835). St. Louis, MO: Mosby.

Waldron, C. A., el-Mofty, S. K., & Gnepp, D. R. (1988). Tumors of the intraoral minor salivary glands: A demographic and histologic study of 426 cases. *Oral Surgery, Oral Medicine, and Oral Pathology*, *66*(3), 323–333. doi:10.1016/0030-4220(88)90240-X PMID:2845326

Skalova, A., & Michal, M. (2005). Cystadenoma. In E. L. Barnes, J. W. Eveson, & D. Sidransky (Eds.), *Pathology and Classification of Head and Neck Tumours* (pp. 273–274). Lyon: IARC.

Gilcrease, M. Z., Nelson, F. S., & Guzman-Paz, M. (1998). Tyrosine-rich crystals associated with oncocytic salivary gland neoplasms. *Archives of Pathology & Laboratory Medicine*, *122*(7), 644–649. PMID:9674547

Brandwein, M., & Huvos, A. (1995). Laryngeal oncocytic cystadenomas. Eight cases and a literature review. *Archives of Otolaryngology--Head & Neck Surgery*, *121*(11), 1302–1305. doi:10.1001/archotol.1995.01890110076014 PMID:7576479

Paparo, F., Massarelli, M., & Giuliani, G. (2016). A rare case of parotid gland lipoma arising from the deep lobe of the parotid gland. *Annals of Maxillofacial Surgery*, *6*(2), 308–310. doi:10.4103/2231-0746.200335 PMID:28299278

Pandey, D., Vats, M., Akhtar, A., & Pathania, O. P. (2015). Sialolipoma of the parotid gland: A rare entity. *BMJ Case Reports*.

Lara-Sánchez, H., Peral-Cagigal, B., Madrigal-Rubiales, B., & Verrier-Hernández, A. (2014). Cavernous hemangioma of the parotid gland in adults. *Journal of Clinical and Experimental Dentistry*, *6*, e592–e594.

Chapter 12
Recurrent Pleomorphic Adenoma

ABSTRACT

This chapter discusses the etiology, clinical presentation, assessment, and treatment of recurrent pleomorphic adenoma. Recurrent tumor following surgery (or any other treatment) usually presents as a recurrent swelling at the primary site, with or without local symptoms. The incidence of recurrence following surgery varies depending on surgical technique, surgeon's experience, duration of follow-up, and clinical integrity. A recurrence rate of less than 1% is generally considered acceptable. The best policy to prevent recurrence of pleopmorphic adenoma is excisional biopsy of the tumor with maximal safe margin and functional neurological preservation. Treatment is determined by the age and physical health of the patient, number of pervious operations, and anatomical extent of the recurrence. Treatment options include observation, local excision, superficial parotidectomy, total conservative parotidectomy, total parotidectomy with resection of the involved nerve and immediate nerve graft (any procedure is followed by radiotherapy), and radiotherapy alone.

DOI: 10.4018/978-1-7998-5603-0.ch012

CAUSES OF RECURRENCE

Multicentricity

Pleomorphic adenomas (PAs) are unifocal disease in the major salivary glands; surgeons and pathologists *no* longer support this theory.

The Bare Area

The tumor capsule may vary in thickness from very thin (a few cells) to very thick; this variation may occur on the surface of the same tumor (Stennert, Guntinas-Lichius, Klaussmann, & Arnold, 2001). Because many PAs have a nodular surface, there is always the possibility of a nodule attached by a narrow stalk becoming separated from the main tumor mass thus giving rise to a recurrence (Webb & Eveson, 2001).

Pseudopodia (microscopic finger-like formations of tumor tissue extending beyond the main mass of tumor) are a significant risk factor for local recurrence of Pas (Chen, 2004; Hendrikisson, 1998). This is known as "*capsule penetration*", which occurs earlier and is more common in the bosselation process (Lawson, 1989). In capsular perforation, the tumor cells perforate the capsule and lie adjacent to the normal parotid tissue. Subcapsular splitting may be no more than a dehiscence resulting from peri-operative handling, and the presence of blood within the split would support this hypothesis. Another publication (McGregor, Burgoyne, & Tan, 1988), confirmed that no tumor has a smooth surface, and all tumors have a "bare- area".

The bare area is *not* always exposed to the facial nerve and may occur at any location along the tumor surface. The surgeon should carry out a wide local excision with the tumor contained within as much normal tissue as is possible. The bare area or deep surface of the tumor can lie against the cartilaginous external auditory meatus, styloid process, facial nerve, or masseter muscle.

Tumor Rupture

Rupture of the tumor, because of overzealous traction, instrument compression, rough handling, or poor surgical technique, with spillage into the surgical wound are factors which have been thought to predispose to recurrence.

The interior of a PA is usually soft and gelatinous, and it is these myxoid and friable cellular tumors that are at highest risk for rupture (McGregor,

Burgoyne, & Tan, 1988). Recent reports suggest that there is no correlation between tumor capsule rupture and recurrence of PA (Hendrikisson, 1998; Duchman, 1994; Notvig, 1994). However, this evidence does not fully explain the most frequent finding of multiple nodules rather than solitary, isolated recurrences. These observations suggest that rupture of the capsule of the tumor and spillage of tumor cells are still the most likely factors contributing to recurrence of tumor. Long-term follow-up, even annual follow-up by mail, may give a more accurate picture of tumor-free disease survival, than hoping that patients who develop a recurrence will come back and consult with their original surgeon.

Extension of Tumor Into Other Areas

Extension of tumor into other areas which may go unrecognized at the time of surgery has been cited (Maran, 1984; Rabinov, 1997) and suggested to be the cause of recurrence. For instance, the tumor may become wedged between the mastoid process and the body of the mandible.

Misdiagnosis

Many clinicians still believe that a small mass in the pre-auricular area is more likely to be a lymph node or a sebaceous cyst than a PA. This belief results in an incisional biopsy or a local enucleation, followed by the discovery days later that the lesion was actually a PA. The clinician often elects to follow a "watch and wait" policy, and the recurrence becomes evident years later.

Enucleation

Local excision or "enucleation" was a practice recommended in the 1970s and 1980s as primary treatment of PA in the parotid gland followed by post-operative radiotherapy (Dawson, 1989; Dawson, 1985). These procedures fell out of favor many years ago but advocates are resurgent again, suggesting that in "expert hands" using *extra-capsular dissection* benign tumors can be removed safely by techniques much less invasive than a formal parotidectomy (McGurk, 2004; McGurk, 2003). However, a recurrence rate of 2% has been associated with this procedure. Other authors continue to discourage minimal margin surgery in the parotid gland (Paris, 2003; Piekarski, 2004; Stennert, 2004; Witt, 2002).

Unfortunately, the capsule surrounding PA is at best a *pseudo-capsule* that allows for bits of satellite tumors to be left behind at enucleation surgery or allows spillage during handling or manipulation during surgery, possibilities that have been discussed by many authors (Armitstead, 1979; Clairmont, 1977; McEvedy, 1976). If the tumor has been enucleated with obvious rupture or documented spillage, then the proper course of treatment is a formal parotidectomy.

Implantation of Tumor Cells

Implantation of tumor cells may take place along the tract of a suction drain or at the point of egress from the skin in cases of tumor rupture. Recurrences tend to be found within the surgical scar or on either side of it, marking the entry and exit points of the suture needle (Maran, MacKenzie, & Stanley, 1984). Soiling and contamination of instruments and gloves from an unrecognized microrupture may also cause recurrence.

Pre-Operative Biopsy

Pre-operative biopsy or intra-operative sampling of the tumor may lead to soiling of the surrounding tissues and create a potential risk of recurrence. A survey of 34 internationally recognized head and neck oncologists concluded that the routine use of fine needle aspiration cytology (FNAC) does not alter the treatment of a discreet mass in the parotid (McGurk & Hussain, 1997).

Poorly Designed Incisions

The incision may be poorly designed, most often in parotid surgery, usually too small limiting complete exposure of the tumor mass, and as a consequence, the surgeon may cut across the posterior border or outer surface of the tumor when the flap is being raised (Touquet, McKenzie, & Carrouth, 1990).

CLINICAL COURSE

In the parotid gland, there is frequently evidence of a formal parotidectomy with a large scar or a smaller scar in the pre-auricular area suggesting local surgery, most commonly involving the lower pole of parotid.

Recurrences are best *classified* clinically as uninodular or solitary isolated lump or multinodular or with multiple nodules extending above and below the scar. Maran et al. (1984) reported 63.2% recurrences of multinodular tumors in their series of recurrent parotid tumors. A solitary palpable single nodule is almost always discovered at microscopy to be a small cluster of grapes (nodules) lacking even the most rudimentary capsule.

The time interval between the first operation and recurrence varies largely between 1 and 7 years (Maran, 1984; Fee, 1987). Assessment of recurrent disease must include CT and/or MRI and probably ultrasound. FNAC is mandatory to ensure that the tumor presenting is still a PA, as errors initially may have occurred or pathological changes may have developed in the interval between original surgery and the current presentation.

ASSESSMENT

The pathological recurrence is usually much bigger and more extensive than clinically suspected and the revision surgery is rather difficult and time consuming. The risk of trauma to the facial nerve is high and may be difficult to identify even with nerve monitoring. If traumatized, the facial nerve may never recover normal function, and even may be permanently paralyzed.

The skin may need to be replaced if recurrences invade or are adherent to the skin. Should the patient have had prior adjuvant radiotherapy or further recurrences, further surgery if offered will be more difficult than anticipated.

TREATMENT

Recurrent pleomorphic adenoma poses a significant treatment challenge, considering its propensity for further recurrence and potential for malignant transformation (Mc Loughlin, 2019; Aro, 2019).

Options of Treatment

The best policy to prevent recurrence of PA is excisional biopsy of the tumor with maximal safe margin; functional neurological preservation is the ultimate goal (Yugueros, Goellner, & Petty, 1998). Treatment of the recurrent PA is determined by the age and physical health of the patient, the number of pervious operations, and the anatomical extent of the recurrence. Pre-operative assessment must include imaging and biopsy. Available options, for recurrences confirmed as benign by FNAC, include:

- *No treatment* for the elderly and infirmed; very small tumors, isolated recurrence, or enormous tumors with complex anatomical involvement;
- *Local excision of a solitary recurrence* including the overlying scar (rarely feasible);
- *Superficial parotidectomy and facial nerve dissection* for the recently enucleated tumor of small size and limited to the superficial lobe in which there has been no attempt to locate the facial nerve (Laskawi, 1998; Leverstein, 1997);
- *Total parotidectomy with facial nerve dissection and preservation*; the overlying scar is excised in continuity (Laskawi, Schott, & Schroder, 1998);
- *Total parotidectomy with resection of the involved nerve and immediate nerve graft* with or without replacement of overlying skin;
- Any of these surgical procedures followed by radiotherapy (Dawson, 1985; Liu, 1995). However, the role of adjuvant radiotherapy in the management of recurrent PA has been reported to be widely debated Mc Loughlin, Gillanders, Smith, & Young, 2019);
- *Radiotherapy alone* after FNAC confirmation of PA may be used, after full patient and family consent.

Results of Treatment

Myssiorek et al. (1990) reported that only 67% of patients with recurrent PAs ultimately achieved tumor-free status after surgery. Although initial recurrence of PA can occur as long as 20 years following the first surgery, most subsequent recurrences are known to develop within 2–5 years (Dawson, 1985; Fee, 1987). In the parotid gland, recurrence deep to the facial nerve, which would include recurrences in the parapharyngeal space, are less likely to be controlled by further surgery than recurrences lateral to the nerve (Carew, Spiro, Singh, & Shah, 1999).

Patients with more than one recurrence were significantly younger than patients who have had only one recurrence (Laskawi, Schott, & Schroder, 1998). Once a patient has a second recurrence the tumor appears to become more aggressive. Subsequent recurrences are more likely and appear more quickly than the initial recurrence (Fee, Goffinet, & Calcaterra, 1987), and the likelihood of histological malignant degeneration is also greater (Dawson, 1985; Leonetti, 2005; Phillips, 1995).

THE FACIAL NERVE

Radical excision with sacrifice of the facial nerve has been advocated for the treatment of recurrent PA, but morbidity is naturally high. Even if the nerve is grafted a House-Brackman grade III is as good a result as one gets (Fleming, 1987; Glas, 2001; Vaughan, 1993). Several authors expressed reservations about forfeiting neural integrity in the presence of benign disease and recommended *parotidectomy with dissection and preservation of the facial nerve* (Myssiorele, 1990; Phillips, 1995).

Facial nerve injury is more likely if the tumor is deep, is in multiple sites, or if extensive scar tissue is present. It also depends on the extent of previous surgery and whether the facial nerve was paralyzed previously but recovered. Facial nerve paralysis after the first operation for recurrent PA is approximately 15%. There is a greater risk of permanent nerve damage with each ensuing operation (30% chance of *permanent* nerve injury after three operations).

The likelihood of a *temporary* facial nerve weakness for 6 months was 27% at the first operation, 14% after the second, and rose to 33% at the third attempt. The likelihood of permanent paralysis rose from 27% after the first surgery to 29% at the second surgery (Fee, Goffinet, & Calcaterra, (1987). A retrospective series of 35 patients treated surgically for first recurrence of a PA of the parotid gland were seen over a 15-year period, with a minimum follow-up of 7 years. Loco-regional control was 77%, and malignant transformation was 5.7% (Maxwell, Hall, & Freeman, 2004).

In a series of 126 patients from the Mayo Clinic, rates of tumor recurrence after one operation were 32.3%, 7.1% after two operations, and 1.6% after three. After all procedures, partial facial nerve paralysis was recorded in 13.5% of patients and total paralysis in 5.5%. In 24 patients who had had multiple operations, the rate of facial nerve paralysis was 53% (38% temporary and 15% permanent) (Phillips & Olsen, 1995). In another series of 42 patients (Leonetti, Marzo, Petruzzelli, & Herr, 2005), all patients had multinodular, non-tender recurrent nodules following one to four prior surgical procedures, and 6 patients had been treated with radiotherapy. In 30 patients the facial nerve was preserved. Ten patients had House-Brackmann Facial Nerve Grading grade I–II, 14 patients had grade III–IV, and 6 patients had grade V–VI. In the 12 patients who had the facial nerve sacrificed, the facial nerve function was grade III–IV in only 5 and grade V–VI in 7.

The use of *loupes* and operating *microscope* as well as *continuous facial nerve monitoring* have greatly helped with minimizing permanent paralysis of the facial nerve after revision surgery for recurrent PA (Dulguerov, 1999; Olsen, 1994). In such cases, facial nerve monitoring resulted in reduced facial nerve deficit and faster recovery (Makeieff, 2005; Zabren, 2005).

RISK OF MALIGNANT TRANSFORMATION

The risk of malignant transformation of recurrent PA is said to increase with time. In the literature, this incidence has varied from less than 10% to as much as 40% (Dawson & Orr, 1985). In a series, 2 out of 36 (6.9%) patients treated for multiple recurrences developed malignant disease. In another series, 2 out of 40 (5%) patients (Jackson, Roland, larke, & Jones, 1993) developed carcinoma ex-pleomorphic adenoma and died of disseminated metastases to the lung and bone (Leonetti, Marzo, Petruzzelli, & Herr, 2005). Thus, patients with recurrent PA require thorough investigation and biopsy to confirm the true nature of the persistent clinical benign disease to exclude malignant change, prior to recommencing treatment (Phillips & Olsen, 1985). It must be remembered that patients who have been treated with radiotherapy for recurrent PA also continue to have a risk of malignancy (Barton, 1992; Renehan, 1996).

Factors associated with a higher change of malignant transformation in PA of the parotid gland (Phillips & Olsen, 1985) (Figure 1: a and b) were age greater than 40 years at initial treatment, male gender, nodules greater than 2 cm in diameter, tumors of the deep lobe (Jackson, Roland, Clarke, & Jones, 1993), solitary nodules, more frequent recurrences (more than 4) (Mann, Beck, & Karatay, 1985), and having had more than one previous operation. Malignant tumors were reported in 9 (7.1%) patients.

An appraisal of adenocarcinoma ex-pleomorphic adenoma or carcinosarcoma confirms that there is a malignant change in both the epithelial and mesenchymal elements (Gnepp, 1993; Olsen, 2001).

The enigma of the metastasizing PA needs to be considered. It seems to be associated with incomplete surgery or enucleation, leading to multiple recurrences that appear to be a prerequisite for the development of distant metastasis (Hoorweg, Hilgers, Keus, Zoetmulder, & Luftus, 1998). The evidence is overwhelming that this is associated with persistent disease at

Figure 1. (a) A 65-year-old lady with a 20-year history of a 7×5 cm mass in the parotid gland with a recent history of rapid increase in size and pain. Parotidectomy revealed carcinoma ex-pleomorphic adenoma. The patient was treated with adjunctive post-operative radiotherapy, had local and regional control, but died of distant metastasis within two years. (b) CT scan of same patient with carcinoma ex-pleomorphic adenoma.

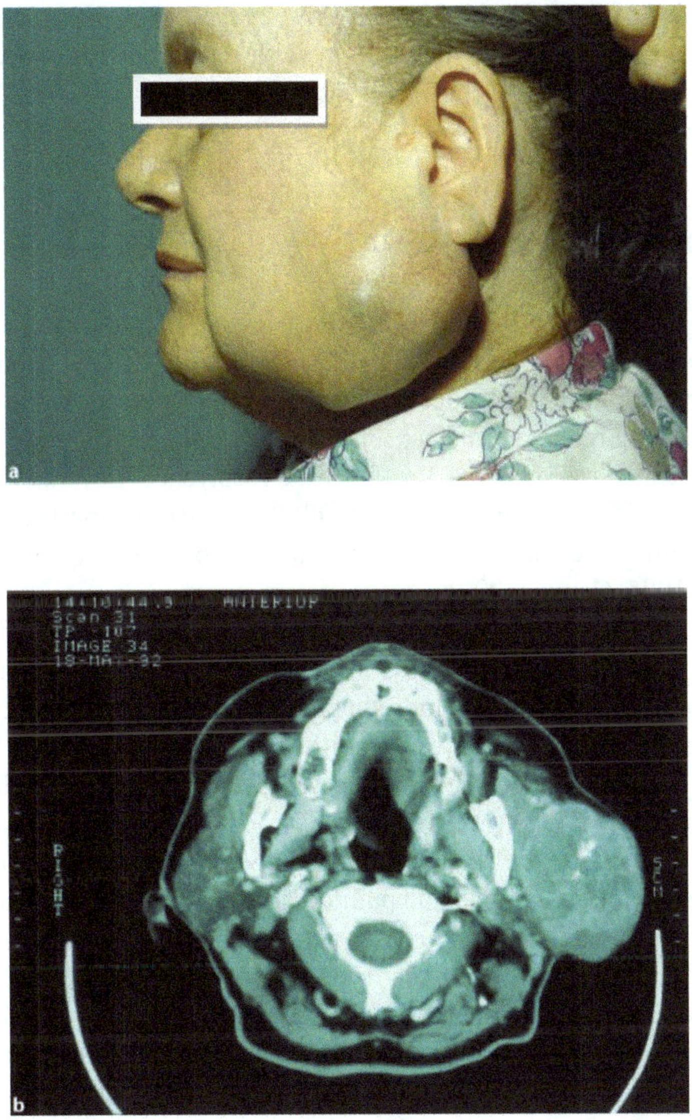

the following sites: 95% associated with the parotid gland followed by the submandibular gland (4%) and minor salivary glands (1%). This should be considered a low-grade malignancy but has lethal potential and can be associated with a fatal outcome (Bradley, 2005). In a case series, 42 patients had sufficient data to analyze. The mean presentation-to-metastasis latency was 16 years. Bone was the most common site for metastases (45%), followed by the head and neck (43%) and lungs (36%). There was significant morbidity and mortality from distant metastases with 5-year disease-specific and disease-free survival of 58% and 50%, respectively (Hodge, Morris, Werning, & Mendenhall, 2005).

THE ROLE OF RADIOTHERAPY

The role of radiotherapy remains controversial in the management of primary or recurrent PA (Natvig, 1994; Laskawi, 1998; Leverstein, 1997). Radiotherapy should be considered if there has been tumor spillage or residual tumor following reoperation (Jackson, 1993; Hodge, 2005). Some surgeons do not treat with radiotherapy for first-time recurrence (Leverstein, Tiwari, Snow, van der Wal, & van der Waal, 1997), because of its ineffectiveness in preventing further recurrences as well as concerns about subsequent morbidity (Dawson, 1985, Carew, 1999).

In a series of patients, a decision was made not to sacrifice the facial nerve in 17 of 21 patients and performed instead a subtotal excision of recurrent PA followed by post-operative radiotherapy. Sixteen of the 17 patients (94%) remained free of clinical recurrence, with an average follow-up of 5.9 years (Samson, Metson, Wang, & Mongomery, 1991). The dose of radiotherapy ranged from 50 to 67 Gy (average 50.5 Gy).

It is to be recommended that certain patients who have undergone surgery and who had ominous clinical and pathological presentations should receive post-operative radiotherapy (Carew, Spiro, Singh, & Shah, 1999).

In a large series of 187 patients from the Christie Hospital, Manchester, UK (Barton, Slevin, & Gleaves, 1992), all had PAs of the parotid gland treated by surgery and post-operative radiotherapy by one of two techniques. Until 1976, *needle implant* was used, to a dose of 60 Gy, and after that time, external beam radiotherapy (*EBRT*) using megavoltage linear accelerators using an inclined plane to avoid the eyes was used. The tumor dose was 50 Gy in 15-16 fractions. This treatment followed surgery for incomplete excision or tumor spillage. The median age was 46 year and the median follow-up for all patients was 14 years. A total of 115 patients had radiotherapy after their first operation, with a recurrence rate of 0.9% (1/115); of the 115 cases there were two cases of radionecrosis, facial palsy, Frey's syndrome, and salivary fistula (one patient each). 72 patients had radiotherapy delayed until one or more recurrences had been surgically treated. Nine of these patients (12.5%) developed yet another recurrence after radiotherapy. There were two cases of radionecrosis, four cases of facial palsy, 16 cases of Frey's syndrome, and one case of malignant change.

Recurrence after radiotherapy continued after 20 years of follow-up. It is recommended that patients having unsatisfactory surgery due to spillage at surgery or residual tumor left behind should have radiotherapy immediately, rather than delaying treatment until local recurrence occurs, because of the increased morbidity and the higher complication incidence of yet further recurrences. A similar treatment plan has been recommended at Princess Margaret Hospital, Toronto, Canada, with treatment to 45 Gy in 20 fractions over 4 weeks, using an ipsilateral technique encompassing the parotid bed. Using this approach, the authors report the long-term control of tumor to be in excess of 90% (Liu et al, 1995).

The use of *neutron radiotherapy* has been recommended for the management of recurrent PA of the parotid gland (Buchholz, 1992; Douglas, 2001). The indications included gross residual disease and multirecurrent multinodular disease. The actuarial 15-year loco-regional control was 76% for patients with gross residual disease versus 100% for those with microscopic disease (Douglas, Einck, & Austin-Seymour, 2001). The use of neutron therapy may be considered an alternative to further surgery when patients present with more than two recurrences, with a functioning facial nerve, and with a tumor less than 5 cm as there is less likely resultant damage to the facial nerve.

The *long-termrisks* of radiotherapy and neutron therapy in the head and neck include osteosarcoma of the mandible, malignant fibrous histiocytoma, synovial fistula of the temporo-mandibular joint, and osteo-necrosis of the temporal bone (Patel, 1999; van der Laan, 1995).

CONCLUSION

- A recurrence rate in surgery for PA of less than 1% is considered acceptable;

- Recurrences may present 15-20 years after initial surgery. Recurrent PA is encountered much less frequently nowadays because of correct primary surgical procedure is being performed initially;
- Recurrences are most commonly due to poor surgical technique rather than tumor biology;
- The original histopathology should be reviewed and FNAC performed before starting further treatment;
- Management of recurrent PA is currently further surgery, aiming at complete local excision with preservation of neurological structures, with consideration to adding adjunctive radiotherapy post-operatively;
- There remains a risk of further recurrence even after apparent successful revision surgery;
- Frequent or persistent PA recurrences may proceed to the metastasizing PA with a potential fatal outcome;
- Radiotherapy should currently be reserved for patients who refuse surgery, if facial nerve is likely to be excised and resultant paralysis is unacceptable in an adjunctive setting following resection of a carcinoma ex-PA;
- Persistent risk of malignant degeneration remains in patients who have PA. Repeated recurrences, whether the patient has had adjunctive radiotherapy or not, carry a life-long risk of malignant degeneration which may result in a fatal outcome.

REFERENCES

Armitstead, P. R., Smiddy, F. G., & Frank, H. G. (1979). Simple enucleation and radiotherapy in the treatment of pleomorphic adenoma of the parotid gland. *British Journal of Surgery*, *66*(10), 716–717. doi:10.1002/bjs.1800661012 PMID:228786

Aro, K., Valle, J., Tarkkanen, J., Mäkitie, A., & Atula, T. (2019). Repeatedly recurring pleomorphic adenoma: A therapeutic challenge. *L'Oto-Rino-Laringologia Italiana*, *39*(3), 156–161. doi:10.14639/0392-100X-2307 PMID:31131834

Barton, J., Slevin, N. J., & Gleaves, E. N. (1992). Radiotherapy for pleomorphic adenoma of the parotid gland. *International Journal of Radiation Oncology, Biology, Physics*, *22*(5), 925–928. doi:10.1016/0360-3016(92)90789-K PMID:1313407

Bradley, P. J. (2005). Metastasizing pleomorphic salivary adenoma should now be considered a low-grade malignancy with a lethal potential. *Current Opinion in Otolaryngology & Head & Neck Surgery*, *13*(2), 123–126. doi:10.1097/01.moo.0000153450.87288.2a PMID:15761289

Buchholz, T. A., Laramore, G. E., & Griffin, T. W. (1992). Fast neutron radiation for recurrent pleomorphic adenoma of the parotid gland. *American Journal of Clinical Oncology*, *15*(5), 441–445. doi:10.1097/00000421-199210000-00009 PMID:1326226

Buchman, G., Stringer, S. P., Mendenhall, W. M., Parsons, J. T., Jordan, J. R., & Cassisi, N. J. (1994). Pleomorphic adenoma: Effect of tumor spill and inadequate resection on tumor recurrence. *The Laryngoscope*, *104*(10), 1231–1234. doi:10.1288/00005537-199410000-00008 PMID:7934593

Carew, J. F., Spiro, R. H., Singh, B., & Shah, J. P. (1999). Treatment of recurrent pleomorphic adenoma of the parotid gland. *Otolaryngology - Head and Neck Surgery*, *121*(5), 539–542. doi:10.1016/S0194-5998(99)70053-7 PMID:10547466

Chen, R. L., Wang, C. M., & Wen, Y. M. (2004). Study of the relative factors of the biological behavior of pleomorphic adenoma of parotid. *Zhonghua Kou Qiang Yi Xue Za Zhi*, *39*, 277–279. PMID:15454008

Clairmont, A. A., Richardson, G. S., & Hanna, D. C. (1977). The pseudocapsule of pleomorphic adenoma (benign mixed tumors). *American Journal of Surgery*, *134*(2), 242–243. doi:10.1016/0002-9610(77)90354-3 PMID:196513

Dawson, A. K. (1989). Radiation therapy in recurrent pleomorphic adenoma of the parotid gland. *International Journal of Radiation Oncology, Biology, Physics*, *16*(3), 819–821. doi:10.1016/0360-3016(89)90501-4 PMID:2537808

Dawson, A. K., & Orr, L. A. (1985). Long-term results of local excision and radiotherapy in pleomorphic adenoma of the parotid gland. *International Journal of Radiation Oncology, Biology, Physics*, *11*(3), 451–455. doi:10.1016/0360-3016(85)90174-9 PMID:2982770

Douglas, J. G., Einck, J., Austin-Seymour, M., Koh, W.-J., & Laramore, G. E. (2001). Neutron radiotherapy for recurrent pleomorphic adenomas of major salivary glands. *Head & Neck, 23*(12), 1037–1042. doi:10.1002/hed.10027 PMID:11774388

Dulguerov, P., Marchal, F., & Lehmann, W. (1999). Post parotidectomy facial nerve paralysis: Possible aetiological factors and results with routine facial nerve monitoring. *The Laryngoscope, 109*(5), 754–762. doi:10.1097/00005537-199905000-00014 PMID:10334226

Fee, W. E. Jr, Goffinet, D. R., & Calcaterra, T. C. (1987). Recurrent mixed tumors of the parotid gland: Results of surgical therapy. *The Laryngoscope, 88*(2), 265–273. doi:10.1288/00005537-197802000-00008 PMID:202823

Fleming, W. B. (1987). Recurrent pleomorphic adenoma of the parotid gland. *The Australian and New Zealand Journal of Surgery, 57*(3), 173–176. doi:10.1111/j.1445-2197.1987.tb01329.x PMID:3039958

Glas, A. S., Vermey, A., Hollema, H., Robinson, P. H., Roodenburg, J. L., Nap, R. E., & Plukker, J. T. (2001). Surgical treatment of recurrent pleomorphic adenoma of the parotid gland: A clinical analysis of 52 patients. *Head & Neck, 23*(4), 311–316. doi:10.1002/hed.1036 PMID:11400233

Gnepp, D. R. (1993). Malignant mixed tumors of the salivary glands: A review. *Pathology Annual, 28*, 279–328. PMID:8380049

Hendrikisson, H. H., Westrin, K. M., Carlsoo, B., & Silfverswärd, C. (1998). Recurrent primary pleomorphic adenomas of salivary origin. *Cancer, 82*, 617–620. doi:10.1002/(SICI)1097-0142(19980215)82:4<617::AID-CNCR1>3.0.CO;2-I PMID:9477091

Hodge, C. W., Morris, C. G., Werning, J. W., & Mendenhall, W. M. (2005). Role of radiotherapy for pleomorphic adenoma. *American Journal of Clinical Oncology, 28*(2), 148–151. doi:10.1097/01.coc.0000144266.48387.02 PMID:15803008

Hoorweg, J. J., Hilgers, F. J. M., Keus, R. B., Zoetmulder, F. A. N., & Luftus, B. M. (1998). Metastasizing pleomorphic adenoma: A report of three cases. *European Journal of Surgical Oncology, 24*(5), 452–455. doi:10.1016/S0748-7983(98)92651-8 PMID:9800983

Jackson, S. R., Roland, N. J., Clarke, R. W., & Jones, A. S. (1993). Recurrent pleomorphic adenoma. *The Journal of Laryngology and Otology*, *103*(6), 546–549. doi:10.1017/S0022215100123667 PMID:8393908

Laskawi, R., Schott, T., & Schroder, M. (1998). Recurrent pleomorphic adenoma of the parotid gland: Clinician evaluation and long-term follow up. *British Journal of Oral & Maxillofacial Surgery*, *36*(1), 48–51. doi:10.1016/S0266-4356(98)90748-3 PMID:9578257

Lawson, H. H. (1989). Capsular penetration and perforation in pleomorphic adenoma of the parotid salivary gland. *British Journal of Surgery*, *76*(6), 594–596. doi:10.1002/bjs.1800760622 PMID:2547497

Leonetti, J. P., Marzo, S. J., Petruzzelli, G. J., & Herr, B. (2005). Recurrent pleomorphic adenoma of the parotid gland. *Otolaryngology - Head and Neck Surgery*, *133*(3), 319–322. doi:10.1016/j.otohns.2005.04.008 PMID:16143173

Leverstein, H., Tiwari, R. M., Snow, G. B., van der Wal, J., & van der Waal, I. (1997). The surgical management of recurrent or residual pleomorphic adenoma of the parotid gland: Analysis and results of 40 patients. *European Archives of Oto-Rhino-Laryngology*, *254*(7), 313–317. doi:10.1007/BF02630721 PMID:9298665

Liu, F.-F., Rotstein, L., Davison, A. J., Pintilie, M., O'Sullivan, B., Payne, D. G., ... Cummings, B. (1995). Benign parotid adenomas: A review of the Princess Margaret Hospital Experience. *Head & Neck*, *17*(3), 177–183. doi:10.1002/hed.2880170302 PMID:7782201

Makeieff, M., Venail, F., Cartier, C., Garrel, R., Crampette, L., & Guerrier, B. (2005). Continuous facial nerve monitoring during pleomorphic adenoma recurrence surgery. *The Laryngoscope*, *115*(7), 1310–1314. doi:10.1097/01.MLG.0000166697.48868.8C PMID:15995527

Mann, W., Beck, C., & Karatay, M. C. (1985). Recurrent benign tumors of the parotid gland and their tendency for becoming malignant. *Laryngology, Rhinology and Otology (Stuttg)*, *64*, 133–135. doi:10.1055-2007-1008101 PMID:2985894

Maran, A. G. D., MacKenzie, I. J., & Stanley, R. E. (1984). Recurrent pleomorphic adenoma of the parotid gland. *Archives of Otolaryngology*, *110*(3), 167–171. doi:10.1001/archotol.1984.00800290031007 PMID:6322731

Maxwell, E. L., Hall, F. T., & Freeman, J. L. (2004). Recurrent pleomorphic adenoma of the parotid gland. *The Journal of Otolaryngology*, *33*(03), 181–184. doi:10.2310/7070.2004.03022 PMID:15841997

Mc Loughlin, L., Gillanders, S. L., Smith, S., & Young, O. (2019). The role of adjuvant radiotherapy in management of recurrent pleomorphic adenoma of the parotid gland: A systematic review. *European Archives of Oto-Rhino-Laryngology*, *276*(2), 283–295. doi:10.100700405-018-5205-z PMID:30426229

McEvedy, B. V., & Ross, W. M. (1976). The treatment of mixed parotid tumors by enucleation and radiotherapy. *British Journal of Surgery*, *63*(5), 341–342. doi:10.1002/bjs.1800630503 PMID:178397

McGregor, A. D., Burgoyne, M., & Tan, K. C. (1988). Recurrent pleomorphic adenoma salivary adenoma: The relevance of age at first presentation. *British Journal of Plastic Surgery*, *41*(2), 177–181. doi:10.1016/0007-1226(88)90048-3 PMID:2832025

McGurk, M. (2004). Benign parotid tumors. *British Medical Journal*, *329*(7478), 1299–1300. doi:10.1136/bmj.329.7478.1299 PMID:15576716

McGurk, M., & Hussain, K. (1997). Role of fine needle aspiration cytology in the management of the discrete parotid lump. *Annals of the Royal College of Surgeons of England*, *79*, 198–202. PMID:9196341

McGurk, M., Thomas, B. L., & Renehan, A. G. (2003). Extracapsular dissection for clinically benign parotid lumps: Reduced morbidity without oncological compromise. *British Journal of Cancer*, *89*(9), 1610–1613. doi:10.1038j.bjc.6601281 PMID:14583757

Myssiorek, D., Ruah, G. B., & Hybels, R. L. (1990). Recurrent pleomorphic adenomas of the parotid gland. *Head & Neck*, *12*(4), 332–336. doi:10.1002/hed.2880120410 PMID:2361864

Natvig, K., & Soberg, R. (1994). Relationship of intraoperative rupture of pleomorphic adenoma to recurrence: 11-25 year follow up study. *Head & Neck*, *16*(3), 213–217. doi:10.1002/hed.2880160302 PMID:8026950

Nouraei, S. A. R., Fergusin, M. S., Clarke, P. M., Sandison, A., Sandhu, G. S., Michaels, L., & Rhys-Evans, P. (2006). Metastasizing pleomorphic salivary adenoma. *Archives of Otolaryngology--Head & Neck Surgery*, *132*(7), 788–793. doi:10.1001/archotol.132.7.788 PMID:16847191

Olsen, K. D., & Daube, J. R. (1994). Intra-operative monitoring of the facial nerve: An aid in the management of parotid gland pleomorphic adenomas. *The Laryngoscope*, *104*, 232–239.

Olsen, K. D., & Lewis, J. E. (2001). Carcinoma ex-pleomorphic adenoma: A clinicopathologic review. *Head & Neck*, *23*(9), 705–712. doi:10.1002/hed.1100 PMID:11505478

Paris, J., Facon, F., & Chrestian, M. A. (2003). Recurrences of pleomorphic adenomas of the parotid: Changing attitudes. *Revue de Laryngologie - Otologie - Rhinologie*, *124*, 229–234. PMID:15038565

Patel, S. G., See, A. C. H., Williamson, P. A., Archer, D. J., & Rhys Evans, P. H. (1999). Radiation induced sarcoma of the head and neck. *Head & Neck*, *21*(4), 346–349. doi:10.1002/(SICI)1097-0347(199907)21:4<346::AID-HED9>3.0.CO;2-B PMID:10376755

Phillips, P. P., & Olsen, K. D. (1995). Recurrent pleomorphic adenoma of the parotid gland: Report of 126 cases and a review of the literature. *The Annals of Otology, Rhinology, and Laryngology*, *104*(2), 100–104. doi:10.1177/000348949510400203 PMID:7857010

Piekarski, J., Nejc, D., Szymczak, W., Wroński, K., & Jeziorski, A. (2004). Results of Extracapsular dissection of pleomorphic adenoma of parotid gland. *Journal of Oral and Maxillofacial Surgery*, *62*(10), 1198–1202. doi:10.1016/j.joms.2004.01.025 PMID:15452805

Rabinov, C. R., Canalis, R. F., Alavi, S., & Lee, E. J. (1997). Recurrent pleomorphic adenoma of the parotid gland involving the osseous external auditory canal. *The Annals of Otology, Rhinology, and Laryngology*, *106*(7), 589–593. doi:10.1177/000348949710600711 PMID:9228861

Renehan, A., Gleaves, E. N., & McGurk, M. (1996). An analysis of the treatment of 114 patients with recurrent pleomorphic adenoma of the parotid gland. *American Journal of Surgery*, *172*(6), 710–714. doi:10.1016/S0002-9610(96)00293-0 PMID:8988685

Samson, M. J., Metson, R., Wang, C. C., & Mongomery, W. W. (1991). Preservation of the facial nerve in the management of recurrent pleomorphic adenomas of the parotid gland. *The Laryngoscope*, *101*(10), 1060–1062. doi:10.1288/00005537-199110000-00006 PMID:1656154

Stennert, E., Guntinas-Lichius, O., Klaussmann, J. P., & Arnold, G. (2001). Histopathology of pleomorphic adenoma in the parotid gland: A prospective unselected series of 100 cases. *The Laryngoscope*, *111*(12), 2195–2200. doi:10.1097/00005537-200112000-00024 PMID:11802025

Stennert, E., Wittekindt, C., Klaussmann, J. P., Arnold, G., & Gunitas-Lichius, O. (2004). Recurrent pleomorphic adenoma of the parotid gland: A prospective histological and immunohistochemical study. *The Laryngoscope*, *114*(1), 158–163. doi:10.1097/00005537-200401000-00030 PMID:14710014

Touquet, R., McKenzie, I. J., & Carrouth, J. A. S. (1990). Management of the parotid pleomorphic adenoma: the problem of exposing tumor tissue at operation: the logical pursuit of treatment policies. *British Journal of Oral & Maxillofacial Surgery*, *28*(6), 404–408. doi:10.1016/0266-4356(90)90040-R PMID:2177656

van der Laan, B. F. A. M., Baris, G., & Gregor, R. T. (1995). Radiation induced tumors of the head and neck. *The Journal of Laryngology and Otology*, *109*, 346–349.

Vaughan, E. D., & Richardson, D. (1993). Facial nerve reconstruction following ablative parotid surgery. *British Journal of Oral & Maxillofacial Surgery*, *31*(5), 274–280. doi:10.1016/0266-4356(93)90060-A PMID:8218080

Webb, A. J., & Eveson, J. W. (2001). Pleomorphic adenomas of the major salivary glands: A study of the capsule form in relation to surgical management. *Clinical Otolaryngology*, *26*(2), 134–142. doi:10.1046/j.1365-2273.2001.00440.x PMID:11309055

Witt, R. L. (2002). The significance of the margin in parotid surgery for pleomorphic adenoma. *The Laryngoscope*, *112*(12), 2141–2154. doi:10.1097/00005537-200212000-00004 PMID:12461331

Yugueros, P., Goellner, J. R., Petty, P. M., & Woods, J. E. (1998). Treating recurrence of parotid pleomorphic adenoma. *Annals of Plastic Surgery*, *40*(6), 573–576. doi:10.1097/00000637-199806000-00001 PMID:9641273

Zabren, P., Tschumi, I., & Nuyens, M. (2005). Recurrent pleomorphic adenoma of the parotid gland. *American Journal of Surgery*, *189*(2), 203–207. doi:10.1016/j.amjsurg.2004.11.008 PMID:15720991

Chapter 13
Malignant Epithelial Tumors of the Parotid Gland

ABSTRACT

Cancer of the parotid gland represents about 20% of all parotid tumors. It either occurs "de-novo" or "on top of pleomorphic adenoma." There is no sex predilection, and the age of developing this cancer is usually above 50 years. Malignant tumors are as varied as their benign counterparts. Certain tumors are "low-grade" (polymorphous low-grade adenocarcinoma, acinic cell carcinoma, epithelial-myoepithelial carcinoma), while others are "high-grade" (salivary duct carcinoma, large cell carcinoma, and small cell carcinoma). The first echelon lymph node (LN) of metastases is the intra- and peri-glandular nodes. The next echelon is level II LNs. Hematogenous spread occurs very late and is mainly to the lungs and bones. However, adenoid cystic carcinoma tends to grow through peri-neural lymphatics with increased risk of nerve involvement, intra-cranial extension, and increased rate of recurrence. In this chapter, characteristic features and management of the individual types of malignant parotid tumors will be discussed.

MALIGNANT TRANSFORMATION OF BENIGN TUMORS

Signs of *malignant transformation* in a pre-existing benign tumor of the parotid gland include rapid rate of growth, harder consistency, or fixation to the underlying muscles or the overlying skin, which may be severe enough to

DOI: 10.4018/978-1-7998-5603-0.ch013

show fungation. The tumor may also show erythema and increased vascularity giving the appearance of a parotid abscess.

The patient may develop pain and tenderness which are usually due infiltration of the auriculo-temporal nerve with the pain being referred to the ipsilateral ear. Trismus due to invasion of the masseter or pterygoid muscles, or due to restricted movements of the temporo-mandibular joint (TMJ) is another finding.

In approximately 10% to 15% of the cases, the facial nerve will be paralyzed. Unequal pulsations of superficial temporal artery may as well be noticed. Manifestations of metastases to regional lymph nodes or distant organs such as the lungs or the liver may ensue. On the first suspicion of any change in the behavior of the pre-existing tumor, FNAC should be done immediately after MRI preferably with a diffusion-weighted and perfusion sequences.

CHARACTERISTIC FEATURES OF MALIGNANT EPITHELIAL TUMORS

Mucoepidermoid Carcinoma (MEC)

This is the *commonest* malignancy of the salivary glands (Foote, 1953; Shafique, 2020) and that of the parotid gland (80% of cases) seems to be less aggressive than that of the submandibular gland (8-13% of cases) and of better prognosis (Waldron & Koh, 1990). It mostly occurs around an age of 50 years, but still, it is the commonest salivary malignancy of the pediatric age group (Waldron, 1990; Browand, 1975). In some series, MEC is more common in women by a ratio of 3:2 while in others there is no sex predominance.

Low-grade and high-grade variants are recognized, where the low-grade one very rarely metastasizes (Boahene, 2004; Gustafsson, 1987). It usually presents as a slowly growing painless mass; however, rapid growth, pain and tenderness may be seen with the high-grade variant (Ogawa, 1992; Terada, 2004) (Figure 2). Metastases occur to LNs, lungs and bones (Waldron, 1990; Browand, 1975). Shafigue et al. (2020) studied the clinicopathological features of MEC using a 3-tier grading system (low, intermediate and high) in 69 patients. They reported that aggressive clinical behavior was seen in the high-grade MEC compared to the intermediate- and low-grade MEC.

Treatment is mucoepidermoid carcinoma (MEC) is surgical resection with neck dissection being reserved for high-grade variants (Boahene et al, 2004).

Figure 1. Malignant tumors of the parotid gland present with a hard, rapidly growing mass (A), that may become fixed to the overlying skin (B), which may be severe enough to show fungation (C). There may be erythema and increased vascularity miming an abscess (D).

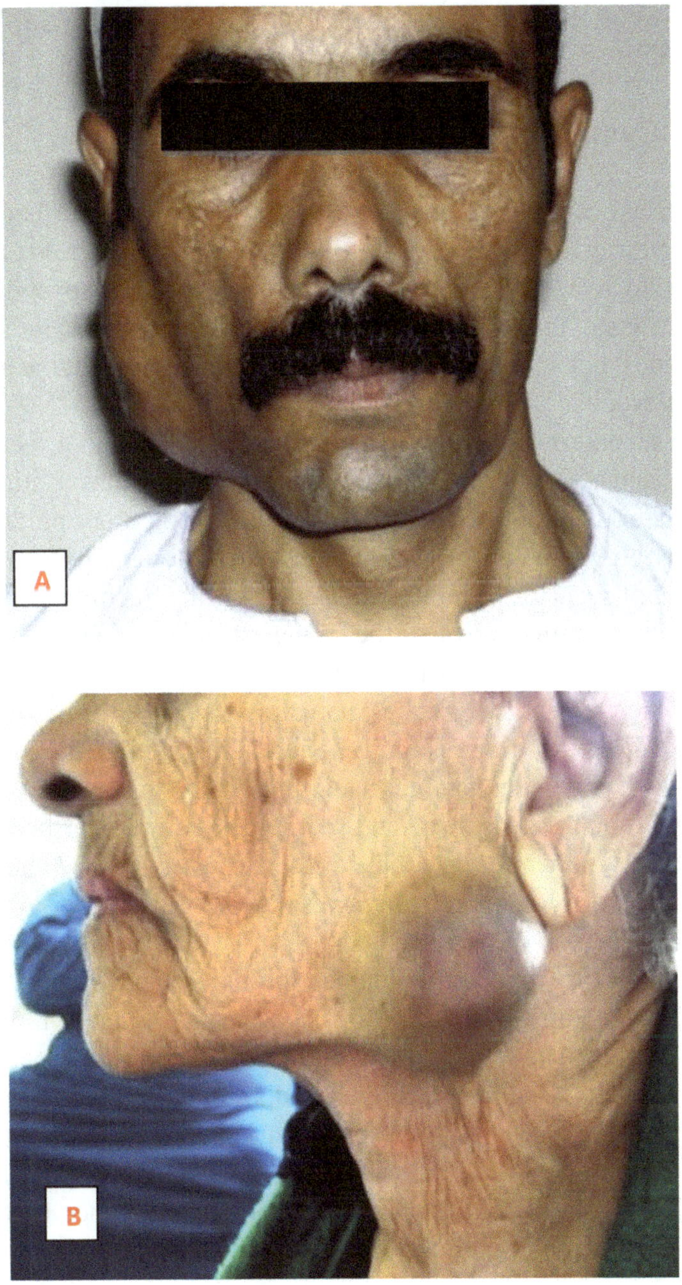

Prognosis is influenced by the grade and stage of the tumor, and patient's age (above 45 years is associated with poor prognosis) and gender. Histological grade is considered one of the most important factors in prognosis. The overall 5-year survival rates range from 92% to 100% for low-grade tumors, and 0% to 43% for high-grade tumors (Smith, Winkler, Perzin, Wazen, & Blitzer, 1985).

Adenoid Cystic Carcinoma (ACC)

This tumor has been given many names since it was first described by *Robin and colleagues* in 1853. From these names, "*cylindroma*" was particularly discouraged to avoid confusion with the benign cutaneous appendage tumor carrying the same name. This tumor arises not only from major and minor salivary glands, but also from sero-mucous glands throughout the body (Lee, 1985; Bradley, 2004).

It is the second most common salivary malignancy and affects patients between 40 and 60 years of age. Although some series have a slight female predominance others show either no sex predilection or a male predominance. It is a slowly growing tumor frequently presenting as a painless mass giving a false sense of security. Lymph node metastases are uncommon but distant metastases occur in up to 60% of the cases, mainly to the liver, lung, bones and brain (Bradley, 2004; Gurrney, 2005). It has a high affinity to *peri-neural invasion*, which results in parasthesia or paralysis of the nerve affected.

Histologically, low-grade (Figure 3) and high-grade (Figure 4) variants are recognized. ACC demonstrates a mixture of three major growth patterns consisting of tubular, cribriform, and solid types. Of these, cribriform is the most common type while the solid type carries an increased risk of nodal metastasis and with it a poorer prognosis (van Weert, van der Waal, Witte, Leemans, & Bloemena, 2015).

Best results of *treatment* are obtained through radical surgery and post-operative radiotherapy. The tumor is radiosensitive but not radiocurable. Although controversial, neck dissection may be reserved for patients with clinically positive LNs (Gurney, 2005; Rapidis, 2005; Gerughty, 1969). Some studies showed that age over 45 years, advanced clinical stage, parasthesia, as well as increased expression of p53 are associated with poor *prognosis* (Bradley, 2004; Gurney, 2005). The prognostic significance of perineural invasion and DNA ploidy remain controversial.

Figure 2. A rapidly growing (high-grade) muco-epidermoid carcinoma (MEC) in a 51-year-old gentle-man (A) that became fixed to the overlying skin (B) within two weeks

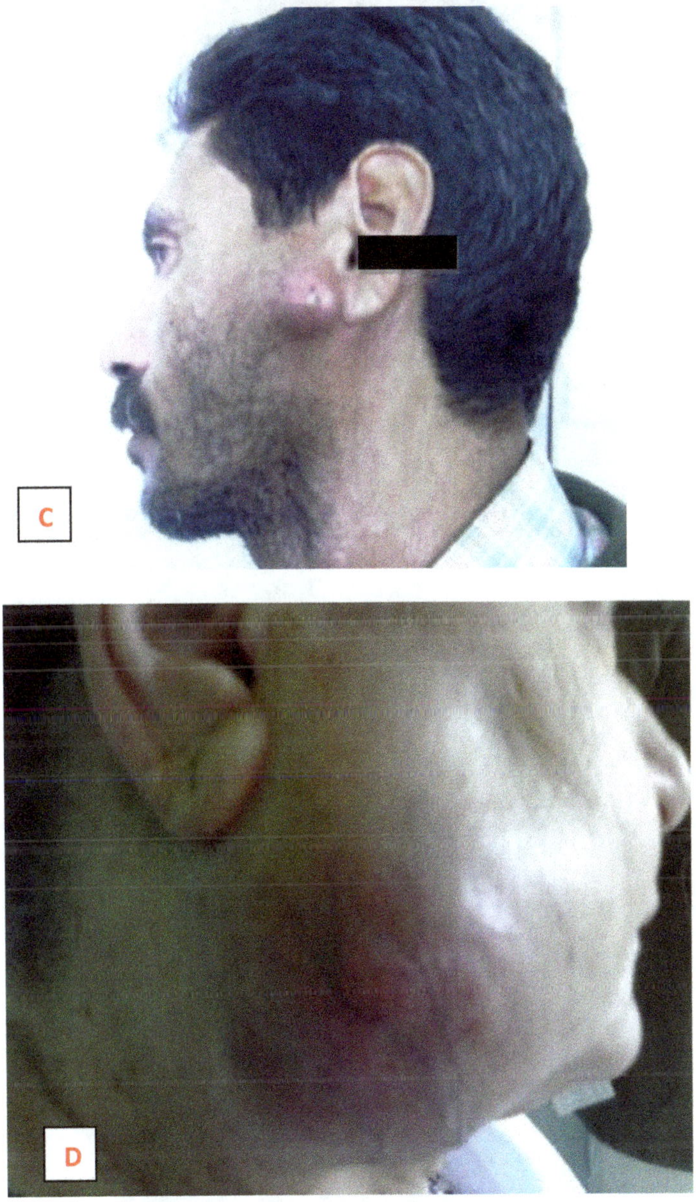

Figure 3. Low-grade adenoid cystic carcinoma (ACC) with a notable cribriform pattern (H&E, X100)

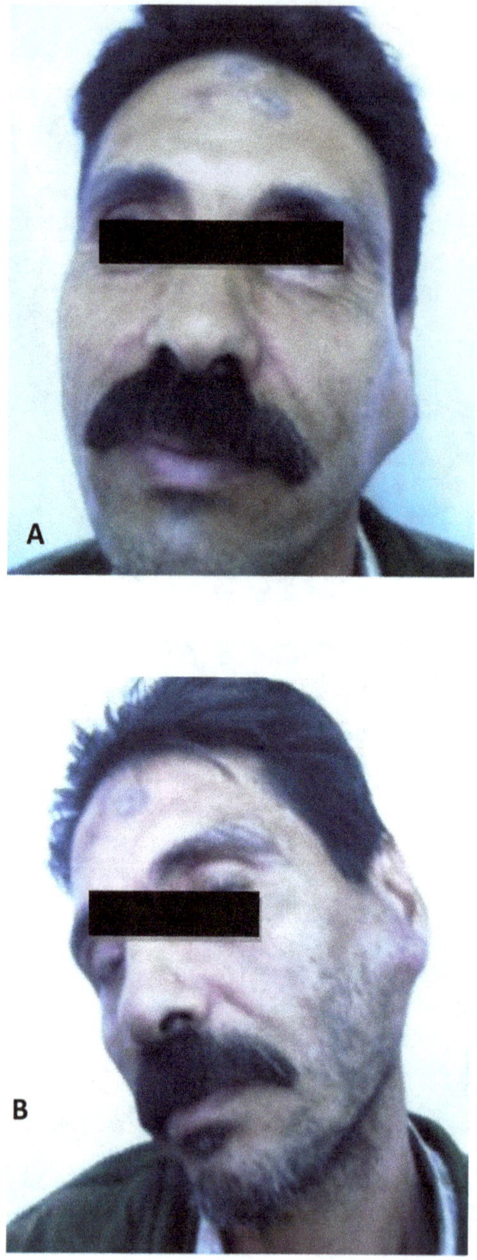

Figure 4. High-grade adenoid cystic carcinoma (ACC) with a pre-dominant (>70%) solid pattern. The lower right corner still depicts tubular structures (H&E, x100).

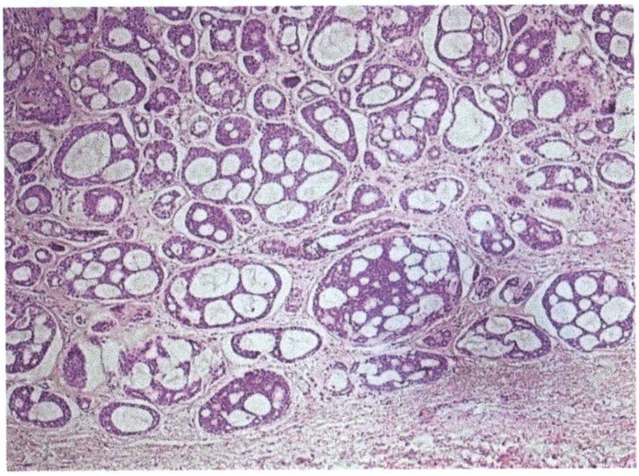

Carcinoma Ex-Pleomorphic Adenoma (CEPA)

This is by definition the malignant transformation of a long-standing PA, which occurs in about 25% of such cases (Gerughty, 1969, 1969; LiVolsi, 1977; Milford, 1989). Although rare, it has been reported to occur in 0.15% of lesions (Valstar et al, 2017). *Clinical features* predictive of *malignant transformation* are age, tumor size, long history, and submandibular location. On *imaging*, new infiltrative margins and rapid enlargement of a preexisting well-circumscribed salivary gland mass are features, highly suggestive of transformation. *Histologically*, the presence of hyalinized stroma is the most predictive parameter for malignant transformation (Zarbo, 2002). The carcinoma is usually a high-grade adenocarcinoma or an undifferentiated carcinoma although numerous other types including SCC, MEC, ACC, myoepithelial carcinoma, clear cell carcinoma, papillary carcinoma, and terminal duct carcinoma have been reported.

Carcinoma Ex-pleomorphic adenoma (CEPA) occurs in the major salivary glands in 80% of the cases, from which again 80% occurs in the parotid gland. The average age at diagnosis is 50–60 years, which is approximately 10 years older than most individuals with PA. It is extremely uncommon in individuals below the age of 20 years (Gerughty, 1969; Gnepp, 1993). Female to male ratio is 1.2 to 3:1. In 12–55% of cases, rapid enlargement will be painful and often associated with facial nerve palsy and fixation to the surrounding soft tissues (Enerotn, 1074).

CEPA metastasizes in up to 70% of the cases to distant sites rather than regionally, with special affinity to the lungs and vertebral column. *Treatment* is surgical resection usually with neck dissection. In- situ variant is that tumor which did not invade the capsule of a PA and thence was diagnosed post-operatively. In this case, the performed standard resection of a PA is curative.

True Malignant Mixed Tumor (TMMT)

True malignant mixed tumor is a very rare neoplasm that may be regarded as *carcino-sarcoma* since both epithelial and stromal components are histologically malignant, and both can metastasize. Such metastases are more commonly via a hematogenous rather than lymphatic route, with the lungs and bones being the most frequent sites (Barnes, 1985; Lwon, 2001). There is a wide range of age affection (14-87 years) and there is no sex predilection (Kwon, 2001; Fowler, 2006). Clinical presentation is similar to that of CEPA. Treatment is surgical resection, combined with radiation and chemotherapy. Even with such radical treatment most patients die within five years (Gnepp, 1993).

Acinic Cell Carcinoma

It is a rare tumor, which is indistinguishable clinically from benign parotid neoplasms being of low-grade malignancy (Lewis, 1991; Mehta, 2004). Yet, it can rarely de-differentiate into an aggressive high-grade tumor. The parotid gland is the most common site (80%) followed by the minor salivary glands (16%) and the submandibular gland (4%). It is second to Warthin's tumor in bilateral incidence (Miki et al, 1999), and second to MEC in pediatric age group involvement (Ellis & Simpson, 2005). Patients typically present with a slowly enlarging painless mass that is not fixed to the surrounding soft tissue or skin. Pain occurs in approximately 22% of patients and facial nerve palsy in nearly 3-8% (Lewis, 1991; Hanson, 1975).

On imaging, acinic cell carcinoma typically presents as a well-circumscribed, homogeneously enhancing, slow-growing mass, similar to other benign or low-grade malignant tumors. Therefore, imaging is rather non-specific and tissue sampling is often necessary to establish diagnosis. As with other malignancies, acinic cell carcinoma may sometimes have a more aggressive appearance, mimicking MEC or ACC. In these cases, careful evaluation for spread of disease is essential (Al-Zaher, Obeid, Al-Salam, & Al-Kayyali, 2009).

Treatment is complete surgical resection. Neck dissection is usually not recommended because of the relatively low incidence of metastases to regional LNs (Lewis, Olsen, & Weiland, 1991). It is usually radio-resistant; however, radiotherapy is resorted to when complete resection is not achieved, in case of peri-neural invasion, and if LNs are affected (Chong1974; Neto, 2005). The recurrence rate averages 10–35% and the distant metastatic rate 13–16% (Lewis, 1991' Miki, 1999). The 5-year survival rate ranges from 78 to 90% (El-Naggar, 1990; Skalova, 1994).

Basal Cell Adenocarcinoma

Basal cell adenocarcinoma is the malignant counterpart of basal cell adenoma (BCA). It is an uncommon low-grade malignancy that accounts for about 1.5% of all salivary gland tumors and 3% of all salivary gland malignancies (Muller & Barnes, 1996). There is no sex predilection (Gross, Maly, Goldfarb, & Eliashar, 2004), and most patients are in their 6th or 7th decade, though cases have been reported in patients as young as 2 months and as old as 92 years (Muller, 1996; Gross, 2004; Jayakrishnan, 2003; Nagao, 1998; Warrick, 2000; deSousa, 2000). The majority of these tumors arises de-novo. Origin in a pre-existing BCA is uncommon and usually involves the membranous subtype (Gross, 2004; Jayakrishnan, 2003; deSousa, 2000). Nearly 90% of tumors arise in the major salivary glands, mostly parotid (Ellis & Wiscovitch, 1990). Patients present with a slowly growing asymptomatic mass; pain and tenderness are uncommon (Seifert, 1996). In 10-15% of cases, it occurs in conjunction with dermal cylindromas and tricho-epitheliomas as compared to 40% of BCA (Chhieng & Paulino, 2002). Treatment is complete surgical excision, with neck dissection being reserved for patients with clinically positive lymph nodes (Savera, 2000; Said, 2005; Foss, 1996).

Myoepithelial Carcinoma

Myoepithelial carcinoma (Malignant Myo-epithelioma) is the malignant counterpart of myoepithelioma. By definition it is composed of myoepithelial cells with an infiltrative growth pattern. It is a rare tumor accounting for only 0.2% of all epithelial salivary gland tumors (Savera, Sloman, Huvos, & Klimstra, 2000), and involving the parotid glands in 75% of cases (Savera,

2000; Said, 2005; Foss, 1996). Approximately 50% of cases arise in a pre-existing BT, usually a PA or a myoepithelioma. Myoepithelial carcinoma is most common in the sixth and seventh decades and occurs with no sex predilection (Savera, Sloman, Huvos, & Klimstra, 2000). A painless mass is usually the only clinical complaint. *Treatment* is complete surgical excision. The clinical behavior of this tumor is unpredictable and unrelated to histological features (Foss, Ellis, & Auclair, 1996).

Cystadenocarcinoma

Cystadenocarcinomas of the salivary glands are low-grade cystic neoplasms, which are twice as common in the major salivary glands as in the minor salivary glands, and most frequently occur in the parotid (Kleinsasser, Klein, & Hubner, 1968). The majority of patients (75%) are over the age of 50 years (Kleinsasser, Klein, & Hubner, 1968). Recognizing these tumors as carcinomas is predicated by finding areas of infiltrative growth. Peri-neural invasion is *not* a feature of this neoplasm. Complete surgical excision is usually curative as these tumors are of low-grade malignancy (Hosal, Fan, Barnes, & Myers, 2003).

Salivary Duct Carcinoma

Salivary duct carcinoma is a rare high-grade tumor thought to arise from the large excretory ducts (Jaehne, Roeser, & Jaekel, 2005). The peak incidence of this tumor occurs in the sixth and seventh decades. It is more common in men than women (2.5:1). It occurs most commonly in the parotid gland (78%) followed by the submandibular gland (12%) and the minor salivary glands (10%) (Hosal, Fan, Barnes, & Myers, 2003).

It comprises about 6-10% of all carcinomas of the parotid (Anderson, Muller, & Piorkowski, 1992). Many patients present with signs and symptoms reflecting the aggressive behavior of this tumor including a rapidly enlarging painful mass and facial nerve paresis or paralysis. In the series by Hosal et al, approximately two-thirds of patients presented with T3 or T4 tumors (Hosal, Fan, Barnes, & Myers, 2003). The presence of calcifications has been reported to be seen on CT scans in also one-third of the patients with salivary duct carcinoma (Brandwei, 1990; Delgado, 1992; Haines, 1984; Lewis, 1996; Murrah, 1994; Ockner, 1994; Smith, 1983).

The differential diagnosis includes metastatic adenocarcinoma from the prostate and metastatic ductal carcinoma of the breast. Immunoperoxidase staining for prostate-specific antigen aids in ruling out metastatic prostate carcinoma (Barnes et al, 1994). Identifying areas of intraductal (in-situ) tumor would serve to distinguish salivary duct carcinoma from both metastatic prostate and breast carcinoma (Hosal, Fan, Barnes, & Myers, 2003).

Because of its aggressive clinical behavior, salivary duct carcinoma is treated by complete surgical excision of the primary combined with neck dissection and adjuvant radiotherapy. Cervical lymph node metastases are present in 60-80% of cases. The incidence of distant metastases ranges from 33% to 66%. Two-thirds of patients die of their disease usually within 4 years of treatment, usually from distant metastases, which occur most commonly to the lungs and bone (Bradwein, 2004; Delgado, 1996).

Primary Squamous Cell Carcinoma (PSCC)

Primary squamous cell carcinomas of the salivary glands (PSSC) are rare, extremely aggressive neoplasms, the majority of patients presenting with advanced disease (Marciani, 1970; Shemen, 1987). In a review of 2,807 salivary gland tumors, PSSC accounted for only 1.9% (Shemen, 1987; Auclair, 1991). About 9% of patients have a history of prior radiation exposure (Shemen, 1987; Auclair, 1991; Cornoy, 1970; Gaughan, 1992; Lee, 2001; Marks, 1987). The parotid gland is involved in over two-thirds of cases and the remaining involves the submandibular gland (Shemen, Huvos, & Spiro, 1987). PSSC is twice as common in men as women (Li, Baloch, Tomaszewski, & LiVolsi, 2000). Although it has been reported in all decades of life, it is most common in the seventh decade. It is extremely uncommon in individuals below the age of 20 years (Nagao et al, 2002). Signs and symptoms include a painful rapidly enlarging mass and facial nerve palsy, although up to 50% of cases may present with an asymptomatic mass (Batsakis, 1983; Gaughan, 1992; Lee, 2001; Marks, 1987; Shemen, 1987).

Differential Diagnosis includes squamous metaplasia, necrotizing sialometaplasia, teratocystoma, high-grade mucoepidermoid carcinoma, and metastatic SCC. *Metastatic SCC* to salivary glands is more common than PSSC, particularly in the parotid with its rich supply of both peri- and intraglandular LNs (Lewis & Olsen, 2005). The presence of a focus of SCC in-situ distinguishes PSSC from metastatic SCC. SCC metastatic to the parotid usually originates from skin lesions of the head and neck. The skin of the frontal and temporal areas, the periorbital region, the cheek, the pinna, the external ear canal, and the pre- and postauricular areas are favored sites.

Treatment: Since this is an aggressive tumor, radical resection with neck dissection is usually indicated. The facial nerve maybe spared if not directly infiltrated by tumor. Up to 75% of patients have histologically positive cervical LNs. There is a significant incidence of local-regional recurrence which has led to the use of post-operative radiation therapy in many instances. Distant metastases occur in 20-30% of patients. The 5-year survival rate is 25%.

PROGNOSTIC FACTORS OF PAROTID CANCER

Recently, Kim et al. (2020) reported their results of investigating the prognostic factors and treatment outcomes of primary parotid carcinoma treated with surgery and post-operative radiotherapy (PORT). They reviewed retrospectively 57 patients with primary parotid carcinoma who were treated with surgery and PORT between 2005 and 2014. Superficial parotidectomy was performed in 19 patients, total parotidectomy in 10, and total parotidectomy with lymph node (LN) dissection in 28. PORT on the tumor bed was performed in 41 patients, and on tumor bed and ipsilateral cervical LNs in 16 patients. With a median follow-up of 66 months, the 5-year overall survival, disease-free survival, locoregional control, and distant control rates were 77.0%, 60.2%, 77.6%, and 72.8%, respectively. The 5-year overall survival by stage was 100%, 100%, 80.0%, and 46.4% in stage I, II, III, and IV, respectively. Recurrences at primary lesions were found in seven patients and at cervical nodes in six. Distant recurrences were developed in 12 patients. No patient with the low and intermediate histologic grade developed distant failure. This study revealed that differentiation grade, histologic grade, pathological T-stage, and lympho-vascular invasion were significant independent prognostic factors on clinical outcomes.

REFERENCES

Al-Zaher, N., Obeid, A., Al-Salam, S., & Al-Kayyali, B. S. (2009). Acinic cell carcinoma of the salivary glands: A literature review. *Hematology/Oncology and Stem Cell Therapy*, *2*(1), 259–264. doi:10.1016/S1658-3876(09)50035-0 PMID:20063555

Anderson, C., Muller, R., Piorkowski, R., Knibbs, D. R., & Vignoti, P. (1992). Intraductal carcinoma of major salivary gland. *Cancer*, *69*(3), 609–614. doi:10.1002/1097-0142(19920201)69:3<609::AID-CNCR2820690302>3.0.CO;2-1 PMID:1309674

Auclair, P. L., & Ellis, G. L. (1991). *Primary Squamous Cell Carcinoma.* In G. L. Ellis, P. L. Auclair, & D. R. Gnepp (Eds.), *Surgical pathology of the Salivary Glands* (pp. 369–378). Philadelphia, PA: WB Saunders Co.

Barnes, L., Appel, B. N., Perez, H., & El-Attar, A. M. (1985). Myoepithelioma of the head and neck: Case report and review. *Journal of Surgical Oncology*, *28*(1), 21–28. doi:10.1002/jso.2930280107 PMID:2982059

Barnes, L., Rao, U., Krause, J., Conti, S. L., Schwartz, A., & Scalamogna, P. (1994). Salivary duct carcinoma. Part I. A clinicopathologic evaluation and DNA image analysis of 13 cases with review of the literature. *Oral Surgery, Oral Medicine, and Oral Pathology*, *78*(1), 64–73. doi:10.1016/0030-4220(94)90119-8 PMID:8078666

Batsakis, J. G. (1983). Primary squamous cell carcinomas of major salivary glands. *The Annals of Otology, Rhinology, and Laryngology*, *92*(1), 97–98. doi:10.1177/000348948309200123 PMID:6824290

Boahene, D. K., Olsen, K. D., Lewis, J. E., Pinheiro, A. D., Pankratz, V. S., & Bagniewski, S. M. (2004). Mucoepidermoid carcinoma of the parotid gland: The Mayo clinic experience. *Archives of Otolaryngology--Head & Neck Surgery*, *130*(7), 849–856. doi:10.1001/archotol.130.7.849 PMID:15262762

Bradley, P. J. (2004). Adenoid cystic carcinoma of the head and neck: A review. *Current Opinion in Otolaryngology & Head & Neck Surgery*, *12*(2), 127–132. doi:10.1097/00020840-200404000-00013 PMID:15167050

Brandwein, M. S., Jagirdar, J., Patil, J., Biller, H., & Kaneko, M. (1990). Salivary duct carcinoma (cribriform salivary carcinoma of excretory ducts). A clinicopathologic and immunohistochemical study of 12 cases. *Cancer*, *65*(10), 2307–2314. doi:10.1002/1097-0142(19900515)65:10<2307::AID-CNCR2820651024>3.0.CO;2-1 PMID:1693309

Brandwein-Gensler, M., Hille, J., Wang, B. Y., & Mark, U. (2004). Low-grade salivary duct carcinoma: Description of 16 cases. *The American Journal of Surgical Pathology*, *28*(8), 1040–1044. doi:10.1097/01.pas.0000128662.66321.be PMID:15252310

Browand, B. C., & Waldron, C. A. (1975). Central mucoepidermoid tumors of the jaws. Report of nine cases and review of the literature. *Oral Surgery, Oral Medicine, and Oral Pathology*, *40*(5), 631–643. doi:10.1016/0030-4220(75)90373-4 PMID:1059064

Chhieng, D. C., & Paulino, A. F. (2002). Cytology of myoepithelial carcinoma of the salivary gland. *Cancer*, *96*(1), 32–36. doi:10.1002/cncr.10314 PMID:11836700

Chong, G. C., Beahrs, O. H., & Woolner, L. B. (1974). Surgical management of acinic cell carcinoma of the parotid gland. *Surgery, Gynecology & Obstetrics*, *138*(1), 65–68. PMID:4809004

Cornog, J. L. (1970). Surgical and Clinical Pathology of Salivary Gland Tumors. In R. Rankow & I. Polayes (Eds.), *Diseases of Salivary Glands* (pp. 92–142). Philadelphia, PA: WB Saunders Co.

de Sousa, S. O., Schwarzschild, M., de Araujo, N. S., & de Araujo, V. C. (2000). Basal cell adenocarcinoma of the palate with squamous metaplasia. *Journal of Clinical Pathology*, *53*(2), 153–156. doi:10.1136/jcp.53.2.153 PMID:10767834

Delgado, R., Klimstra, D., & Albores-Saavedra, J. (1996). Low grade salivary duct carcinoma. A distinctive variant with a low-grade histology and a predominant intraductal growth pattern. *Cancer*, *78*(5), 958–967. doi:10.1002/(SICI)1097-0142(19960901)78:5<958::AID-CNCR4>3.0.CO;2-8 PMID:8780532

Delgado, R., Vuitch, F., & Albores-Saavedra, J. (1992). High grade salivary duct carcinoma. *Modern Pathology*, *5*, 71A.

El-Naggar, A. K., Batsakis, J. G., Luna, M. A., McLemore, D., & Byers, R. M. (1990). DNA flow cytometry of acinic cell carcinomas of major salivary glands. *The Journal of Laryngology and Otology*, *104*(5), 410–416. doi:10.1017/S0022215100158578 PMID:2370468

Ellis, G., & Simpson, R. (2005). Acinic cell carcinoma. In L. Barnes, J. Eveson, P. Reichart, & D. Sidransky (Eds.), *Pathology and Genetics Head and Neck Tumours* (pp. 216–218). Lyon, France: IARC Press.

Ellis, G. L., & Wiscovitch, J. G. (1990). Basal cell adenocarcinomas of the major salivary glands. *Oral Surgery, Oral Medicine, and Oral Pathology*, *69*(4), 461–469. doi:10.1016/0030-4220(90)90380-B PMID:2326038

Eneroth, C. M., & Zetterberg, A. (1974). Malignancy in pleomorphic adenoma. A clinical and microspectrophotometric study. *Acta Oto-Laryngologica*, *77*(6), 426–432. doi:10.3109/00016487409124645 PMID:4365171

Foote, F. W. Jr, & Frazell, E. L. (1953). Tumors of the major salivary glands. *Cancer*, *6*(6), 1065–1133. doi:10.1002/1097-0142(195311)6:6<1065::AID-CNCR2820060602>3.0.CO;2-0 PMID:13106826

Foss, R. D., Ellis, G. L., & Auclair, P. L. (1996). Salivary gland cystadenocarcinomas. A clinicopathologic study of 57 cases. *The American Journal of Surgical Pathology*, *20*(12), 1440–1447. doi:10.1097/00000478-199612000-00002 PMID:8944036

Fowler, M. H., Fowler, J., Ducatman, B., Barnes, L., & Hunt, J. L. (2006). Malignant mixed tumors of the salivary gland: A study of loss of heterozygosity in tumor suppressor genes. *Modern Pathology*, *9*(3), 350–355. doi:10.1038/modpathol.3800533 PMID:16400327

Gaughan, R. K., Olsen, K. D., Lewis, J. E., & Richtsmeier, W. J. (1992). Primary squamous cell carcinoma of the parotid gland. *Archives of Otolaryngology--Head & Neck Surgery*, *118*(8), 798–801. doi:10.1001/archotol.1992.01880080020006 PMID:1642829

Gerughty, R. M., Scofield, H. H., Brown, F. M., & Hennigar, G. R. (1969). Malignant mixed tumors of salivary gland origin. *Cancer*, *24*(3), 471–486. doi:10.1002/1097-0142(196909)24:3<471::AID-CNCR2820240309>3.0.CO;2-0 PMID:4310021

Gnepp, D. R. (1993). Malignant mixed tumors of the salivary glands: A review. *Pathology Annual*, *28*(1), 279–328. PMID:8380049

Gross, M., Maly, B., Goldfarb, A., & Eliashar, R. (2004). Basal cell adenocarcinoma in a buccal minor salivary gland. *Acta Oto-Laryngologica*, *124*(2), 213–216. doi:10.1080/00026480410016243 PMID:15072428

Gurney, T. A., Eisele, D. W., Weinberg, V., Shin, E., & Lee, N. (2005). Adenoid cystic carcinoma of the major salivary glands treated with surgery and radiation. *The Laryngoscope*, *115*(7), 1278–1282. doi:10.1097/01.MLG.0000165381.64157.AD PMID:15995521

Gustafsson, H., Dahlqvist, A., Anniko, M., & Carlsoo, B. (1987). Mucoepidermoid carcinoma in a minor salivary gland in childhood. *The Journal of Laryngology and Otology*, *101*(12), 1320–1323. doi:10.1017/S0022215100103779 PMID:3323383

Haines, K., & Murad, T. (1989). Infiltrating salivary duct carcinoma of the parotid. *Laboratory Investigation*, *60*, 36A.

Hanson, T. A. (1975). Acinic cell carcinoma of the parotid salivary gland presenting as a cyst. Report of two cases. *Cancer*, *36*(2), 570–575. doi:10.1002/1097-0142(197508)36:2<570::AID-CNCR2820360236>3.0.CO;2-0 PMID:50876

Hosal, A. S., Fan, C., Barnes, L., & Myers, E. N. (2003). Salivary duct carcinoma. *Otolaryngology - Head and Neck Surgery*, *129*(6), 720–725. doi:10.1016/S0194-5998(03)01386-X PMID:14663441

Jaehne, M., Roeser, K., Jaekel, T., Schepers, J. D., Albert, N., & Löning, T. (2005). Clinical and immunohistologic typing of salivary duct carcinoma: A report of 50 cases. *Cancer*, *103*(12), 2526–2533. doi:10.1002/cncr.21116 PMID:15900577

Jayakrishnan, A., Elmalah, I., Hussain, K., & Odell, E. W. (2003). Basal cell adenocarcinoma in minor salivary glands. *Histopathology*, *42*(6), 610–614. doi:10.1046/j.1365-2559.2003.01651.x PMID:12786899

Kim, Y. H., Chung, W. K., Jeong, J. U., Cho, I. J., Yoon, M. S., Song, J. Y., ... Lim, S. C. (2020). *Evaluation of Prognostic Factors for the Parotid Cancer Treated With Surgery and Postoperative Radiotherapy. Clinical and Experimental Otorhinolaryngology*, *13*(1), 69–76.

Kleinsasser, O., Klein, H. J., & Hubner, G. (1968). Salivary duct carcinoma. A group of salivary gland tumors analogous to mammary duct carcinoma. *Archiv fur Klinische und Experimentelle Ohren- Nasen- und Kehlkopfheilkunde*, *192*(1), 100–105. doi:10.1007/BF00301495 PMID:4301301

Kwon, M. Y., & Gu, M. (2001). True malignant mixed tumor (carcinosarcoma) of parotid gland with unusual mesenchymal component: A case report and review of the literature. *Archives of Pathology & Laboratory Medicine*, *125*(6), 812–815. PMID:11371238

Lee, D. J., Smith, R. R., Spaziani, J. T., Rostock, R., Holliday, M., & Moses, H. (1985). Adenoid cystic carcinoma of the nasopharynx. Case reports and literature review. *The Annals of Otology, Rhinology, and Laryngology*, *94*(3), 269–272. PMID:2990313

Lee, S., Kim, G. E., Park, C. S., Choi, E. C., Yang, W. I., Lee, C. G., ... Suh, C.-O. (2001). Primary squamous cell carcinoma of the parotid gland. *American Journal of Otolaryngology*, *22*(6), 400–406. doi:10.1053/ajot.2001.28068 PMID:11713725

Lewis, J. E., McKinney, B. C., Weiland, L. H., Ferreiro, J. A., & Olsen, K. D. (1996). Salivary duct carcinoma. Clinicopathologic and immunohistochemical review of 26 cases. *Cancer*, *77*(2), 223–230. doi:10.1002/(SICI)1097-0142(19960115)77:2<223::AID-CNCR1>3.0.CO;2-N PMID:8625227

Lewis, J. E., & Olsen, K. D. (2005). *Tumors of Salivary Glands.* In E. L. Barnes, J. Eveson, P. Reichart, & D. Sidransky (Eds.), *Pathology and Genetics Head and Neck Tumors* (pp. 245–246). Lyon: IARC.

Lewis, J. E., Olsen, K. D., & Weiland, L. H. (1991). Acinic cell carcinoma. Clinicopathologic review. *Cancer*, *67*(1), 172–179. doi:10.1002/1097-0142(19910101)67:1<172::AID-CNCR2820670129>3.0.CO;2-X PMID:1985714

Li, S., Baloch, Z.W., & Tomaszewski, J.E., & LiVolsi, V.A. (2000). Worrisome histologic alterations following fine-needle aspiration of benign parotid lesions. *Archives of Pathology & Laboratory Medicine*, *124*, 87–91. PMID:10629137

Livolsi, V. A., & Perzin, K. H. (1977). Malignant mixed tumors arising in salivary glands. I. Carcinomas arising in benign mixed tumors: A clinicopathologic study. *Cancer*, *39*(5), 2209–2230. doi:10.1002/1097-0142(197705)39:5<2209::AID-CNCR2820390540>3.0.CO;2-8 PMID:192443

Loy, T. S., McLaughlin, R., Odom, L. F., & Dehner, L. P. (1989). Mucoepidermoid carcinoma of the parotid as a second malignant neoplasm in children. *Cancer*, *64*(10), 2174–2177. doi:10.1002/1097-0142(19891115)64:10<2174::AID-CNCR2820641032>3.0.CO;2-F PMID:2804906

Marciani, R. D., Trodahl, J. N., Dauchess, V. G., & Cantas, M. S. (1976). Squamous cell carcinoma of the submandibular gland. *Journal of Oral Surgery*, *34*, 646–650. PMID:1064715

Marks, M. W., Ryan, R. F., Litwin, M. S., & Sonntag, B. V. (1987). Squamous cell carcinoma of the parotid gland. *Plastic and Reconstructive Surgery*, *79*(4), 550–554. doi:10.1097/00006534-198704000-00006 PMID:3823246

Mehta, R. P., Faquin, W. C., & Deschler, D. G. (2004). Pathology quizcase 1. Acinic cell carcinoma of the parotid gland with ductal extension. *Archives of Otolaryngology--Head & Neck Surgery*, *130*(6), 790–793. doi:10.1001/archotol.130.6.790 PMID:15210565

Miki, H., Masuda, E., Ohata, S., Komaki, K., Hirokawa, M., Uehara, H., ... Monden, Y. (1999). Late recurrence of acinic cell carcinoma of the parotid gland. *Journal of Investigative Medicine*, *46*(3-4), 213–216. PMID:10687318

Milford, C. A., Mugliston, T. A., O'Flynn, P., & McCarthy, K. (1989). Carcinoma arising in a pleomorphic adenoma of the epiglottis. *The Journal of Laryngology and Otology*, *103*(3), 324–327. doi:10.1017/S0022215100108837 PMID:2539422

Muller, S., & Barnes, L. (1996). Basal cell adenocarcinoma of the salivary glands. Report of seven cases and review of the literature. *Cancer*, *78*(12), 2471–2477. doi:10.1002/(SICI)1097-0142(19961215)78:12<2471::AID-CNCR4>3.0.CO;2-N PMID:8952553

Murrah, V. A., & Batsakis, J. G. (1994). Salivary duct carcinoma. *The Annals of Otology, Rhinology, and Laryngology*, *103*(3), 244–247. doi:10.1177/000348949410300315 PMID:8122843

Nagao, T., Serizawa, H., Iwaya, K., Shimizu, T., Sugano, I., Ishida, Y., ... Ibihara, Y. (2002). Keratocystoma of the parotid gland: A report of two cases of an unusual pathologic entity. *Modern Pathology*, *15*(9), 1005–1010. doi:10.1097/01.MP.0000026053.67284.A3 PMID:12218219

Nagao, T., Sugano, I., Ishida, Y., Hasegawa, M., Matsuzaki, O., Konno, A., ... Nagao, K. (1998). Basal cell adenocarcinoma of the salivary glands: Comparison with basal cell adenoma through assessment of cell proliferation, apoptosis, and expression of p53 and bcl-2. *Cancer*, *82*(3), 439–447. doi:10.1002/(SICI)1097-0142(19980201)82:3<439::AID-CNCR3>3.0.CO;2-K PMID:9452259

Neto, A. G., Pineda-Daboin, K., Spencer, M. L., & Luna, M. A. (2005). Sinonasal acinic cell carcinoma: A clinicopathologic study of four cases. *Head & Neck*, *27*(7), 603–607. doi:10.1002/hed.20186 PMID:15900565

Ockner, D. M., Mills, S. E., Swanson, P. E., & Wick, M. R. (1994). Salivary duct carcinoma: An immunohistologic comparison with invasive ductal carcinoma of the breast. *Laboratory Investigation*, *70*, 100A.

Ogawa, I., Nikai, H., Takata, T., & Yasui, R. (1992). Clear-cell variant of mucoepidermoid carcinoma: Report of a case with immunohistochemical and ultrastructural observations. *Journal of Oral and Maxillofacial Surgery*, *50*(8), 906–910. doi:10.1016/0278-2391(92)90289-C PMID:1378889

Rapidis, A. D., Givalos, N., Gakiopoulou, H., Faratzis, G., Stavrianos, S. D., Vilos, G. A., ... Patsouris, E. (2005). Adenoid cystic carcinoma of the head and neck. Clinicopathological analysis of 23 patients and review of the literature. *Oral Oncology*, *41*(3), 328–335. doi:10.1016/j.oraloncology.2004.12.004 PMID:15743696

Said, S., & Campana, J. (2005). Myoepithelial carcinoma ex pleomorphic adenoma of salivary glands: A problematic diagnosis. *Oral Surgery, Oral Medicine, Oral Pathology, Oral Radiology, and Endodontics*, *99*(2), 196–201. doi:10.1016/j.tripleo.2003.11.014 PMID:15660092

Seifert, G. (1996). Classification and differential diagnosis of clear and basal cell tumors of the salivary glands. *Seminars in Diagnostic Pathology*, *13*(2), 95–103. PMID:8734415

Shafique, K., Zhang, P. J., Montone, K. T., Song, S., Livolsi, V. A., & Baloch, Z. (2020). Pathologic grading of mucoepidermoid carcinomas of the salivary gland and its effect on clinicopathologic follow-up: An institutional experience. *Human Pathology*. doi:10.1016/j.humpath.2020.02.001

Shemen, L. J., Huvos, A. G., & Spiro, R. H. (1987). Squamous cell carcinoma of salivary gland origin. *Head & Neck Surgery*, *9*(4), 235–240. doi:10.1002/hed.2890090407 PMID:3667298

Skalova, A., Leivo, I., Von Boguslawsky, K., & Saksela, E. (1994). Cell proliferation correlates with prognosis in acinic cell carcinomas of salivary gland origin. Immunohistochemical study of 30 cases using the MIB 1 antibody in formalin-fixed paraffin sections. *The Journal of Pathology*, *173*(1), 13–21. doi:10.1002/path.1711730104 PMID:7931834

Smith, A., Winkler, B., Perzin, K. H., Wazen, J., & Blitzer, A. (1985). Mucoepidermoid carcinoma arising in an intraparotid lymph node. *Cancer*, *55*(2), 400–403. doi:10.1002/1097-0142(19850115)55:2<400::AID-CNCR2820550218>3.0.CO;2-4 PMID:3965095

Smith, J. A., Warhol, M. J., & Brodsky, G. L. (1983). An immunohistochemical study of a carcinoma of the parotid gland exhibiting both ductal and acinic cell differentiation. *Oral Surgery, Oral Medicine, and Oral Pathology*, *55*(3), 267–273. doi:10.1016/0030-4220(83)90326-2 PMID:6188085

Terada, T., Ikeuchi, S., Inomoto, C., & Shimamura, K. (2004). Mucoepidermoid carcinoma of the palate composed exclusively of clear cells (clear cell variant). *Virchows Archiv*, *445*(5), 541–543. doi:10.100700428-004-1086-1 PMID:15517374

Valstar, M. H., de Ridder, M., van den Broek, E. C., Stuiver, M. M., van Dijk, B. A., van Velthuysen, M. L., ... Smeele, L. E. (2017). Salivary gland pleomorphic adenoma in the Netherlands: A nationwide observational study of primary tumor incidence, malignant transformation, recurrence, and risk factors for recurrence. *Oral Oncology*, *66*, 93–99. doi:10.1016/j.oraloncology.2017.01.004 PMID:28249655

van Weert, S., van der Waal, I., Witte, B. I., Leemans, C. R., & Bloemena, E. (2015). Histopathological grading of adenoid cystic carcinoma of the head and neck: Analysis of currently used grading systems and proposal for a simplified grading scheme. *Oral Oncology*, *51*(1), 71–76. doi:10.1016/j.oraloncology.2014.10.007 PMID:25456010

Waldron, C. A., & Koh, M. L. (1990). Central mucoepidermoid carcinoma of the jaws: Report of four cases with analysis of the literature and discussion of the relationship to mucoepidermoid, sialodontogenic, and glandular odontogenic cysts. *Journal of Oral and Maxillofacial Surgery*, *48*(8), 871–877. doi:10.1016/0278-2391(90)90349-7 PMID:2197385

Warrick, P. D., Irish, J. C., Mancer, K., Dardick, I., Pynn, B. R., & Gullane, P. (2000). Basal cell adenocarcinoma: A rare malignancy of the salivary glands. *The Journal of Otolaryngology*, *29*(2), 102–109. PMID:10819109

Chapter 14
Parotid Gland Lymphoma

ABSTRACT

Lymphoma accounts for 15% of malignant salivary gland tumors. The parotid gland is the most commonly affected salivary gland (80%). It is generally seen in older men and women. It is associated with human immunodeficiency virus (HIV) infection and in approximately 6% of patients with Sjogrin's syndrome. There are two types: Hodgkin lymphoma and Non-Hodgkin lymphoma. Parotid lymphoma may be primary or secondary (far more common). Primary lymphoma first involves the parotid gland and later other parts of the body including lymph nodes and bone marrow. Secondary lymphoma involves other parts of the body first, such as peripheral blood, lymph nodes, bone marrow, and other organs. Treatment depends upon stage, overall health, age, and subtype of lymphoma. It includes chemotherapy, total or radical parotidectomy, and radiotherapy. If there is no response, or the chance of recurrence is high, then bone marrow transplantation or stem cell transplantation can be considered.

PATHOLOGY

Parotid lymphoma can either be a B-cell lymphoma (far more common) or a T-cell lymphoma. There is increased number of intra-parotid lymph nodes with infiltrative characteristics. There are various (histological) subtypes of parotid gland lymphomas and some of these include (Lennert, 2013):

DOI: 10.4018/978-1-7998-5603-0.ch014

- MALT (mucosa associated lymphoid tissue) lymphoma of the salivary gland (most common subtype);
- Diffuse large B-cell lymphoma (rare subtype);
- Follicular lymphoma (rare subtype).

RISK FACTORS / ETIOLOGY

Risk (Predisposing) Factors

Sjögren's syndrome patients have a 44-fold excess risk for the development of non-Hodgkin's lymphoma particularly mucosa-associated lymphoid tissue (MALT) lymphoma, prevalently affecting the major salivary glands (Titsinides, Nikitakis, Piperi, & Sklavounou, 2017). However, the exact cause of the condition is generally unknown. No specific risk factors have been identified for parotid lymphoma. However, the condition is known to be associated with the following factors:

- Autoimmune disorders;
- Sjögren's syndrome (inflammatory disorder);
- Lymphoepithelial sialadenitis;
- Hepatitis C virus (HCV) infection;
- Advanced age;
- Immunodeficiency;
- Family history of immune disease;
- Smoking;
- Exposure to radiation and industrial chemicals;
- Chemotherapy;
- Viruses (rare): Epstein-Barr virus (EBV) infection;
- Profession involving radiation exposure, which may include nuclear plant workers, pilots, astronauts, etc.;
- Certain medications and drugs.

International Prognostic Index (IPI)

According to some scientists, the IPI may not be very helpful in evaluating lymphoma of salivary gland. However, some scientists believe that it is helpful in some cases, to determine prognosis. The IPI for aggressive non-Hodgkin lymphoma (NHL) lists a few factors that determine the overall risk:

- Age over 60 years;
- Elevated level of serum lactate dehydrogenase (LDH);
- Performance status, which could range from being fully active (low risk) to being completely disabled (very high risk);
- Individuals who have already suffered from lymphoma or other types of blood cancers may have a relapse or a recurrence;
- Presence of an immunodeficiency syndrome such as AIDS is a high risk factor;
- Those infected with EBV.

PATHOGENESIS

It is believed that the abnormal development of lymphocytes gives rise to cancerous cells leading to the formation of lymphoma. Nevertheless, how this occurs and the factors that cause it remain under investigation.

There may be certain genetic defects, such as translocation, which is a juxtaposition of regions of the chromosomes. This may result in:

- Change of regulatory elements of certain cancer-causing genes (oncogenes), which can lead to increased production of their mRNA (over-expression), thus increasing their protein levels;
- Exchange of protein coding regions of the gene, giving rise to new proteins that can stimulate the inappropriate growth of cells.

CLINICAL PRESENTATION

The signs and symptoms of parotid depend on whether it is a primary or a secondary condition. In a majority of primary lymphomas, if the tumor is small, it may be usually asymptomatic and the individuals will not have any significant symptoms. The symptoms also depend upon the extent of lymphoma involvement in other parts of the body.

The signs and symptoms of lymphoma of the parotid gland may include the following:

- Presence of a lump in the face, which may be accompanied by pain;
- Swelling of the face;
- Facial palsy (usually by large tumors);
- Difficulty during eating, drinking, or even opening the mouth;
- Dryness of mouth;
- Foul taste or smell from the mouth;
- Unintentional weight loss; changes in appetite;
- Fatigue and weakness, headache;
- Anemia;
- Frequent infections;
- Hypotension.

When organs other than the parotid gland are involved, then, the signs and symptoms may be based on the specific organs that are affected.

DIAGNOSIS' INVESTIGATIONS

In addition to obtaining a complete medical history and performing a thorough physical examination, diagnosis is generally performed by obtaining biopsy samples. There are other tests and procedures that could help in the diagnosis and these include the following.

Laboratory Tests

Blood tests that may include: complete blood cell count (CBC), absolute lymphocyte count on peripheral blood, liver function tests (LFT) and lactate dehydrogenase (LDH) blood test.

Imaging

Imaging may be performed specific to location of the involved organ, and to determine the extent of lymphoma in the body including plain X-ray US, CT scan of the neck (Figure 1), whole body bone scan, whole body CT-PET (positron emission tomography) scans to determine how far the lymphoma has spread, and brain MRI (if neurological symptoms are present).

Figure 1. CT scan of the neck showing lymphoma of the parotid glands (arrows)

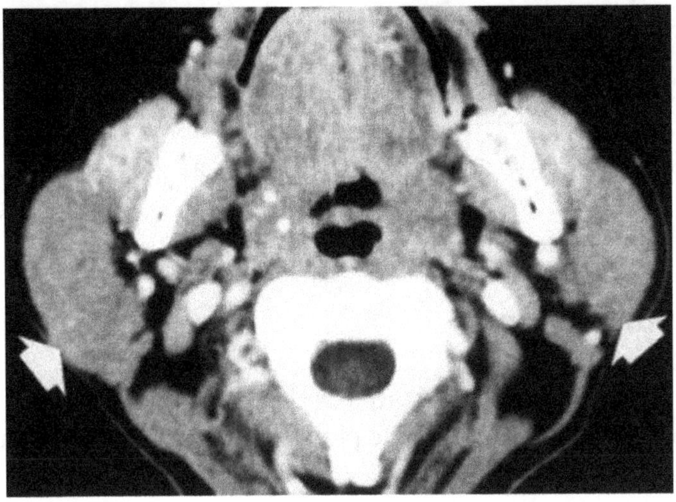

Tissue Biopsy

Tissue biopsy from the affected salivary gland is considered to be gold standard in arriving at a conclusive diagnosis, either through a fine needle aspiration biopsy (FNAB) or core-needle biopsy. Biopsy specimens are studied initially using Hematoxylin and Eosin (H&E) staining. Sometimes, the pathologist may perform special studies, which may include immunohistochemical (IHC) stains, molecular testing, flow cytometric analysis and very rarely, electron microscopic studies, to assist in the diagnosis.

Bone Marrow Aspiration and Biopsy

Bone marrow aspiration and biopsy may be needed to determine if the bone marrow is involved. However, a bone marrow biopsy is not needed in the early stages of the condition.

Flow Cytometry

Flow cytometry measures the number and percentage of cells in a blood sample, and cell characteristics such as size, shape, and the presence of biomarkers on the cell surface. This method helps to sub-classify the condition and also to detect residual levels of disease after treatment. This tool can help in diagnosing relapse and restart treatment as needed.

Fluorescence in-Situ Hybridization (FISH)

Fluorescence in-situ hybridization (FISH): It is a cytogenetic analysis test performed on blood or bone marrow cells to detect chromosome changes (genetic) abnormalities) in blood cancer cells.

Immunophenotyping

Immunophenotyping may be resorted in order to identify a specific type of cell in a sample, which can help determine the best treatment course to be prescribed to the patient.

Polymerase Chain Reaction (PCR)

Polymerase chain reaction (PCR): It is used to measure the presence of certain biomarkers in blood or bone marrow cells. The test is ultrasensitive and detects extremely low amounts of biomarkers remaining in blood, which can be missed by cytogenetic methods, such as FISH, karyotype, or flow cytometry. Thus, PCR allows a more sensitive follow-up of patients in remission and can help determine whether additional treatment is necessary.

Exploratory (Diagnostic) Laparoscopy

Exploratory laparoscopy (diagnostic laparoscopy) may be required, if gastrointestinal symptoms are present. A diagnostic laparoscopy is also helpful in staging of the tumor. Nevertheless, this procedure is not very much used.

COMPLICATIONS

Complications due to *parotid lymphoma* include:

- Involvement of local and distant organs: It can lead to systemic or disseminated disease in some cases;

- Loss of function of the organ/area to which cancer has spread due to systemic involvement;
- Acute difficulty while eating, swallowing, or speaking;
- Immunosuppression, which can become more severe during treatment. Consequently, patients are more vulnerable to infections;
- Occasionally, the tumor can transform into a more aggressive form or subtype of lymphoma;
- Complications related to *chemotherapy* used for treatment may include dizziness, vomiting, loss of appetite, mouth ulcers, hair loss, infertility (in men and women), secondary infections, and secondary cancers such as skin cancer.

TREATMENT

Treatment depends upon the stage, overall health, age, and subtype of lymphoma. It includes the following.

Chemotherapy

This approach uses a combination of drugs or target therapy, and can be used for all stages of the tumor. Many lymphomas can be resistant to chemotherapy and there can be severe side effects including infertility, immunosuppression, secondary infections, and secondary cancers.

Surgery

Surgical excision of the lymphoma of the parotid gland entails total parotidectomy or radical (non-conservative) parotidectomy if the facial nerve cannot be preserved.

Radiotherapy

Radiation therapy is generally used for early stage lymphomas. It is most commonly used in combination with chemotherapy. The side effects of radiation therapy include nausea, vomiting, fatigue, pain, risk of cancer later in life, and risk of heart disease.

Supportive Treatment

Steroids, blood transfusions, anti-nausea medications, and antibiotics, may be used as supportive therapy. In combination with other treatment measures, these can help combat the symptoms of immunodeficiency. Undertaking treatment of underlying infection/disorder should be done as warranted (Adler, 2005).

Transplantation

If salivary gland lymphoma is not fully responsive to treatment, or if the chance of recurrence is high, then *bone marrow transplantation* or *stem cell transplantation* can be considered.

PREVENTION

Currently, it is not possible to prevent lymphoma of salivary gland. However, controlling certain factors may help lower one's risk for the condition as follows:

- Healthy diet and exercise, as well as avoidance of unnecessary exposure to chemicals, may help decrease its risk;
- Avoiding smoking;
- Undertaking appropriate and early treatment of any condition that affects the salivary gland;
- Using appropriate protective gear while working with X-rays and other radioactive source;
- In order to avoid a relapse, or be prepared for a recurrence, the entire diagnosis, treatment process, drugs administered, etc. should be well-documented and follow-up measures initiated;
- Regular medical screening at periodic intervals with blood tests, scans, and physical examinations, are mandatory. Often several years of active vigilance are crucial and necessary.

PROGNOSIS (OUTCOMES / RESOLUTIONS)

Lymphoma of salivary glands is a slow-growing malignancy with a generally good prognosis with early diagnosis and treatment. Prognosis depends on many factors including the subtype and stage of lymphoma, progression of the condition, response to treatment, and overall health of the individual (Adler & Page, 2008):

- **Stage of Tumor:** With lower-stage tumors, when the tumor is confined to site of origin, the prognosis is usually excellent with appropriate therapy. In higher-stage tumors, such as tumors with metastasis, the prognosis is poor;
- **Overall Health of The Individual:** Individuals with overall excellent health have better prognosis compared with those with poor health;
- **Age of The Individual:** Older patients generally have poorer prognosis than younger ones;
- **Size of The Tumor:** Individuals with small-sized tumors fare better than those with large-sized ones. Individuals with bulky disease have a poorer prognosis;
- **Involvement of Vital Organs:** May complicate the condition;
- **Surgical Respectability:** Of the tumor - a rare option;
- **Recurrent Tumors:** Have worse prognosis compared to tumors that do not recur;
- **Response to Treatment:** Tumors that respond to treatment have better prognosis compared to those that do not. Tolerance to chemotherapy sessions is a positive influencing factor;
- **Progression of the Condition:** Makes the outcome worse (progressive salivary gland lymphoma). Progression to bone marrow failure is usually associated with short survival.

REFERENCES

Adler, E. M. (2005). *Living with Lymphoma A Patient's Guide*. Baltimore, MD: Johns Hopkins University Press.

Adler, N. E., & Page, A. E. (Eds.). (2008). *Cancer Care for the Whole Patient: Meeting Psychosocial Health Needs*. Washington, DC: National Academies Press.

Lennert, K. (2013). *Histopathology of Non-Hodgkin's Lymphomas: Based on the Kiel Classification*. Berlin: Springer-Verlag.

Titsinides, S., Nikitakis, N., Piperi, E., & Sklavounou, A. (2017). MALT Lymphoma of Minor Salivary Glands in a Sjögren's Syndrome Patient: a Case Report and Review of Literature. *Journal of Oral Maxillofacial Research*, *31*(1), e5.

Chapter 15
Cancer Metastatic to the Parotid Gland

ABSTRACT

Carcinoma metastatic to the parotid gland is a region-specific disorder. History usually reveals a previous cutaneous squamous cell carcinoma (SCC) or melanoma. Physical examination may show scars of previous operations, current head and neck lesions, associated lymphadenopathy, and altered sensation. Investigations include fiberoptic naso-endoscopy, fine needle aspiration cytology, computed tomography scan, magnetic resonance imaging, and positron emission tomography. Treatment options include surgery (ablative/reconstructive), radiotherapy (indicated for SCC and melanoma), chemotherapy (indicated for SCC), chemo-immunotherapy (may have a role for melanoma). Complications to avoid include (1) wound-related complications (skin flap necrosis and skin flap "button-hole" formation), (2) tumor-related complications (inappropriate surgery due to inadequate preoperative investigation or omitting neck dissection in patients with concomitant neck disease, tumor rupture, and local tumor recurrence), (3) gland-related complications (salivary fistula and sialocele), and (4) nerve-related complications (facial nerve injury, Frey's syndrome or gustatory sweating, and great auricular nerve neuroma).

DOI: 10.4018/978-1-7998-5603-0.ch015

INTRODUCTION

Metastatic involvement of the salivary glands is relatively rare, but most commonly seen in the parotid gland. Although many malignancies have been implicated, metastasis is typically due to cutaneous squamous cell carcinoma (SCC) and melanoma (Clark & Wang, 2016). The major mechanism through which this occurs is via lymphatic spread into intra-parotid lymph nodes (LNs). The presence of lymphatic tissue within the parotid gland is a unique feature and results from incorporation of lymphoid tissue due to late encapsulation of the parotid gland during embryogenesis. Intra-parotid LNs act as the major drainage pathway of the ocular adnexa and the cutaneous surfaces of the forehead and lateral aspect of the head (Kashiwagi et al, 2016). Therefore, identification of abnormal-appearing intra-parotid LNs should warrant close inspection of these regions for a primary malignancy.

On imaging, metastases to intra-parotid LNs appear similar to metastatic LNs elsewhere in the head and neck region. Progressive enlargement, central necrosis, and ill-defined margins are all imaging features, suggestive of lymphatic metastasis. In clinical practice, differentiating metastatic intra-parotid LNs from primary salivary cancer is very difficult and *biopsy* is often necessary. Kashiwagi et al. (2016) reported that metastatic involvement most commonly occurs in the parotid tail and pretragal region of the superficial lobe. Thus, identification of a lesion in one of these areas in a patient with known cutaneous SCC or melanoma should raise the suspicion for metastatic involvement.

PATHOLOGY OF CANCER METASTATIC TO THE PAROTID GLAND

Carcinoma metastatic to the parotid gland is a region-specific disorder where the relative incidence of the various histopathological types is dependent on geographical location as shown in Table 1. In Australia, metastatic cutaneous squamous cell carcinoma (SCC) is the most common malignancy seen in the parotid, including primary cancer of the parotid gland (Bron, Traynor, McNeil, & O'Brien, 2003). This contrasts with North America and Europe where primary cancer of the parotid gland is more frequent (Woods, Chong, & Beahrs, 1975). Although metastatic cancer to the parotid is relatively infrequent worldwide, in 40% of patients with this disease it will be the first manifestation of skin cancer (Malata, Camilleri, McLean, Piggott, & Soames, 1998).

Squamous Cell Carcinoma (SCC)

It is estimated that 5% of cutaneous SCCs metastasize to regional lymph node (LN) basins, including the parotid (O'Brien, McNeil, & McMahon, 2001). Current evidence suggests that between 25% and 50% of patients with nodal metastases to the parotid from SCC will also have cervical nodal disease (O'Brien, McNeil, & McMahon, 2001). Clinico-pathological features that increase the risk of nodal metastases are listed in Table 2. In high-risk SCC the associated risk of nodal metastases is up to 20% (Audet et al, 2004). Overall mortality for cutaneous SCC is low at 3.4% but increases substantially in patients with regional metastatic disease (Joseph, Zulueta, & Kennedy, 1992). In a multicenter study of 325 patients with metastatic SCC to the parotid there was a 27% rate of synchronous neck disease and overall survival was 72% at 5 years (Andruchow et al, 2006). Loco-regional control in metastatic SCC of the parotid is high with the exception of patients with highly invasive disease (bone or other deep structures) or extensive peri-neural invasion. Cutaneous SCC has a high predilection for peri-neural invasion, which may affect both motor (facial) and sensory (auriculotemporal nerve, CN-V) nerve within the parotid and surrounding tissue.

Table 1. Pathology of metastatic cancer to the parotid

Cutaneous and Mucosal Primary	Solid Organ	Lymphoproliferative
- SCC - Melanoma - Merkel cell carcinoma - Sinonasal carcinoma - Nasopharyngeal carcinoma - Other rare (dermato-fibrosarcoma, metastatic BCC)	- Renal cell carcinoma - Lung - Other rare	Lymphoma

Melanoma

Approximately, 10% to 20% of cutaneous melanoma arises in the head and neck (Myers, 1999) and nearly 20% of patients develop regional metastases (Mack & McKinnon, 2004). Patients with clinically palpable metastatic

Table 2. Clinicopathological features that increase risk of nodal metastases

High Risk SCC
- Size > 2 cm - Invasion into subcutaneous fat - Depth > 5 mm - Poorly differentiated tumors - Peri-neural invasion - Lympho-vascular invasion - Site: ear or lip - Incomplete excision - Local recurrence - Immunosuppression

melanoma in the parotid have a high rate of occult neck disease, ranging from 28% to 58% (O'Brien, 2001; Barr, 1994; Caldwell, 1988). The overall mortality for cutaneous melanoma of the head and neck is high, with 10-year survival rates ranging from 45% to 72%. This falls to 34% for patients with proven nodal metastases and further decreases with increasing number of positive nodes (O'Brien, 1995; O'Brien, 1993). Clinico-pathological features predictive of nodal disease and mortality are listed in Table 3.

Table 3. Clinico-pathological features that predict nodal disease and metastases

High Risk Cutaneous Melanoma
- Tumor thickness (> 1 mm) - Tumor ulceration - Site (scalp) - Level of invasion (Clark level IV) - Gender (male) - Age (increasing age)

Other Primary Malignancies

Merkel cell carcinoma is a rare, aggressive neuro-endocrine cutaneous malignancy. The largest reported series of head and neck Merkel cell carcinoma showed nodal metastases in 48 of 110 patients. Loco-regional control is most effective when surgery is combined with radiotherapy (Clark, 2007; Veness, 2005). There is no evidence to support routine use of adjuvant chemotherapy (Poulsen, 2004).

Mucosal cancer, including SCC, infrequently metastasizes to the parotid gland. *Naso-pharyngeal* cancer has been reported as a primary site (King wet al, 20000) and extensive sinonasal cancers involving the subcutaneous tissue of cheek and orbit may disseminate to the parotid gland. Advanced oro-pharyngeal cancers may also invade directly through the para-pharyngeal space to involve the parotid gland. *Renal cell carcinoma* is the most common solid organ cancer to metastasize to the parotid (Coppa & Oszczakiewicz, 1990).

INVESTIGATIONS AND STAGING OF CANCER METASTATIC TO THE PAROTID GLAND

Clinical Assessment

For patients with cancer metastatic to the parotid, all potential *cutaneous and mucosal sites* need examination. This includes fiberoptic examination of the nasopharynx and oropharynx. Particular care is necessary when inspecting potential cutaneous sites since cutaneous malignancies may be small relative to the bulk of regional disease. Inconspicuous lesions hiding in the hair, behind the ear, nasal vestibule, and in the external auditory canal are easily overlooked. *Non-pigmented* nodular lesions are difficult to diagnose and may represent amelanotic melanoma or Merkel cell cancer.

Examination should include assessment of fixation, parapharyngeal extension, synchronous cervical disease, and facial nerve grading as standard. The great auricular nerve may be involved directly causing ear lobule/angle of mandible dysesthesia and the trigeminal nerve may be involved via branches of the auriculotemporal nerve. Hence sensation in the distribution of both these nerves should also be assessed.

A thorough history of previous cutaneous surgery is essential. Pathology reports should be obtained and the original pathology slides may need to be reviewed by an experienced pathologist to confirm unusual primary lesions such as poorly differentiated SCC, Merkel cell carcinoma, spindle cell tumors, and even melanoma.

Investigations

Fine-needle aspiration biopsy (FNAB) is recommended for all parotid tumors and is useful for planning the extent of surgery and stratifying urgency for intervention (Seethala, LiVolsi, & Baloch, 2005). All clinically malignant parotid tumors need cytological confirmation and FNA is reliable in the detection of metastatic SCC (Alphs, Eisele, & Westra, 2006).

Imaging with high resolution multislice computed tomography (CT) scanning with intravenous contrast is recommended in patients with and without fixed disease. This allows assessment of the parotid and surrounding structures, including the parapharyngeal space. Bone windows are used to determine cranial or mandibular invasion. CT examines both potential mucosal sites and the neck to detect subclinical synchronous nodal disease. A dedicated temporal bone CT is obtained where there is fixation or facial nerve deficit.

Magnetic resonance imaging (MRI) can be substituted for CT and is particularly useful in patients with parapharyngeal extension and neurotrophic cancers and is equivalent to CT scan in cervical LN assessment. However, it is more expensive; less readily obtained, poorly tolerated by patients, and provides poor cortical bone definition.

Ultrasound (US) has been reported to be highly specific and sensitive for cervical node disease in selected series (Stuckensen, Kovacs, Adams, & Baum, 2000) and can be combined with US-guided FNA. However, is inferior to CT or MRI in patients with extensive parotid disease, in particular those with facial paresis.

There are few data examining the role of *positron emission tomography* (PET) in metastatic cancer to the parotid gland. PET or PET-CT is being used more frequently as a standard investigation and has a role in the assessment of regional and distant metastatic disease. PET is more likely to be positive in patients with melanoma where distant disease is common. 18F-FDGPET is superior to other modalities in the detection of distant metastases and in patients with recurrent disease where the sensitivity and specificity ranges from 70% to 100% (Belhocine, Scott, Even-Sapir, Urbain, & Essner, 2006). However, PET is relatively insensitive (0-40%) in the detection of regional metastases in patients with early-stage disease when compared to sentinel node biopsy.

Detection of distant metastases has both prognostic and therapeutic value, since isolated distant diseases amenable to surgical resection (Essner, 2003). Regardless of distant disease status, loco-regional control is of value for symptomatic relief since the rate of disease progression is unpredictable.

Staging of Cutaneous Metastatic SCC

The current staging system stages all patients with cutaneous squamous cell carcinoma (SCC) and nodal metastases to the parotid as N1 regardless of the extent or volume of disease (Bell & Gaillard, 2003). O'Brien (2006) has proposed a revised staging system, which has demonstrated prognostic value as shown in Table 4.

Table 4. Revised staging of Metastatic SCC (O'Brien, 2006)

Parotid		Neck	
P0	No clinical parotid disease	**N0**	No clinical neck disease
P1	Metastatic node < 3 cm	**N1**	Single ipsilateral neck node < 3 cm
P2	Metastatic node > 3 cm but < 6 cm Multiple parotid nodes	**N2**	Single node > 3 cm Multiple or contralateral neck LNs
P3	Metastatic node > 6 cm Multiple or contralateral neck nodes		

Staging of Melanoma

Staging for melanoma is listed in Table 5. Parotid metastases are included as regional nodal disease. There is no separate staging for parotid disease.

Table 5. AJCCS staging of Cutaneous Melanoma

Tumor		Node		Metastasis	
T1	< 1 mm thick	**N1**	Single nodal or parotid metastases	**M1a**	Distant skin, SC or distant nodal mets
T2	1–2 mm thick	**N2**	2–3 nodal metastases	**M1b**	Lung metastases
T3	2–4 mm thick	**N3**	> 3 nodal metastases	**M1c**	Other visceral mets or any distant mets with ↑ LDH
T4 a **b**	> 4 mm thick No ulceration Ulceration	**a** **b**	Micronodal metastases Macronodal metastases		

SURGERY FOR CANCER METASTATIC TO THE PAROTID GLAND

Ablative Surgery

The extent of surgery in both the parotid and the neck is an ongoing area of controversy as shown in Table 6). Current evidence does not indicate that more extensive surgery is associated with either improved disease control or survival (Eicher, Clayman, Myers, & Gillenwater, 2002). This may reflect the frequent use of adjuvant radiotherapy (O'Brien, 1997), which is effective for control of microscopic nodal disease in both the parotid and neck. This is applicable for both SCC and melanoma, although melanoma traditionally is considered to be radio-resistant (Ballo & Ang, 2003).

Table 6. Ablative surgery for metastatic cancer to the parotid gland

Parotidectomy	Neck Dissection (Elective and Therapeutic)
Limited parotidectomy Superficial parotidectomy Total parotidectomy with nerve preservation Radical parotidectomy Extended parotidectomy - Skin resection - Mandibulectomy - Lateral temporal bone resection	Selective Comprehensive Extended

Superficial parotidectomy is the standard procedure. There is no evidence that a limited or more aggressive approach is preferable. Parotid lymphatics and LNs are present throughout the parotid substance, both superficial and deep. However, superficial lymph nodes are more numerous and more likely to harbor metastatic disease. McKean et al. (1985) reported up to 22 nodes in the superficial lobe compared with less than 5 in the deep lobe.

Total parotidectomy with facial nerve sacrifice (*radical parotidectomy*) is highly morbid with aesthetic and functional consequences (Table 7) and current trends are toward more conservative surgery where possible (Veness, Morgan, Palme, & Gebski, 2005). More extensive dissection is indicated in invasive parotid metastases or recurrent disease and may necessitate facial nerve sacrifice ± temporal bone resection and resection of adjacent structures involved by the cancer such as skin, mandible, and skull base.

Table 7. Functional and aesthetic consequences of radical parotidectomy

Functional	Aesthetic
- Visual disturbance (brow ptosis - frontalis) - Corneal exposure and ulceration (orbicularis oculi) - Oral incompetence (orbicularis oris, depressor - anguli oris, depressor labii inferioris) - Speech impairment (buccinator, orbicularis oris)	- Contour defect - Brow ptosis - Eyelid paralysis - Ectropion - Nasal collapse - Upper lip asymmetry - Lower lip asymmetry

Resection of skin is relatively simple and can be restored using a number of standard techniques such as a cervico-facial rotation flap (Moore, Wine, & Netterville, 005) or free flap where indicated. In more advanced disease the likelihood of local control needs to be balanced against the morbidity of surgery. As more radical procedures are undertaken the rate of positive surgical margins also increases (Khurana et al, 1995) hence more radical surgery does not necessarily confer disease control. An argument can be made for more radical parotid surgery where radiotherapy is contraindicated, such as recurrent disease, or where radiotherapy may be avoided by adequate surgery, such as single small nodal metastasis with no extra-capsular extension or neck disease.

Neck dissection may be combined with parotidectomy as an elective or therapeutic procedure. Therapeutic neck dissection is appropriate to maximize disease control (Khurana et al, 1995) and should incorporate all at risk nodal basins. This depends on the location of the primary and the extent of nodal metastasis. In general, neck dissection of levels I to V is standard; however, in low volume neck disease a selective dissection of levels II to V is appropriate for posterior primaries or levels I to IV for anterior lesions (O'Brien, 2006). Resection of non-lymphatic structures, such as the sternomastoid muscle (SCM) and internal jugular vein (IJV) is indicated where disease is suspected to involve them directly.

Consideration needs to be given to nodal groups that are not traditionally encompassed in neck dissection for mucosal SCC. This includes external jugular LNs, which are at high risk for any malignancy involving the parotid and should be included routinely (O'Brien, 2006). Level IIb should be routinely dissected. Occipital and retroauricular LNs are at high risk in posterior scalp malignancy and lesions involving the pinna. Peri-facial LNs are at high risk in cheek, lip, and nasal primaries.

Elective neck dissection has not been shown to confer improved disease control or survival despite the substantial rate of occult neck disease.

Presumably this is due to the frequent use of adjuvant radiotherapy (O'Brien, 2001); Pedraza, 2001). *Selective neck dissection* of levels II and III may be appropriate as a staging procedure in selected patients; however, this depends on the location of the primary. In patients where adjuvant radiotherapy is not possible a more comprehensive neck dissection should be combined with parotidectomy.

Elective parotidectomy in patients with cervical disease is not generally employed. However parotid nodes are frequently involved in patients with cervical disease from primary cutaneous malignancy, in particular primary melanoma and SCC of the ear, face, and anterior scalp. Shah et al. (1995) reported that 33 of 57 elective parotidectomies for neck disease had melanoma involving the parotid and adjacent nodes. This is supported by the high rate of sentinel nodes biopsies occurring in the peri-parotid region (Chao et al, 2003); however, other series have not replicated this high rate of positive metastases to the parotid (Vaglini, Belli, Santinami, & Cascinelli, 1990). There may be a role for lymphoscintigraphy to determine whether the parotid contains any sentinel nodes for the primary. Potential complications that may occur after parotid surgical procedures for the treatment of metastatic malignancy to the parotid gland are summarized in Table 8.

Table 8. Complications of parotid surgery for metastatic malignancy

Facial nerve palsy: - Facial nerve paralysis or paresis - increased in malignancy
Other complications - Lip depressor weakness — increased when combined with neck dissection - Great auricular neuroma or dysesthesia - Frey's syndrome - Sialocele - Salivary fistula - Wound infection or necrosis

Reconstructive Surgery

Reconstruction following radical parotid surgery is frequently required. The most common structure sacrificed is *skin* followed by *facial nerve*. Cutaneous reconstruction depends on the extent of cutaneous defect, type of neck dissection, other structures sacrificed, and whether radiotherapy has been given previously. In moderate-sized defects, a cervico-facial rotation flap

(Tan & MacKinnon, 2006) is an excellent method, particularly for elderly patients not concerned about the contour deformity that arises from extensive parotid surgery. The *cervico-facial flap* (Tan & MacKinnon, 2006) is favored in patients where the facial artery is preserved due to its reliability and lesser dissection. The *submental island flap* is also very useful due to the excellent color match with the cheek (Pistre, Pelissier, Martin, Lim, & Baudet, 2001); however, it requires planning with regards to incisions and the pedicle needs to be carefully dissected (Figures 1 and 2).

Figure 1. (a) Metastatic SCC right parotid involving overlying skin. (b) Design of excision and cervicofacial rotation flap. (c) Limited parotidectomy with cervicofacial rotation flap raised. (d) Inset cervicofacial flap.

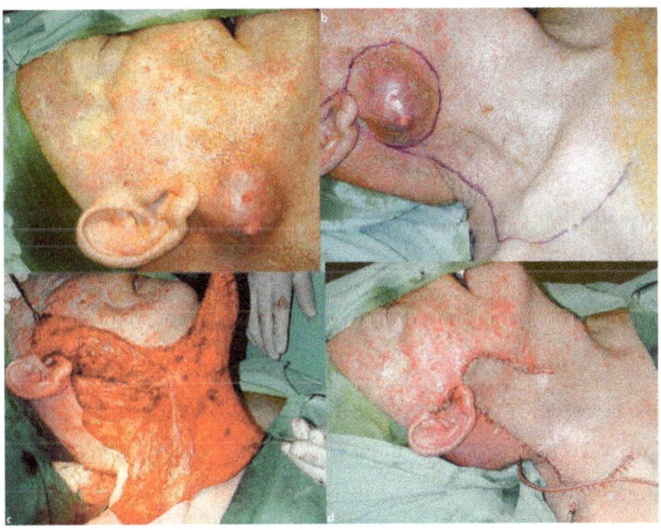

Many patients are best managed with *free tissue reconstruction*, in particular, those with prior irradiation or extensive cutaneous defects where a cervico-facial flap is insufficient or likely tofail. This is important in patients with exposed bone and where post-operative radiotherapy or chemo-radiation is planned and marginal flap necrosis will delay the onset of radiotherapy, which should be commenced within six weeks after surgery. Reliable free flaps such as the *radial forearm* have a low failure rate of<1% (Bae, 2006; Disa, 2001). However, morbidity of this donor site is substantial if large flaps are harvested, and the color match with the head and neck is poor. Color

Figure 2. (a) Retroauricular metastatic SCC involving tail of parotid. Design of deep plane cervicofacial flap based on perforators from facial artery. (b) Inset deep plane cervicofacial flap following parotidectomy and neck dissection.

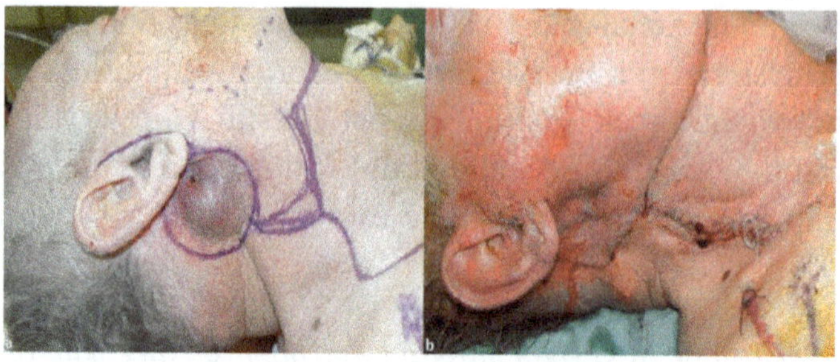

match is important in the face and is best obtained by using flaps located in proximity of the head and neck.

Following radical parotidectomy there are several components to optimal reconstruction which can be performed primarily (ideally) or secondarily. These include the cutaneous defect (if present), contour defect, bone defect, facial nerve, brow ptosis, eyelid paralysis, ectropion, and lip paralysis. There are many options in reconstructing these complex problems depending on individual or institutional expertise.

Facial Nerve

Where the proximal facial nerve can be accessed in the temporal bone without disease, a cable nerve graft can be performed using sural, saphenous, or antebrachial cutaneous nerve. Facial nerve function following neurorrhaphy is unlikely to be better than a House Rickman grade III and some synkinesis is unavoidable (Tulley et al, 2000).

Contour

The contour defect is well corrected using a *de-epithelialized fascio-cutaneous free flap* such as para-scapular or antero-lateral thigh. A *temporo-parietal flap* can be used as a pedicled flap for small defects. Muscle flaps should be avoided since the ultimate volume is unpredictable.

Table 9. Standard radiation therapy for metastatic SCC to the parotid gland

Clinical target volume (CTV)	The volume including the site of resected gross disease, surgical bed/scar, and next echelon of draining lymph nodes with a minimum of a 0.5-cm margin in all dimensions
Planning target volume	Defined as CTV 1 with a minimum of a 1.0-cm margin in all dimensions
Radiation dose	50–60 Gy in 25–30 fractions, 2 Gy per fraction, 5 fractions per week

Static Reconstruction

The *upper eyelid* is managed using a gold weight and the *lower eyelid* using a tendon sling to prevent ectropion with or without canthoplasty. Using this combination, a *lateral tarsorrhaphy*, which is aesthetically inferior, is usually unnecessary. The *oral commissure* is lateralized using a woven tendon sling (plantaris or palmaris). This is favored over fascia lata, which tends to stretch over time. The commissure and lip is suspended from the zygomatic arch using multiple passes to recreate the appropriate vectors. The lip is over-corrected initially (lateralized) to create a more natural lip position in the long-term. The lower lip can be everted and depressed using the anterior belly of digastric as a semi-dynamic reconstruction (Tulley et al, 2000).

All of the above-mentioned components are undertaken primarily. Other minor corrections can be performed secondarily such as a brow lift, revision canthoplasty, or tarsorrhaphy and flap revision to remove excess bulk.

ADJUVANT THERAPY FOPR CANCER METASTATIC TO THE PAROTID GLAND

Squamous Cell Carcinoma (SCC)

Adjuvant therapy for metastatic SCC to the parotid includes: radiotherapy, concurrent chemotherapy.

Radiotherapy (RT)

Traditionally, the parotid was regarded as *radio-resistant* and there is limited data regarding *primary* RT treatment for metastases to the parotid. One such study reported a 2-year local control rate of 50% in14 patients (Krengli,

Pisani, & Pia, 1993). After 5 years the figure dropped to 20%. The sole use of radiotherapy should be restricted to those in whom surgery is not possible. In patients with bulky disease, radiotherapy is likely to be palliative only.

Currently, in patients with metastatic SCC to the parotid, the vast majority will undergo *adjuvant* radiotherapy. Local failure rates with combined therapy are approximately one third of those with surgery alone. Guillamondegui et al. (1975) showed a reduction in local recurrence from 30% to 9% and Taylor et al. (1991) from 27% to 11%. Various radiation schedules have been used for metastatic cancer to the parotid; however, standard fractionation has been advocated as described below in Table 9 (Trans-Tasman Radiation Oncology Group, 2005).

Data from MD Anderson demonstrated that for high-risk SCC of the head and neck, increasing the post-operative dose beyond a biologically effective dose of 60 Gy increased the risk of late complications, with no increased benefit in loco-regional control (Peters et al, 1993). Where parotid metastases shave occurred 12 months or more following definitive treatment to the index lesion, consideration should be given to including the primary site and intervening dermal lymphatics in the treatment volume.

Concurrent Chemo-Radiotherapy

Concurrent radiotherapy and chemotherapy is superior over radiotherapy alone for advanced mucosal SCC. Recent data have also demonstrated improved loco-regional control and survival with concurrent chemo-radiation in the post-operative setting for high-risk mucosal cancer, albeit at the cost of a substantial increase in both early and late adverse effects. At present, there is no compelling data to suggest that the same benefit is present in cutaneous SCC and this is the subject of several trials (Cooper, Pajak, Forastiere, & Jacobs, 2004).

Current therapeutic agents have included *cisplatin* and *fluorouracil* in conjunction with radiotherapy. Brizel et al. (1998) reported on hyper-fractionated irradiation with or without concurrent chemotherapy. For mucosal cancer, Cisplatin was given for 5 days at a dose of 12 mg/m2 of body surface area/day and 600 mg/m2 of fluorouracil/day during weeks 1 and 6 of irradiation. Two cycles of cisplatin and fluorouracil were given after the completion of radiotherapy. Loco-regional control at 3 years was 70% in the combined group and 44% in radiotherapy alone. There was no statistically significant difference in overall complications of the two groups, although the rates of nasogastric feeding or gastrostomy feeding tubes were higher in the combined treatment group.

More recently, trials using *carboplatin* rather than cisplatin have been used in an attempt to minimize the toxicity, particularly for elderly patients who are most commonly affected by advanced cutaneous disease. For the Post-Operative Skin Trial (POST) trial, carboplatin is given once per week for six weeks, 30 minutes prior to radiotherapy. The dose is calculated according to Calvert formula and based on glomerular filtration rate (GFR).

Melanoma

Adjuvant therapy for metastatic melanoma includes: radiotherapy, chemo-immunotherapy.

Radiotherapy (RT)

Patients receiving RT have improved locoregional control, but not overall survival (Overgaard, 1986). Despite the high incidence of distant metastases, loco-regional control is a vital component in the management plan. Parotid metastases fall into the high-risk group for regional relapse (Table 10).

Table 10. Significant risk of regional disease

Significant Risk of Regional Disease
> 1 parotid node > 2 neck or axillary nodes > 3 groin nodes

Hypo-fractionated schedules are thought to improve the therapeutic ratio for melanoma (Bentzen et al, 1989). In one such study, indications for RT included microscopically involved or close surgically resected margins, neurotrophic desmoplastic histopathology, perineural spread, or tumor satellites. With a starting date for the majority of patients less than six weeks post-surgery, they received 30-36 Gy in six fractions over 18 days. Parotid and neck lymph node fields were treated with direct electron fields or photon wedge pair fields. In-field recurrence was the only significant predictor of survival (Stuckensen et al, 2000).

A randomized clinical trial proposed a schedule of 48 Gy delivered in 20 fractions over 30 days. Outcome measures included regional metastasis, as well as morbidity, patterns of relapse, and overall survival (Trans-Tasman Radiation Oncology Group, 2003).

Chemo-Immunotherapy

The role of chemotherapeutic agents and immunotherapy has yet to be established in the treatment of locally advanced or metastatic melanoma. It is proposed that *interferon-alfa* (IFN-α) may interfere with the growth of tumor cells (ECOG Trial National Cancer Institute Sponsor, 2005).

Also being investigated is whether there may be a synergistic role with IFN-α and *interleukin-2* (IL-2) in combination. IL-2 is thought to stimulate white blood cells to mount a response to melanoma cells (SWOG Trial National Cancer Institute Sponsor, 2005). It is hoped that colony-stimulating factors such as *sargramostim* may result in increased immune cells in bone marrow and peripheral blood, and also the use of vaccines has been postulated.

REFERENCES

Alphs, H. H., Eisele, D. W., & Westra, W. H. (2006). The role of fine needle aspiration in the evaluation of parotid masses. *Current Opinion in Otolaryngology & Head & Neck Surgery*, *14*(2), 62–66. doi:10.1097/01.moo.0000193184.38310.0a PMID:16552260

Andruchow, J., Veness, M. J., Morgam, G. T., Gao, K., Clifford, A., Shannon, K. F., ... O'Brien, C. J. (2006). Implications for clinical staging of metastatic cutaneous squamous carcinoma of the head and neck based on a multicenter study of treatment outcomes. *Cancer*, *106*(5), 1078–1083. doi:10.1002/cncr.21698 PMID:16444748

Audet, N., Palme, C., Gullane, P., Gilbert, R., Brown, D., Irish, J., & Neligan, P. (2004). Cutaneous metastatic squamous cell carcinoma to the parotid gland: Analysis and outcome. *Head & Neck*, *26*(8), 727–732. doi:10.1002/hed.20048 PMID:15287040

Bae, Y. C., Zuker, R. M., Manktelow, R. T., & Wade, S. (2006). A comparison of commissure excursion following gracilis muscle transplantation for facial paralysis using a cross face nerve graft versus the motor nerve to the masseter nerve. *Plastic and Reconstructive Surgery*, *117*(7), 2407–2413. doi:10.1097/01.prs.0000218798.95027.21 PMID:16772949

Ballo, M. T., & Ang, K. K. (2003). Radiation therapy for malignant melanoma. *The Surgical Clinics of North America*, *83*(2), 323–342. doi:10.1016/S0039-6109(02)00096-8 PMID:12744612

Barr, L. C., Skene, A. I., Fish, S., & Thomas, J. M. (1994). Superficial parotidectomy in the treatment of cutaneous melanoma of the head and neck. *British Journal of Surgery*, *81*(1), 64–65. doi:10.1002/bjs.1800810121 PMID:8313124

Belhocine, T. Z., Scott, A. M., Even-Sapir, E., Urbain, J.-L., & Essner, R. (2006). Role of nuclear medicine in the management of cutaneous malignant melanoma. *Journal of Nuclear Medicine*, *47*, 957–967. PMID:16741305

Bell, D. J., & Gaillard, F. (2003). *UICC, TNM Staging*. Radiopaedia.

Bentzen, S. M., Overgaard, J., Thames, H. D., Overgaard, M., Hansen, P. V., von der Maase, H., & Meder, J. (1989). Clinical radiobiology of malignant melanoma. *Radiotherapy and Oncology: Journal of the European Society for Therapeutic Radiology and Oncology*, *16*(3), 169–182. doi:10.1016/0167-8140(89)90017-0 PMID:2587808

Brizel, D., Albers, M., Fisher, S., Scher, R., Richtsmeier, W. J., Hars, V., ... Prosnitz, L. R. (1998). Hyperfractionated irradiation with or without concurrent chemotherapy for locally advanced head and neck cancer. *The New England Journal of Medicine*, *338*(25), 798–1804. doi:10.1056/NEJM199806183382503 PMID:9632446

Bron, L., Traynor, M. D., McNeil, E., & O'Brien, C. J. (2003). Primary and metastatic cancer of the parotid: Comparison of clinical behavior in 232 cases. *The Laryngoscope*, *113*, 1070–1075. doi:10.1097/00005537-200306000-00029 PMID:12782825

Caldwell, C. B., & Spiro, R. H. (1988). The role of parotidectomy in the treatment of cutaneous head and neck melanoma. *American Journal of Surgery*, *156*(4), 318–322. doi:10.1016/S0002-9610(88)80303-9 PMID:3177759

Chao, C., Wong, S. L., Edwards, M. J., Ross, M. I., Reintgen, D. S., Noyles, R. D., ... McMasters, K. M. (2003). Sentinel lymph node biopsy for head and neck melanomas. *Annals of Surgical Oncology*, *10*(1), 21–26. doi:10.1245/ASO.2003.06.007 PMID:12513955

Clark, J., & Wang, S. (2016). Metastatic cancer to the parotid. *Advances in Oto-Rhino-Laryngology*, *78*, 95–103. doi:10.1159/000442129 PMID:27092549

Clark, J. R., Veness, M. J., Gilbert, R., O'Brien, C. J., & Gullane, P. J. (2007). Merkel cell carcinoma of the head and neck: Is adjuvant radiotherapy necessary? *Head & Neck*, *29*(3), 249–257. doi:10.1002/hed.20510 PMID:17163472

Cooper, J., Pajak, T., Forastiere, A., Jacobs, J., Campbell, B. H., Saxman, S. B., ... Fu, K. K. (2004). Postoperative concurrent radiotherapy and chemotherapy for high risk squamous cell carcinoma of the head and neck. *The New England Journal of Medicine*, *350*(19), 1937–1944. doi:10.1056/NEJMoa032646 PMID:15128893

Coppa, G. F., & Oszczakiewicz, M. (1990). Parotid gland metastasis from renal carcinoma. *International Surgery*, *75*(3), 198–202. PMID:2242976

Disa, J. J., Pusic, A. L., Hidlago, D. H., & Cordeiro, P. G. (2001). Simplifying microvascular reconstruction: A rational approach to donor site selection. *Annals of Plastic Surgery*, *47*(4), 385–389. doi:10.1097/00000637-200110000-00004 PMID:11601572

ECOG Trial National Cancer Institute Sponsor. *US ECOG-* 1697, 2005.

Eicher, S., Clayman, G., Myers, J., & Gillenwater, A. (2002). A prospective study of intraoperative lymphatic mapping for head and neck cutaneous melanoma. *Archives of Otolaryngology--Head & Neck Surgery*, *128*(3), 241–246. doi:10.1001/archotol.128.3.241 PMID:11886337

Essner, R. (2003). Surgical treatment of malignant melanoma. *The Surgical Clinics of North America*, *83*(1), 109–156. doi:10.1016/S0039-6109(02)00205-0 PMID:12691453

Guillamondegui, O. M., Byers, R. M., Luna, M. A., Chiminazzo, H. Jr, Jesse, R. H., & Fletcher, G. H. (1975). Aggressive surgery in treatment for parotid cancer; the role of adjuvant postoperative radiotherapy. *American Journal of Roentgentology*, *123*(1), 49–53. doi:10.2214/ajr.123.1.49 PMID:164132

Joseph, M. G., Zulueta, W. P., & Kennedy, P. J. (1992). Squamous cell carcinoma of the skin of the trunk and limbs: The incidence of metastases and their outcome. *The Australian and New Zealand Journal of Surgery*, *62*(9), 697–701. doi:10.1111/j.1445-2197.1992.tb07065.x PMID:1520151

Kashiwagi, N., Murakami, T., Toguchi, M., Nakanishi, K., Hidaka, S., Fukui, H., ... Tomiyama, N. (2016). Metastases to the parotid nodes: CT and MR imaging findings. *Dento Maxillo Facial Radiology*, *45*(8), 20160201. doi:10.1259/dmfr.20160201 PMID:27635667

Khurana, V. G., Mentis, D. H., O'Brien, C. J., Hurst, T. L., Stevens, G. N., & Packham, N. A. (1995). Parotid and neck metastases from cutaneous squamous cell carcinoma of the head and neck. *American Journal of Surgery*, *170*(5), 446–450. doi:10.1016/S0002-9610(99)80326-2 PMID:7485729

King, A. D., Ahuja, A. T., Leung, S. F., Wynnie, W. M., Jeo, P., Chan, Y.-L., & Metrwelli, C. (2000). Neck node metastases from nasopharyngeal carcinoma: MR imaging patterns of disease. *Head & Neck*, *22*(3), 275–281. doi:10.1002/(SICI)1097-0347(200005)22:3<275::AID-HED10>3.0.CO;2-N PMID:10748451

Krengli, M., Pisani, P., & Pia, F. (1993). Exclusive radiotherapy of parotid metastases. Results in 14 cases. *La Radiologia Medica*, *86*(5), 684–686. PMID:8272555

Mack, L., & McKinnon, G. (2004). Controversies in the management of metastatic melanoma to regional lymphatic basins. *Journal of Surgical Oncology*, *86*(4), 189–199. doi:10.1002/jso.20080 PMID:15221926

Malata, C., Camilleri, I., McLean, N., Piggott, T., & Soames, J. (1998). Metastatic tumors of the parotid gland. *British Journal of Oral & Maxillofacial Surgery*, *36*(3), 190–195. doi:10.1016/S0266-4356(98)90496-X PMID:9678884

McKean, M. E., Lee, K., & McGregor, I. A. (1985). The distribution of lymph nodes in and around the parotid gland: An anatomical study. *British Journal of Plastic Surgery*, *38*(1), 1–5. doi:10.1016/0007-1226(85)90078-5 PMID:3967103

Moore, B. A., Wine, T., & Netterville, J. L. (2005). Cervicofacial and cervicothoracic rotation flaps in head and neck reconstruction. *Head & Neck*, *27*(12), 1092–1101. doi:10.1002/hed.20252 PMID:16265654

Myers, J. N. (1999). Value of neck dissection in the treatment of patients with intermediate–thickness cutaneous malignant melanoma of the head and neck. *Archives of Otolaryngology--Head & Neck Surgery*, *125*(1), 110–115. doi:10.1001/archotol.125.1.110 PMID:9932599

O'Brien, C. J. (2006). The parotid gland as a metastatic basin for cutaneous cancer. *Archives of Otolaryngology--Head & Neck Surgery*, *131*(7), 551–555. doi:10.1001/archotol.131.7.551 PMID:16027274

O'Brien, C. J., Coates, A. S., Petersen-Schaefer, K., & McCarthy, W. H. (1993). Experience with 998 cutaneous melanomas of the head and neck. *Cancer*, *71*, 751–758.

O'Brien, C. J., McNeil, E. D., McMahon, J. D., Pathak, I., & Lauer, C. S. (2001). Incidence of cervical node involvement in metastatic cutaneous malignancy involving the parotid gland. *Head & Neck*, *23*(9), 744–748. doi:10.1002/hed.1106 PMID:11505484

O'Brien, C. J., Petersen-Schaefer, K., Ruark, D., Menzie, S. J., & Harrison, R. I. (1995). Radical, modified and selective neck dissection for cutaneous malignant melanoma. *Head & Neck*, *17*(3), 232–241. doi:10.1002/hed.2880170311 PMID:7782208

O'Brien, C. J., Peterson-Schaefer, K., Stevens, G., Bass, P. C., Tew, P., Gebski, V. J., ... McCarthy, W. H. (1997). Adjuvant radiotherapy following neck dissection and parotidectomy for metastatic malignant melanoma. *Head & Neck*, *19*(7), 589–594. doi:10.1002/(SICI)1097-0347(199710)19:7<589::AID-HED5>3.0.CO;2-3 PMID:9323147

Overgaard, J. (1986). The role of radiotherapy in recurrent and metastatic malignant melanoma: A clinical radiobiological study. *International Journal of Radiation Oncology, Biology, Physics*, *12*(6), 867–872. doi:10.1016/0360-3016(86)90378-0 PMID:2424880

Pedraza, V., Guerrero, M. R., & Luna, J. D. (2001). Time-doseresponse relationship in postoperatively irradiated patients with head and neck squamous cell carcinomas. *Radiotherapy and Oncology: Journal of the European Society for Therapeutic Radiology and Oncology*, *60*(2), 137–145. doi:10.1016/S0167-8140(01)00381-4 PMID:11439208

Peters, L. J., Goepfert, H., Ang, K. K., Byers, R. M., Maor, M. H., Guillamondegui, O., ... Brown, B. W. (1993). Evaluation of the dose for post-operative radiation therapy of head and neck cancer: First report of a prospective randomized trial. *International Journal of Radiation Oncology, Biology, Physics*, *26*(1), 3–11. doi:10.1016/0360-3016(93)90167-T PMID:8482629

Pistre, V., Pelissier, P., Martin, D., Lim, A., & Baudet, J. (2001). Ten years experience with the submental flap. *Plastic and Reconstructive Surgery*, *108*(6), 1576–1581. doi:10.1097/00006534-200111000-00021 PMID:11711930

Poulsen, M. (2004). Merkel-cell carcinoma of the skin. *The Lancet. Oncology*, *5*(10), 593–599. doi:10.1016/S1470-2045(04)01593-1 PMID:15465461

Seethala, R. R., LiVolsi, V. A., & Baloch, Z. W. (2005). Relative accuracy of fine-needle aspiration and frozen section in the diagnosis of the parotid gland. *Head & Neck*, *27*(3), 217–223. doi:10.1002/hed.20142 PMID:15672359

Shah, J. P., Kraus, D. H., Dubner, S., & Sarkar, S. (1991). Patterns of regional lymph node metastases from cutaneous melanomas of the head and neck. *American Journal of Surgery*, *162*(4), 32–323. doi:10.1016/0002-9610(91)90140-9 PMID:1951882

Stuckensen, T., Kovacs, A. F., Adams, S., & Baum, R. P. (2000). Staging of the neck in patients with oral cavity squamous cell carcinomas: A prospective comparison of PET, ultrasound, CT and MRI. *Journal of Cranio-Maxillo-Facial Surgery*, *28*(6), 319–324. doi:10.1054/jcms.2000.0172 PMID:11465137

SWOG Trial National Cancer Institute Sponsor. *SWOG* S0008, 2005.

Tan, S. T., & MacKinnon, C. A. (2006). Deep plane cervicofacial flap: A useful and versatile technique in head and neck surgery. *Head & Neck*, *28*(1), 46–55. doi:10.1002/hed.20317 PMID:16302190

Taylor, B. W., Brant, T. A., Mendenhall, N. P., Mendenhall, W. M., Cassisi, N. J., Stringer, S. P., & Million, R. R. (1991). Carcinoma of the skin metastatic to parotid area lymph nodes. *Head & Neck*, *13*(5), 427–433. doi:10.1002/hed.2880130510 PMID:1938361

Trans-Tasman Radiation Oncology Group. (2005, March). TROG 05.01. Post-operative concurrent chemo-radiotherapy versus post-operative radiotherapy in high-risk cutaneous squamous cell carcinoma of the head and neck. *Version*, *1*, 11.

Trans-Tasman Radiation Oncology Group Inc. Australia and New Zealand melanoma trials group. A randomized clinical trial of surgery versus surgery plus adjuvant radiotherapy for regional control in patients with completed resected macroscopic nodal metastatic melanoma TROG 02.01 ANZMTG Trial 1–02 July 2003.

Tulley, P., Webb, A., Chana, J. S., Tan, S. T., Hudson, D. A., Grobbelaar, A. O., & Harrison, D. U. (2000). Paralysis of the marginal mandibular branch of the facial nerve: Treatment options. *British Journal of Plastic Surgery*, *53*(5), 378–385. doi:10.1054/bjps.2000.3318 PMID:10876273

Vaglini, M., Belli, F., Santinami, M., & Cascinelli, N. (1990). The role of parotidectomy in the treatment of nodal metastases from cutaneous melanoma of the head and neck. *European Journal of Surgical Oncology*, *16*, 28–32. PMID:2307240

Veness, M., Morgan, G., Palme, C., & Gebski, V. (2005). Surgery and Adjuvant radiotherapy in patients with cutaneous head and neck squamous cell carcinoma metastatic to lymph nodes: Combined treatment should be considered best practice. *The Laryngoscope*, *115*(5), 870–875. doi:10.1097/01.MLG.0000158349.64337.ED PMID:15867656

Veness, M. J., Morgan, G. J., & Gebski, V. (2005). Adjuvant locoregional radiotherapy as best practice in patients with Merkel cell carcinoma of the head and neck. *Head & Neck*, *27*(3), 208–216. doi:10.1002/hed.20134 PMID:15627249

Woods, J. E., Chong, G. C., & Beahrs, O. H. (1975). Experience with 1360 primary parotid tumors. *American Journal of Surgery*, *130*(4), 460–462. doi:10.1016/0002-9610(75)90484-5 PMID:1166937

Chapter 16
Parotidectomy

ABSTRACT

In this chapter, the history of parotidectomy is provided, and indications, contraindications, pre-operative planning, and the different techniques of parotidectomy procedures are described. These include different types of parotidectomy (superficial or lateral parotidectomy, radical parotidectomy, and extended total parotidectomy), limited procedures (partial superficial parotidectomy and extra-capsular dissection), and enucleation (extra-capsular and intracapsular). Indications include neoplasms, inflammatory lesions, salivary duct stones, and sialorrhea. Post-operative complications are discussed. These are either early complications (facial nerve palsy, bleeding/hematoma, surgical site infection, skin flap necrosis, salivary fistula/sialocele, seroma, external otitis, and trismus) or late complications (Frey's syndrome, hypertrophic scar/keloid, unsightly scar, soft tissue defect, and recurrence).

HISTORY OF THE PROCEDURE

Salivary gland surgery dates back to the sixteenth century. The anatomy of the parotid gland and the role of the main ducts were described in the mid-seventeenth century. The earliest references to parotid swellings or "para-auricular swellings," as the Greeks called them, described the findings associated with calculi and inflammation.

Between 1650 and 1750, salivary gland surgery was limited to the treatment of ranulas and oral calculi. The concept of surgical excision of a parotid tumor has been attributed to *Bertrandi* in 1802. The initial applications of this

DOI: 10.4018/978-1-7998-5603-0.ch016

surgery included an extensive approach, which caused serious disfigurement and disability.

In about the 1850s, the focus shifted toward dissection and the intimate relationship between the facial nerve and the parotid gland. Attempts were made to perform the surgery with nerve preservation. In 1846, *John C. Warren*, a physician, was the first to use ether inhalation anesthesia during resection of a parotid tumor in Boston. In 1892, *Codreanu* (a Romanian native) performed the first total parotidectomy with facial nerve preservation.

Before the 1940s, *enucleation* of benign neoplastic processes (e.g. pleomorphic adenoma) was the most common extirpative procedure; however, it was associated with high recurrence rates (RR) reaching up to 43%. This high RR was attributed at that time to "multicentricity" of the tumor. The reason to perform enucleation rather than removal of the gland was concern regarding injury to the facial nerve. *Janes* (1940) and *Bailey* (1941) performed *superficial parotidectomy* and reported a lower RR than enucleation albeit at the expense of increased facial nerve complications.

Martin (1952) and Patey (1958) reported that the reason for recurrence after enucleation was the incomplete capsule of the lesion (tumor satellites).

In 1958, *Beahrs and Adson* eloquently described the relevant anatomy and surgical technique of current parotid gland surgery. They stressed the importance of surgical landmarks for avoiding injury to the facial nerve and advocated complete removal of the superficial portion of the parotid gland for non-invasive lesions confined to that location.

Recently, the introduction of *bipolar diathermy, magnifying loups and nerve stimulator* in parotid surgery resulted in better results and allowed limited resections such as *partial superficial parotidectomy* (PSP) and *extra-capsular dissection* (ECD) with low RRs and less facial nerve complications (injury – Frey's syndrome).

TYPES OF PAROTID PROCEDURES

Throughout history, many different types and techniques have been developed in order to complete a parotidectomy and consequently, many different names have been associated with each type. However, there are really only two main distinctions to be made in parotidectomies (McGurk & Combes, 2013):

1. Specific nerve(s) to be dissected or not dissected?
2. The amount of gland excised / recurrence?

The various and main techniques associated with parotid surgery are summarized in Table 1.

Table 1. Parotid surgery techniques

Parotidectomy	Limited Surgery	Enucleation
- Superficial (Lateral) parotidectomy - Total parotidectomy - Radical parotidectomy - Extended total parotidectomy	- Partial superficial parotidectomy (PSP) - Extra-capsular dissection (ECD)	- Extra-capsular - Intra-capsular

Superficial) (Lateral) Parotidectomy

It entails excising the superficial lobe of the gland lateral to the facial nerve. There are two types; formal and partial:

- **Formal superficial parotidectomy:** Superficial parotidectomy where the main trunk of the facial nerve and its 2 divisions (cervico-facial and temporo-facial) and their branches are dissected;[2]
- **Partial superficial parotidectomy (PSP):** It is similar to superficial parotidectomy but only the portion of the gland surrounding the neoplasm is excised. The main trunk of the facial nerve and only one division with its branches are dissected during this procedure (Alexander, 2013).

Total Parotidectomy

It entails total removal of both lobes of the parotid gland. It is typically performed if the neoplasm is affecting the deep part of parotid gland. The surgeon tries to remove the gland apart from the facial nerve, yet dissecting all branches of the facial nerve (Howe, Yu, Wai, Tsang, & William 2012).

Radical (Non-Conservative) Parotidectomy

Radical or non-conservative parotidectomy is typically performed if the malignant neoplasm is impinging on the facial nerve, which is excised in addition to the parotid gland i.e. in addition to total parotidectomy (Motamed, Laugharne, & Bradley, (2003).

Extended Total Parotidectomy

It means total parotidectomy plus excision of adjacent structures such as the overlying skin, the underlying mandible, temporal bone and external auditory canal, or the deep musculature of the para-pharyngeal space.

Extra-Capsular Dissection (ECD)

In this limited resection procedure, only the tumor and a surrounding cuff of normal parotid tissue (about 2-3 mm) are excised. In such case, neither the main trunk of the facial nerve nor its 2 divisions or terminal branches are dissected (Figure 1).

Figure 1. Extra-capsular dissection (ECD)

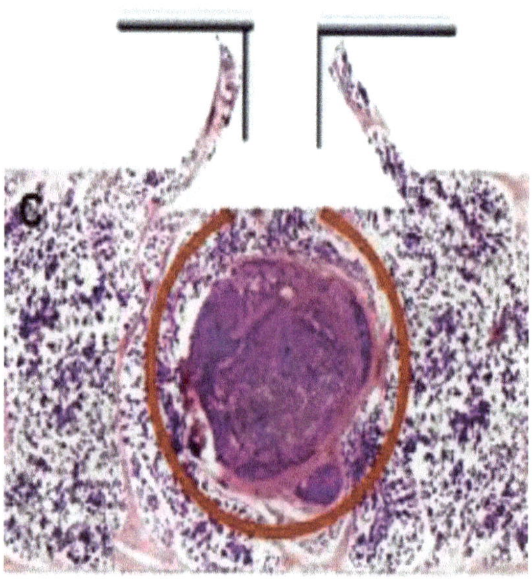

Enucleation

It was the most common extirpative procedure for benign neoplastic lesions (e.g. pleomorphic adenoma) before the 1940s. It is of two types:

- **Extra-capsular Enucleation:** In this procedure, the tumor with its capsule is enucleated from the rest of the parotid tissue (Figure 2);

Figure 2. Extra-capsular enucleation

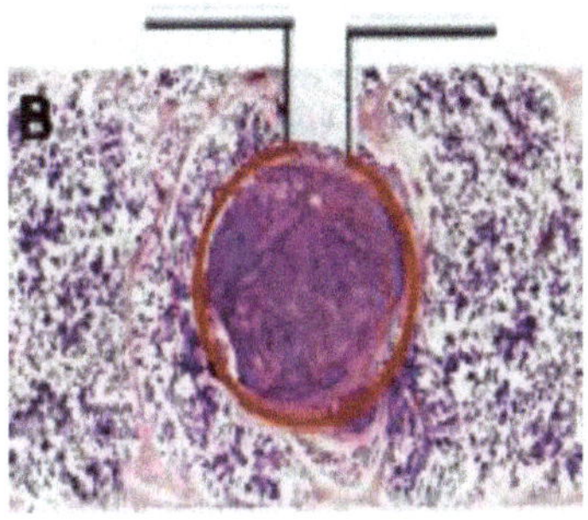

- **Intra-capsular Enucleation:** In this procedure, the tumor is enucleated from within its capsule (Figure 3).

Figure 3. Intra-capsular enucleation

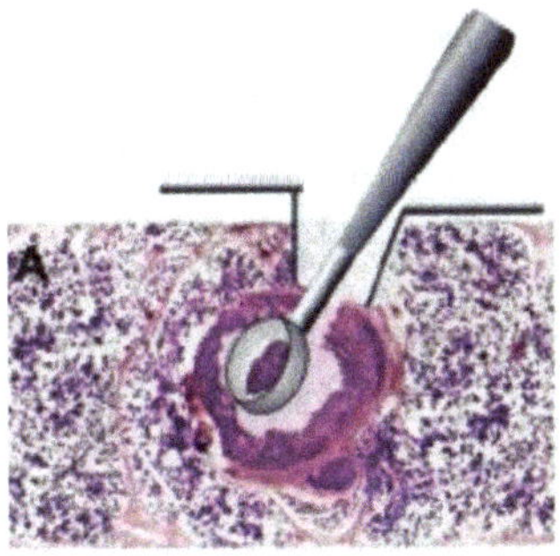

INDICAITONS OF PAROTIDECTOMY

Indications of parotidectomy include the following.

Neoplasms are the most common indication for parotidectomy. The vast majority of primary parotid tumors are benign, but approximately 20% are found to be malignant. In addition, regional and distant disease can metastasize to the parotid and necessitate removal for diagnosis or cure.

Inflammatory processes (e.g. chronic parotitis, deep salivary calculi, or parotid abscess) are occasionally treated with total parotidectomy, with the recognition that surgery in an inflamed gland probably carries a higher risk of post-operative facial nerve dysfunction (Motamed, Laugharne, & Bradley, 2003).

Salivary duct stones may be approached through minimal external parotid incisions, and are aided by sialendoscopy when possible.

Sialorrhea (excessive salivation) is rarely treated with parotidectomy; more often, it is medically managed with anti-sialagogues or botulinum toxin or treated with duct ligation.

CONTRAINDICATIONS OF PAROTIDECTOMY

Patients with benign tumors of the parotid gland who are at *high anesthetic risk* may be observed on a case-by-case basis.

Patients with *multiple parotid cysts* should be tested for human immunodeficiency virus (HIV) before undergoing surgical excision. Benign lymphoepithelial cysts are relatively common in the HIV-positive population but otherwise uncommon. Because these cysts are usually multiple and tend to recur, they are typically managed by means of repeated aspiration or sclerotherapy rather than parotidectomy; they may also respond to anti-retroviral therapy (Dave, Pernas, & Roy, 2007).

PERI-PROCEDURAL CARE

Pre-Procedural Planning

Measures that may be considered before parotidectomy include diagnostic imaging, fine-needle aspiration (FNA), and neck dissection.

Pre-Operative Imaging

Both computed tomography (CT) and magnetic resonance imaging (MRI) can be helpful in operative planning, but they may not be necessary in patients with small, mobile tumors of the parotid tail. Any clinical feature suggestive of malignancy (eg, lymphadenopathy, fixation to surrounding structures, or preoperative facial nerve weakness) warrants radiographic evaluation of the parotid gland and nodal basins in the neck.

Imaging can provide useful clues to the relation between the tumor and the facial nerve. If the tumor lies in a plane inferior to the stylomastoid foramen, the nerve will probably lie on the superior surface of the tumor; likewise, if the tumor is high in the gland, the nerve may pass inferiorly. If the tumor occupies the most superficial portion of the gland, with a significant area of parotid tissue deep to it, the nerve is likely to be deep to the tumor; similarly, a deep tumor abutting the mandible should have the nerve on its superficial surface.

Fine-Needle Aspiration (FNA)

Fine-needle aspiration (FNA) can be used to diagnose parotid tumors preoperatively with a high degree of sensitivity and specificity.[6] With small, mobile tumors of the tail of the parotid, preoperative histological diagnosis may not be required, but even in this setting; such diagnosis can contribute to patient counseling and informed consent. If a malignant tumor is suspected on the basis of radio graphical evaluation or physical examination, FNA should be done to establish the diagnosis and help guide operative planning. If pre-operative FNA is non-diagnostic, intra-operative frozen-section evaluation can be used to establish the diagnosis in most cases (Seethala, LiVolsi, & Baloch, 2005).

Neck Dissection

Removal of all palpable or radiographically suspicious lymph nodes (LNs) via selective neck dissection is appropriate in the setting of malignancy. Elective neck dissection is controversial and usually is performed only for high-grade malignancies in the N0 neck (Kawata, 2010; Emerick, 2007).

Equipment

Some surgeons use a *facial nerve monitor* to facilitate identification of the facial nerve. This device consists of electromyography (EMG) electrodes that are placed, at a minimum, in the orbicularis oris and the orbicularis oculi. Stimulation of the cervico-facial and temporo-facial divisions of the facial nerve causes the respective muscles to contract. In addition to the stimulation inherent in manipulation of the nerve, a probe can be connected to the monitor to permit direct stimulation of suspected nerve branches.

At present, there is no substantial evidence to suggest that continuous EMG facial nerve monitoring prevents injury to the facial nerve (Grosheva, 2009; Sood, 2015). Moreover, intra-operative abnormalities on the facial nerve monitor have not been shown to predict post-operative dysfunction (Meier, Wenig, Manders, & Nenonene, 2006).

The facial nerve can also be monitored through simple observation of facial twitching, although such monitoring requires a vigilant observer during facial nerve dissection. When identification of the facial nerve is in question, the nerve can be directly stimulated with a handheld nerve stimulator to elicit twitching.

TECHNICAL CONSIDERATIONS

Positive identification and preservation of the *facial nerve* are essential for preventing inadvertent facial nerve injury. A thorough understanding of the anatomy of the stylomastoid foramen, the facial nerve, and the parotid gland and its surrounding structures underlies identification and preservation of the nerve. Whenever possible, a normal cuff of parotid tissue should be resected around a tumor to prevent recurrence (Witt, 2002). In the setting of a benign tumor, if a facial nerve branch is found directly on the tumor capsule, the nerve should be gently dissected off the tumor. In the setting of a malignancy, consideration should be given to sacrificing as opposed to preserving the nerve.

Raw gland surface contributes to post-operative salivary leakage (*sialocele or salivary fistula*). In addition, raw gland apposed to skin provides a ready pathway for post-ganglionic parasympathetic fibers to migrate from the salivary tissue and cross-innervate facial sweat glands, resulting in gustatory sweating (Frey syndrome). Efforts should be made to close the parotid capsule after removal of a parotid tumor or a portion of the gland. If closure of the capsule is not feasible, consideration should be given to interposing tissue (eg, dermal fat graft) (Honeybrook, Athavale, Rangarajan, Rohde, & Netterville, 2017) or implantable biologic material (eg, acellular dermis) between the raw gland and the skin.

Injury to the posterior branch of the *greater auricular nerve* (GAN), which supplies sensation to the ear, is often avoidable. If the nerve must be cut, it can be marked with a stitch to facilitate reapproximation at the conclusion of the operation. Patients should be warned to expect at least temporary earlobe numbness and should take precautions to prevent heat or cold injury to the insensate area (eg, frostbite or curling iron burns).

Closed suction drainage is used in most cases to prevent post-operative hematoma or seroma.

PATIENT PREPARATION

Anesthesia

Parotidectomy is typically performed with the patient under *general anesthesia*. To allow adequate monitoring of the facial nerve, paralytics should not be used beyond the induction of anesthesia. It is important to confirm that the patient has regained full motor function (as determined by twitch monitoring) before attempting to dissect out the facial nerve and its branches.

Positioning

The patient is placed in the supine position with the head turned as far as possible away from the side of the operation. A shoulder roll can help with neck extension and thereby facilitate surgical exposure.

The eye on the side to be operated on is lubricated and closed with either a transparent dressing (the authors' preference) or a fine suture that approximates the lids (the so-called tarsorrhaphy stitch). If continuous facial nerve monitoring is to be performed, monitoring electrodes are placed (at a minimum) in the orbicularis oris and the orbicularis oculi, and grounding electrodes are placed outside the field. Incisions are marked (see Technique), and local anesthetic with epinephrine is injected into the skin.

The face may be covered in a transparent dressing or may be prepared, with particular care taken around the eyes and mouth. The remainder of the operative field is prepared, including the temple, the ear, the preauricular and postauricular areas, and the neck. A cotton ball can be placed in the ear canal during prepping to prevent cleaning solution from collecting and causing postoperative irritation (if cleaning solution does get into the canal, it should be washed out with room temperature water or saline at the conclusion of the procedure).

SUPERFICIAL PAROTIDECTOMY

Incision

Skin incisions should be camouflaged in normal facial contours and should be placed with consideration of whether a neck dissection is necessary.

The anterior skin incision can be placed either in the pre-auricular crease or hidden post-tragally, in the manner of a face-lift procedure (Bianchi, Ferri, Ferrari, Copelli, & Sesenna, 2011). The position of the ear lobe should be precisely marked for repositioning at the conclusion of the procedure.

A *modified Blair (Lazy-S) incision* is planned in the pre-auricular skin crease just in front of the external auditory meatus (EAM). It then courses around the ear lobule to the base of the mastoid process, and then into an upper neck crease (Figure 4).

Figure 4. Standard incision: Blair incision (intra-operative and diagramatic presentation)

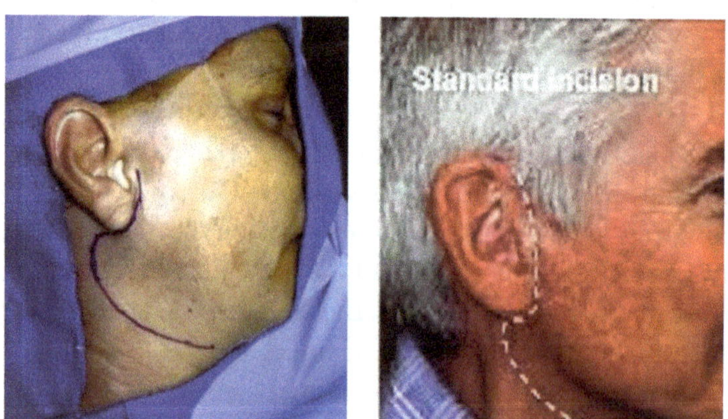

An alternative incision is a *modified face-lift incision*, which starts behind the tragus down to the lobule of the ear, then behind the ear in the crease and then curved in the hair line for a short distance as indicated. It may be extended into the hairline for cosmesis or curved down to a prominent neck crease to allow a neck dissection (Figure 5).

Figure 5. Modified face-lift incision (intra-operative and diagramatic presentation)

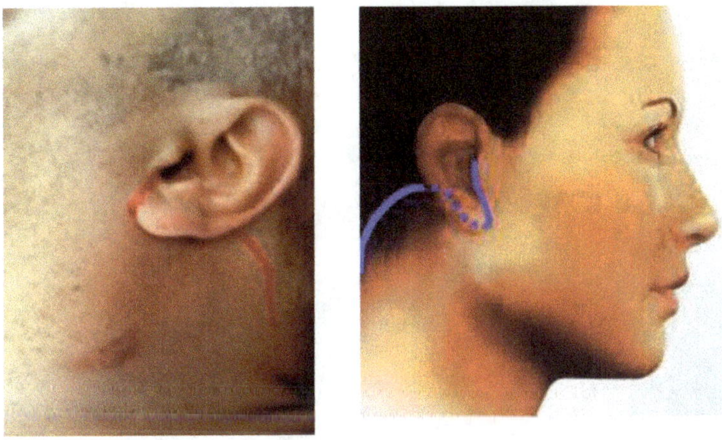

Technique (Steps of the Procedure)

Flap Creation

The skin incision is carried down through the subcutaneous (SC) tissues and platysma muscle. An anterior subplatysmal/subsuperficial musculo-aponeurotic system (SMAS) flap is made by using the natural plane on the surface of the parotid gland. This thick flap is elevated superficial to the GAN (which is preserved whenever possible) and the parotid fascia. Elevation of the flap is carried beyond the extent of the tumor to completely expose parotid fascia anterior to the tissue to be removed. Great caution is exercised in approaching the zygomatic arch, the anterior border of the parotid gland, and the submandibular fascia, all of which are areas where distal branches of the facial nerve emerge from the gland.

A posterior flap is then raised at the level of the sternocleidomastoid (SCM) fascia. At the uppermost end of the SCM, some muscle fibers are inserted into the skin and these must be transected. The GAN branches and

Figure 6. Greater auricular nerve has been transected near junction of parotid gland and sternocleidomastoid (SCM). Junction is marked with dotted line. Proximal nerve is left enveloped in fascia of SCM to aid in reapproximation at end of case. Posterior branch of greater auricular nerve can be seen crossing SCM more superiorly and was left intact. Image is courtesy of Dr. Alexander Langerman and Dr. James Netterville.

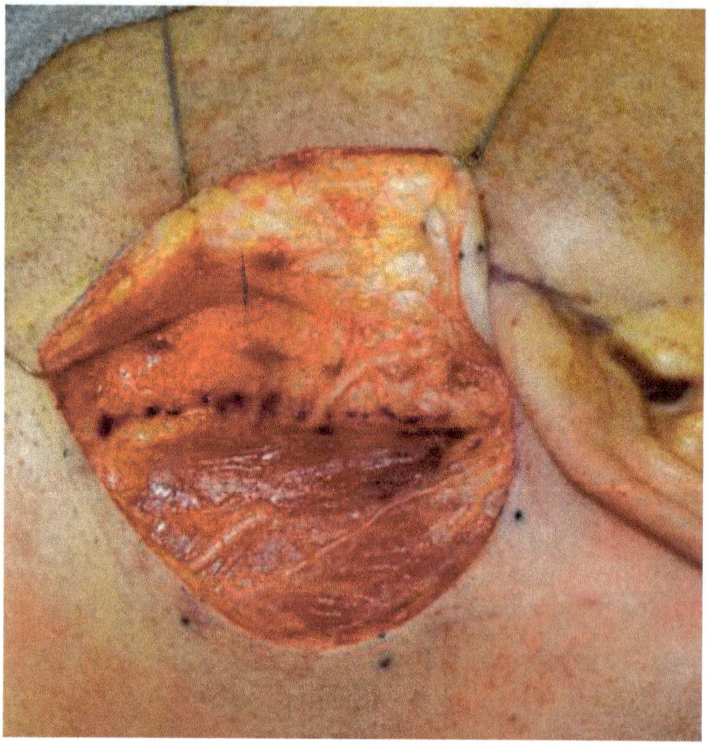

the external jugular vein (EJV) are identified, and the plane is developed superficial to these structures. At this point, if necessary, the anterior branch of the GAN is transected sharply and tagged for reanastomosis. The proximal end is left enveloped in SCM fascia to facilitate re-approximation at the end of the case (Figure 6). It is often necessary to ligate the EJV. The flaps are retracted with silk sutures or self-retaining hooks.

The tail of the parotid gland is elevated off the SCM until the posterior belly of the digastric muscle is seen. During this maneuver, one should watch for the small nerve branch to the posterior belly of the digastric muscle, which is not always seen but can provide a clue to the location of the facial nerve. More important in this area is to avoid the cervical and marginal branches, which usually pass over the facial veins and in the submandibular fascia. If the main trunk is to be identified, the posterior gland is then separated from the cartilage of the tragus and the external auditory canal, with care taken to preserve the perichondrium. This elevation is continued deep to the bony-cartilaginous junction. Once this step is accomplished, attention is turned to identification of the facial nerve.

Identification and Dissection of the Facial Nerve

The basic principle of facial nerve dissection is to avoid any unnecessary stimulation of the nerve. Specific tools used in dissection vary from surgeon to surgeon and include cold, bipolar electro-cauterization, and ultrasonic dissection. Most surgeons caution against the use of a monopolar cautery in close proximity to the facial nerve.

The nerve can be identified in any of the following six ways:

- The *tympano-mastoid suture line* can be followed to the stylo-mastoid foramen;
- The so-called *tragal pointer* is a triangular extension of cartilage inferiorly off the tragus and suggests the location of the facial nerve in the direction of its infero-anterior point;
- The *posterior belly of the digastric muscle* crosses the SCM approximately 1 cm inferior and 1 cm superficial to the location of the nerve; it is highly useful as a marker of the depth of the facial nerve;
- Any *peripheral branch*, including the branch to the digastric muscle, can be followed back to the main trunk, which is then dissected in the usual fashion;
- The *styloid process* can be exposed bluntly from a superior approach, and the nerve is found inferolateral to it. This is an especially useful approach in the setting of revision surgery, because the plane superior to the styloid process is typically not previously dissected;
- The *mastoid* can be drilled to allow identification of the facial nerve in settings of severely abnormal anatomy, complicated revision surgery, or large tumors abutting the stylomastoid foramen;
- If complete dissection of the nerve is planned, once the main trunk is identified it is traced to the pes anserinus, the structure marking the separation of the cervico-facial (lower) and temporofacial (upper) divisions (Figure 7);
- Smaller branches are then followed carefully with the aim of mapping their relation to the tumor. The typical approach is to start at the

Figure 7. Main trunk of facial nerve (asterisk) has been exposed to pes anserinus, branch point of upper (U) and lower (L) divisions. Image courtesy of Dr. Alexander Langerman.

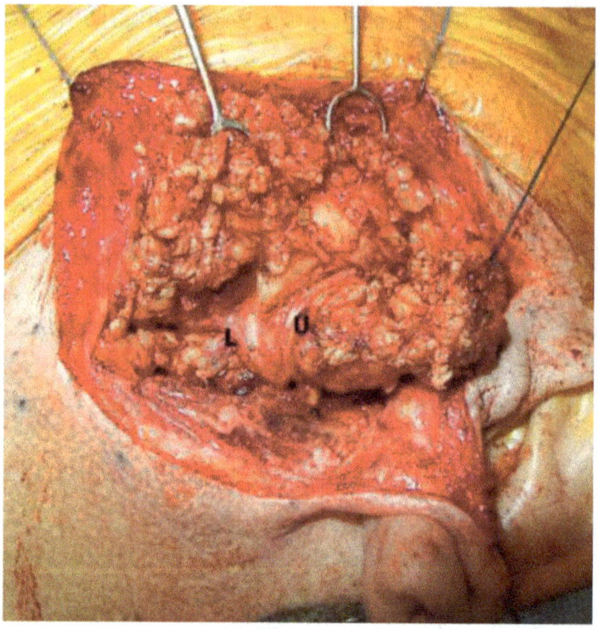

uppermost branch of the upper division or the lowermost branch of the lower division and follow the branch out to a point where it is well clear of the tumor. The next branch is then followed, and so forth, until all branches in the area of the tumor are dissected free and the tumor is mobilized for removal.

A common technique for nerve dissection is to use a small, fine hemostat or a non-locking, smooth-jawed, right-angle dissector (McCabe facial nerve dissector) to gently elevate the parotid tissue in the natural plane just superficial to each nerve. The tissue lateral to and between the tines of the instrument is sealed with a bipolar cautery and divided. Very cautious and gentle traction of the nerve can be accomplished with gauze held in a forceps (Figure 8).

In the setting of malignancy, especially if pre-operative facial nerve dysfunction is present, consideration is given to severing the nerves involved with the tumor and tagging them with non-absorbable sutures for immediate re-approximation, interposition or other grafting as appropriate either at the

Figure 8. Branch of facial nerve is dissected in natural plane just superficial to nerve with McCabe dissector. Gentle back traction is applied with small gauze sponge, and free gland is pulled away by clamp to provide forward traction.

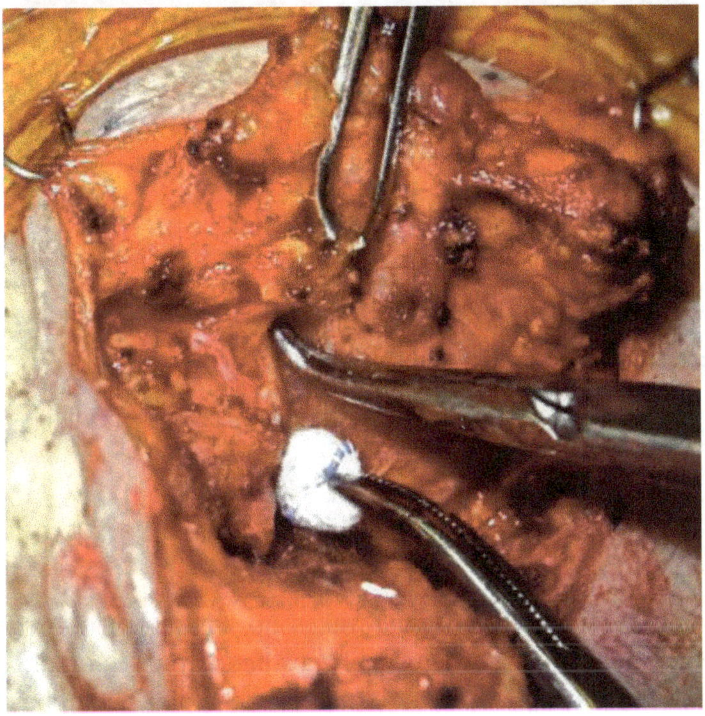

conclusion of the tumor removal or at a later time. Facial nerve repair is discussed in another chapter.

Removal of Parotid Tissue

If the whole superficial lobe of the parotid gland is to be removed (formal superficial parotidectomy), all of the facial nerve branches are dissected and mobilized. Any bleeding that occurs related to division of the gland is carefully controlled under vision.

Once tissue removal is complete, the facial nerve can be tested with a hand-held stimulator or monitor probe to confirm that it is unharmed. Repeated unnecessary stimulation of the nerve; however, is to be avoided out of concern for potential injury.

After the patient is gently awakened and has recovered from anesthesia, the face is examined for motor nerve function. If the facial nerve was not

Figure 9. The facial trunk is dissected and followed peripherally to expose and preserve the two divisions and terminal branches before removing the specimen

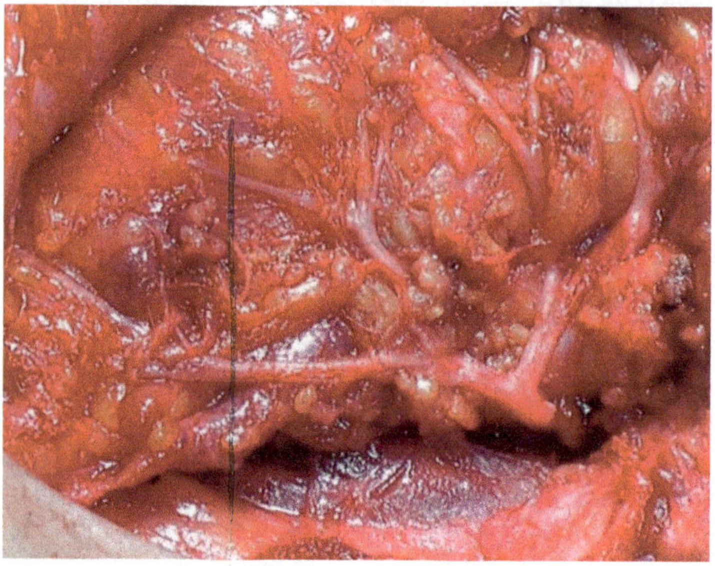

identified as intact and the patient wakes up with a dense paralysis that persists beyond the effects of any local anesthetic, re-exploration should be considered. If the nerve is known to be intact, the patient can be reassured that mild post-operative facial nerve weakness will usually resolve completely.

Reconstruction and Closure

Once the resection is complete and any necessary repair or grafting of the facial nerve has been performed, attention is turned to closure. The primary goals of reconstruction are (1) to cover any raw gland surface remaining, (2) to restore normal facial contours, and (3) to provide coverage of the facial nerve and a reliable plane of dissection in the event that reoperation proves necessary.

Many techniques are used for reconstruction. In small resections, the parotid capsule can often be closed *primarily*. In larger resections, the defect can be filled with autologous *buccal or abdominal fat* (Figure 10) or *acellular dermis* (Figure 11).

The digastric muscle can be cut at the intermediate tendon and the posterior belly rotated into the defect, or a superiorly based flap that includes a portion of the SCM can be used in a similar manner. However, muscle reconstruction

Figure 10. Abdominal fat with attached dermis has been implanted in parotidectomy defect. Fat maintains bulk well over time if handled atraumatically, and dermis allows closure of capsule.

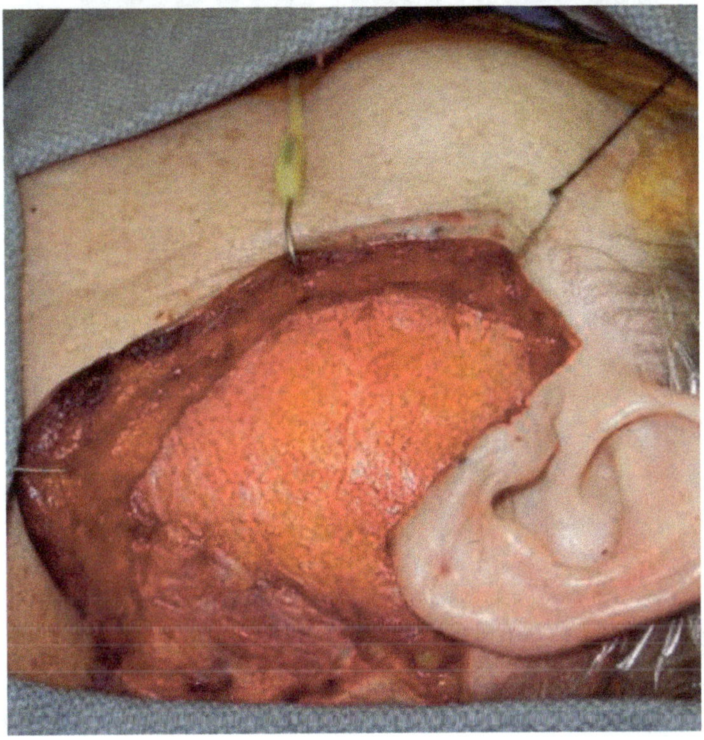

tends to lose volume over time. In massive resections involving removal of mandible or skin, options include skin such as the cervico-facial, myocutaneous (e.g. pectoralis major), and free flaps.

To reconstruct the GAN, the fascia next to the opposing ends of the cut nerve are sutured together to allow tension-free neurorrhaphy. Interrupted 8-0 or 9-0 nylon sutures are then placed in the perineurium to reapproximate the nerve. If the nerve cannot be re-approximated, some authors advocate clipping or burying the proximal end to prevent neuroma formation, although evidence for the effectiveness of these techniques is lacking.

Once reconstruction is complete, closed suction drains are placed through stab incisions in the posterior neck or hairline. The skin is then closed in layers in an interrupted fashion. To prevent a pixie-ear deformity, care is taken not to put excessive tension on the earlobe.

Figure 11. Rolled acellular dermis used to fill small defect after removal of parotid tumor

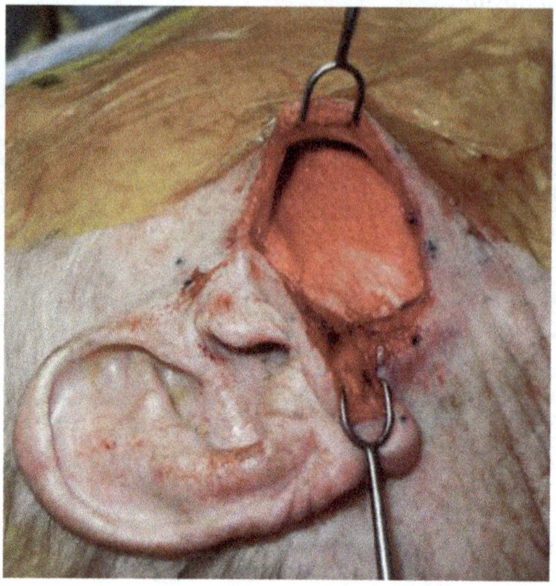

Post-Operative Care and Follow-Up

Duration of post-operative hospitalization is subject to change from patient to patient, with most patients being discharged within 24 hours after surgery (Davidson & Robind, 2013). For benign tumors and slow growing cancers, surgery typically provides a complete cure or remission with no evidence of disease (Davidson & Robind, 2013).

The drain is usually removed on the first post-operative day and the skin sutures are removed within one week. Long-term follow-up depends on the results of pathology. Most patients with benign tumors are followed every 3-6 months for two years and yearly thereafter. Patients with malignant tumors may be followed every 2-3 months for two years, and then every 6 months for 5 years after procedure (Davidson & Robind, 2013).

Mild facial numbness and weakness are normal immediately after a parotidectomy, with symptoms usually subsiding within a few months. Most patients regain full facial function within one year of the procedure (Davidson & Robind, 2013). Patients with facial nerve weakness should thus be regularly monitored and watched for improvement or stabilization; plans should be made for re-animation as necessary.

If a mass develops lateral to the SCM in the location of the GAN, a greater auricular neuroma should be considered. Such masses tend to be painful with manipulation. In the setting of benign disease, reassurance and treatment are both reasonable. Confirmation of this diagnosis with FNA or excision should be considered in the setting of a previous malignancy.

Main Complications of the Procedure

Early and late complications of superficial parotidectomy may occur. There is a reported 25-50% risk of facial nerve palsy directly after parotidectomy and a 1-2% risk of permanent weakness (Fyke & Sherk, 2013). Frey's syndrome may occur in up to 90% of patients (Fyke & Sherk, 2013). Risk of mortality is very low in reference to the surgery. Survival rates due to malignancy depend on the patient and extent of disease. A 10-year survival ranges from 32-83% (Fyke & Sherk, 2013).

PARTIAL SUPERFICIAL PAROTIDECTOMY (PSP)

Technique

Partial superficial parotidectomy (PSP) is started as superficial parotidectomy (SP) by identification of the main trunk of facial nerve and its bifurcation. The branch related to the tumor is completely identified and dissected depending on the tumor site whether in the lower part or in the upper part of the gland. A small part of the superficial parotid lobe containing the tumor with at least 1cm of healthy tissue around the tumor is stripped out from the branch of the facial nerve, related to the tumor. The procedure is completed in a similar fashion to formal SP.

Why Perform PSP?

Partial superficial parotidectomy (PSP) has been proposed as an alternative to formal superficial parotidectomy in certain situations for the following reasons; (1) about 50-60% of parotid tumors are in contact with only one division of the facial nerve, (2) the facial nerve can be preserved (protected) by minimal dissection at the interface between nerve branches and the tumor, and (3) the rate of recurrence can be minimized by dissection away from the parotid tumor (at least one-cm margin).

Tumors Amenable to PSP (Indications)

Not all parotid tumors are amenable to partial superficial parotidectomy. Only benign parotid tumors located in the superficial lobe in relation to upper (Figure 12 or lower (Figure 13) division of the facial nerve and/or its branches can be excised using this technique.

Figure 12. Parotid tumor in the superficial lobe in relation to the upper division of the facial nerve (amenable to PSP)

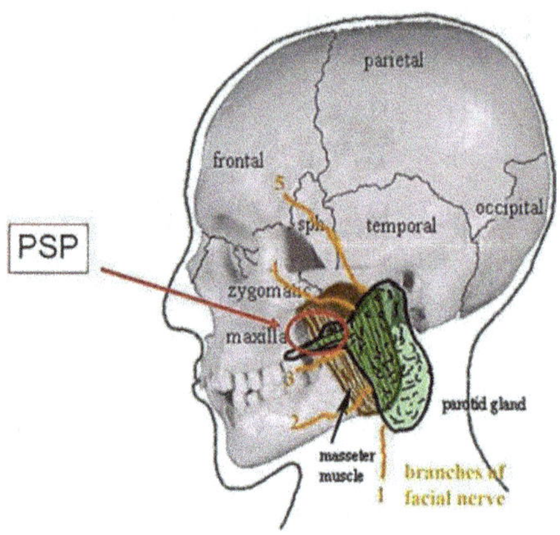

Figure 13. Parotid tumor in the parotid tail of the superficial lobe in relation to the lower division of the facial nerve (amenable to PSP)

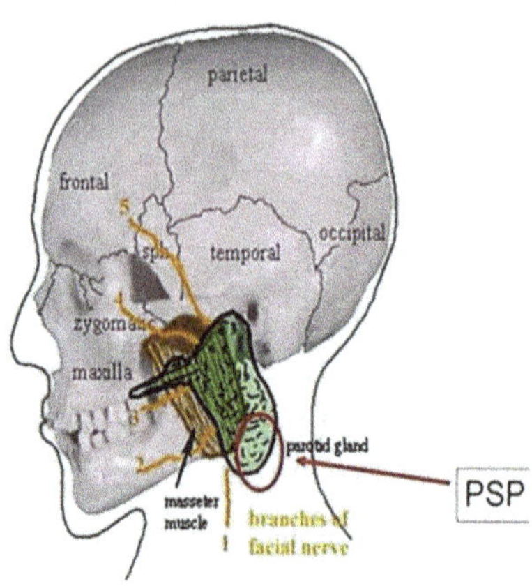

Figure 14. Large tumor (> 3 cm) involving most of the parotid gland. Not amenable to PSP. A formal superficial parotidectomy (SP) should be performed.

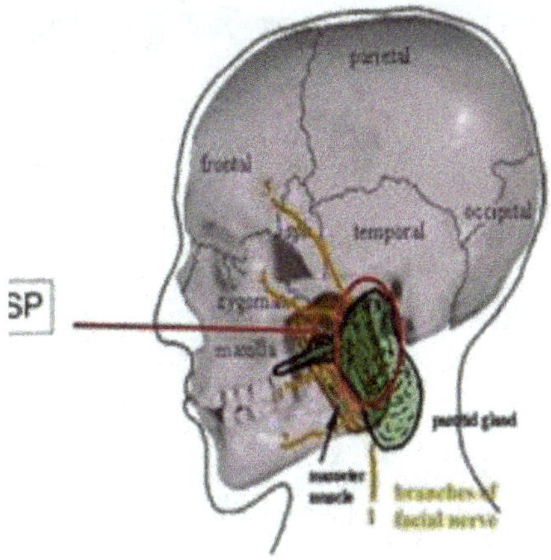

Contraindications

Partial superficial parotidectomy is contraindicated in the following conditions:

- Large tumors (> 3 cm) involving most of the parotid gland (Figure 15);
- Centrally-located tumors irrespective of size (Figure 16);
- Malignant tumors and suspicious tumors by FNAC;
- Previous parotid surgery;
- Deep lobe tumors;
- Facial nerve palsy;
- Scarring in or irradiation to the parotid area.

Results

Partial superficial parotidectomy (PSP) is an adequate and safe procedure for treatment of small benign parotid tumors located in the superficial lobe and related to only one division of the facial nerve. With PSP there is a considerable reduction of operative time and blood loss; at the same time, there is no increase in post-operative morbidity.

Figure 15. A centrally - located tumor in the superficial lobe of the parotid gland. Not amenable to PSP. A formal superficial parotid-ectomy (SP) should be performed.

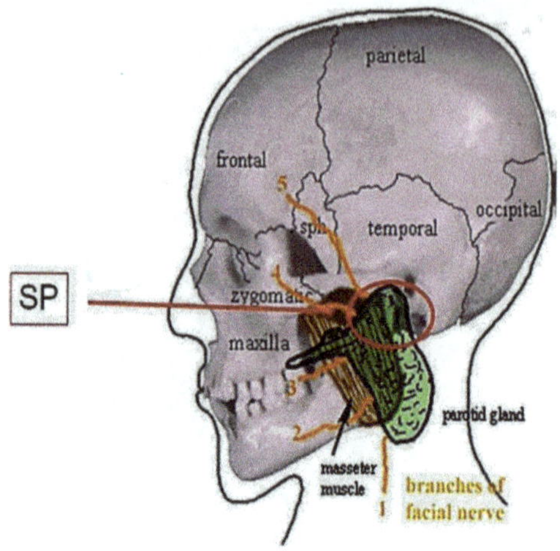

TOTAL PAROTIDECTOMY

While superficial parotidectomy entails removal of the lateral (superficial) portion of the parotid gland with preservation of the facial nerve, total parotidectomy entails complete removal of the superficial and deep lobes of the parotid. In such cases, all of the facial nerve branches are dissected and mobilized, and the deep parotid tissue is then removed from between the branches. If a tumor must be removed from the deep lobe via a lateral approach (as with a tumor invading between nerve branches from the superficial lobe), some authors advocate selective division of some nerve branches with immediate reanastomosis after tumor removal to avoid stretching branches and causing permanent dysfunction.

Total parotidectomy is typically performed if the *benign tumor* is affecting the deep part of parotid gland. should be performed for *malignant tumors* in the following situations: (1) metastasis to a superficial parotid lymph nodes (LNs) from a primary parotid tumor or an extra-parotid malignancy, (2) any parotid malignancy with metastatic involvement of cervical LNs, and (3) any high-grade parotid malignant tumor with a high risk of metastasis, (4) primary parotid malignant tumors originating in the deep lobe, and (5) primary malignancies that extend outside the parotid gland. Total parotidectomy is also performed for multifocal tumors, such as oncocytomas, to ensure complete resection. The operation may involve sparing or sacrificing the facial nerve branches or trunk depending on tumor extent to the nerve.

RADICAL PAROTIDECTOMY

Radical or non-conservative parotidectomy is typically performed if the malignant tumor is impinging on or infiltrating the facial nerve. In such cases, the facial nerve is excised in addition to the parotid gland i.e. in addition to total parotidectomy (Howe, Yu, Wai. Tsang, & William 2012).

EXTENDED TOTAL PAROTIDECTOMY

Excision of the superficial and deep lobes of the parotid gland (total parotidectomy) may also be extended to involve adjacent structures such as the overlying skin, the underlying mandible, the temporal bone and external auditory canal, or the deep musculature of the para-pharyngeal space. Such extensions are dictated by tumor growth and behavior.

Patients with extensive parotid malignancies should be counseled regarding the possibility of extended resections and the resulting functional and cosmetic morbidity. A neck dissection is performed for clinically positive LNs. For the clinically negative neck, the first echelon nodes are inspected. Enlarged or suspicious LNs are examined and a neck dissection is performed if metastatic disease is confirmed by frozen section.

COMPLICATIONS OF PAROTIDECTOMY

Early and late complications of superficial parotidectomy are summarized in Table 2.

Facial Nerve Injury

Unintentional injury to the facial nerve is the most devastating complication of parotid surgery. In a study of surgery for benign disease, temporary postoperative weakness was reported in 18-65% and permanent weakness in 0-19% (Koch, Zenk, & Iro, 2010). This risk must be explicitly discussed

Table 2. Complications following parotidectomy

Early Complications	Late Complications
- Facial nerve palsy - Bleeding/hematoma - Surgical site infection - Skin flap necrosis - Salivary fistula/sialocele - Seroma - External otitis - Trismus	- Frey's syndrome - Hypertrophic scar / keloid - Unsightly scar - Soft tissue defect - Recurrence

with every patient undergoing parotid surgery. Even with ostensibly perfect technique, facial nerve injury can occur for unknown reasons.

The nerve at most risk for injury during is the marginal mandibular branch resulting in deviation of the angle of the mouth towards the normal (sound) side (Figure 16) (Reilly, 2003; Witt, 1999; Dulguerov, 1999). If the motor supply to the orbicularis oculi is weak or absent, aggressive eye care must be instituted to prevent corneal drying and injury. Such care includes the use of lubricants, taping the eye shut at night, and moisture chambers during the day. If long-term paralysis occurs, static facial rehabilitation techniques may be used, including brow lift, gold weight insertion and canthoplasty, and facial slings. Dynamic techniques or nerve repair may also be appropriate.

Figure 16. Deviation of the angle of the mouth towards the sound side (left side) due to injury of the right marginal mandibular branch of the facial nerve

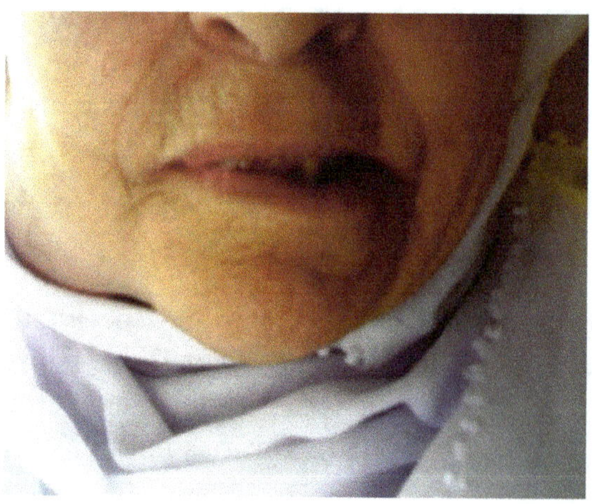

Temporary paresis of the facial nerve usually resolves from weeks to months post-operatively. To achieve the best results, nerve transection requires immediate micro-surgical repair.

Frey's Syndrome (Gustatory Sweating)

Frey's syndrome is now considered an inevitable long-term complication following parotidectomy unless preventive measures are taken (Eisele, 1992). It has been reported in 2-80% of patients, depending on the method of diagnosis (Koch, Zenk, & Iro, 2010); an acceptable incidence would be the lower end of this range when efforts are made to close the parotid capsule or reconstruct the parotid defect (Curry et al, 2009). The incidence of Frey's syndrome may be correlated with the amount of gland removed. It has been suggested that the greater the quantity of parotid tissue removed, the greater the amount of raw surface available to provide aberrant innervation to the skin.

Gustatory sweating results from aberrant re-innervation of cholinergic sympathetic sweat glands in the skin with post-ganglionic fibers from the auriculo-temporal nerve (ATN) that have been exposed following parotidectomy. Thus, a stimulus intended for saliva stimulation, evokes hyperesthesia and sweating. The patient complains of facial sweating and hotness on smell or taste of food, which might sometimes be associated with pain. Diagnosis can be confirmed with starch iodine test.

Preventive measures include SCM flap, temporalis fascial flap and insertion of an artificial membrane or autologous tissue between the skin and the parotid bed. If Frey's syndrome develops, *treatment options* include topical application of anti-perispirant or topical anti-cholinergics (1% glycopyrrolate), and surgical interposition of tissue (eg, temporo-parietal fascia or SCM), or implantable material (eg, acellular dermis). Surgical approaches carry the risks associated with reoperative surgery but are usually effective in minimizing or eliminating Frey syndrome. Recently, local intra-dermal injection of botulinum toxin has yielded good results. Botulinum toxin blocks the release of acetylcholine from pre-synaptic neurons. It is postulated to provide long-term results due to poor re-innervation of the skin's cholinergic sweat glands. It is performed as an out-patient.

Salivary Leakage (Salivary Sialocele or Fistula)

Raw gland surface can result in a collection of saliva below the skin (sialocele) or leakage of saliva from the wound (salivary fistula) in 1-14% of patients (Koch, 2010; Wax, 1991). Salivary leakage is usually mild and self-limited.

A *sialocele* is usually treated with repeated needle aspirations or drainage plus pressure dressings. Salivary *fistula* can be treated with local wound revision if low-flow leakage is present. Botulinum toxin, by blocking the release of acetylcholine from post-ganglionic parasympathetic fibers, results in decreased salivary flow and has been reported to be remarkably effective in several small series (Marchese-Ragona, 2006; Vargas, 2000; Ellies, 2004). A chronic salivary fistula is rare following superficial parotidectomy. Recalcitrant salivary leakage may necessitate surgical reexploration.

Ear Numbness

Hyposthesia in the distribution of the GAN occurs in almost all patients undergoing parotid surgery. The numbness lessens over time in some patients. Its incidence may be reduced by making efforts to preserve the GAN (Witt, 2002). When it must be sacrificed, neurorrhaphy at the conclusion of the case should be performed (tried).

Facial Asymmetry

The significance of the defect and the resulting facial asymmetry after parotidectomy is related to the amount of gland removed and thinness of the patient. Those with more subcutaneous fat may be better able to hide small defects than thin patients are and therefore may not require reconstruction.

Acellular dermis rolled and implanted in the defect, can both reconstruct normal facial contours and serve to close the parotid capsule and cover raw gland surface. Local *rotation* of the posterior belly of the digastric muscle can fill moderate defects and does not result in significant morbidity. An *abdominal fat graft* can be used to fill large defects and maintains volume over the long term if carefully and atraumatically harvested.[(13)]

Skin-Flap Necrosis

Skin-flap necrosis is an uncommon complication. The distal tip of the post-auricular skin flap is the most common location of flap necrosis. Appropriate design of skin incisions can minimize distal flap necrosis. Smoking, prior radiation therapy and diabetes mellitus may contribute to this complication by impairing the blood supply to the flap. If flap necrosis does occur, treatment entails conservative debridement of necrotic tissue and appropriate local wound care.

Mild Trismus

Mild trismus may occur following superficial parotidectomy and may be related to inflammation and fibrosis of the masseter muscle. It usually resolves with range of motion exercises of the jaw.

Hemorrhage / Hematoma

Hemorrhage or hematoma is uncommon after parotidectomy and is usually related to incomplete hemostasis during the procedure. Treatment consists of hematoma evacuation and surgical control of any identified bleeding vessels under general anesthesia.

Infection

Infection is also an uncommon complication after superficial parotidectomy due to the rich vascular supply to the parotid region. It is avoided by the use of aseptic techniques and careful handling of tissues. Peri-operative antibiotics are generally not used. Treatment of infection consists of appropriate antibiotics. Abscess formation is rare and requires surgical incision and drainage together with the appropriate antibiotics.

External Otitis

External otitis may occur post-operatively and may be related to intra-operative blood collection in the external auditory canal (EAC). Treatment consists of just cleaning the EAC and instillation of antibiotic ear drops.

Tumor Recurrence

Parotid tumors can recur as a result of positive margins, micro-satellite disease, or unrecognized nerve invasion. A few basic principles should be followed to ensure adequate extirpation and minimize recurrence:

- If the facial nerve or branch is grossly invaded, sacrifice of the nerve should be considered to ensure complete removal;
- Every effort should be made to keep tumor capsules intact in both benign and malignant disease. If tumor spillage occurs, then copious irrigation is wise;
- Capsular dissection can lead to incomplete excision as a result of failure to recognize microscopic extensions of tumor; therefore, a cuff of healthy gland should be removed with these tumors;
- Capsular dissection of pleomorphic adenomas is controversial; classic teaching is to remove a cuff of healthy tissue around the tumor, but modern data suggest that capsular dissection may not increase recurrence rates; a balance must be made between taking a cuff of healthy tissue and minimizing dissection of facial nerve branches. The cuff of normal parotid does not need to be large and wide margins are not needed for benign disease (Witt, 2002);
- Large-bore needle or incisional biopsies should *not* be performed; if they have been performed, the biopsy tract should be removed in continuity with the surgical specimen whenever possible.

REFERENCES

Alexander, L. (2013). *Parotidectomy*. WebMD LLC.

Bianchi, B., Ferri, A., Ferrari, S., Copelli, C., & Sesenna, E. (2011). Improving esthetic results in benign parotid surgery: Statistical evaluation of facelift approach, sternocleidomastoid flap, and superficial musculoaponeurotic system flap application. *Journal of Oral and Maxillofacial Surgery*, *69*(4), 1235–1241. doi:10.1016/j.joms.2010.03.005 PMID:20708323

Curry, J. M., King, N., Reiter, D., Fisher, K., Heffelfinger, R. N., & Pribitkin, E. A. (2009). Meta-analysis of surgical techniques for preventing parotidectomy sequelae. *Archives of Facial Plastic Surgery*, *11*(5), 327–331. doi:10.1001/archfacial.2009.62 PMID:19797095

Dave, S. P., Pernas, F. G., & Roy, S. (2007). The benign lymphoepithelial cyst and a classification system for lymphocytic parotid gland enlargement in the pediatric HIV population. *The Laryngoscope*, *117*(1), 106–113. doi:10.1097/01.mlg.0000246196.35413.35 PMID:17202938

Davidson, B., & Robind, S. (2013). *Parotidectomy"*. MedStar Georgetown University Hospital.

Dulguerov, P., Marchal, F., & Lehmann, W. (1999). Postparotidectomy facial nerve paralysis: Possible etiologic factors and results with routine facial nerve monitoring. *The Laryngoscope*, *109*(5), 754–762. doi:10.1097/00005537-199905000-00014 PMID:10334226

Eisele, D. W. (1992). Simple method for the assessment of Frey's syndrome. *The Laryngoscope*, *102*(5), 583–584. doi:10.1288/00005537-199205000-00021 PMID:1573957

Ellies, M., Gottstein, U., Rohrbach-Volland, S., Arglebe, C., & Laskawi, R. (2004). Reduction of salivary flow with botulinum toxin: Extended report on 33 patients with drooling, salivary fistulas, and sialadenitis. *The Laryngoscope*, *114*(10), 1856–1860. doi:10.1097/00005537-200410000-00033 PMID:15454785

Emerick, K. S., Fabian, R. L., & Deschler, D. G. (2007). Clinical presentation, management, and outcome of high-grade mucoepidermoid carcinoma of the parotid gland. *Otolaryngology - Head and Neck Surgery*, *136*(5), 783–787. doi:10.1016/j.otohns.2006.11.045 PMID:17478216

Fyke, M. K., & Sherk, S. D. (2013). *Parotidectomy*. Advameg, Inc.

Grosheva, M., Klussmann, J. P., Grimminger, C., Wittekindt, C., Beutner, D., Pantel, M., ... Guntinas-Lichius, O. (2009). Electromyographic facial nerve monitoring during parotidectomy for benign lesions does not improve the outcome of postoperative facial nerve function: A prospective two-center trial. *The Laryngoscope*, *119*(12), 2299–2305. doi:10.1002/lary.20637 PMID:19718745

Honeybrook, A., Athavale, S. M., Rangarajan, S. V., Rohde, S. L., & Netterville, J. L. (2017). Free dermal fat graft reconstruction of the head and neck: An alternate reconstructive option. *American Journal of Otolaryngology*, *38*(3), 291–296. doi:10.1016/j.amjoto.2017.01.026 PMID:28215817

Howe, V. S., Yu, J., Wai, J., Tsang, R. K., & William, W. I. (2012). Review of Salivary Gland Neoplasms. *ISRN Otolaryngology*, 872–982. PMID:23724273

Kawata, R., Koutetsu, L., Yoshimura, K., Nishikawa, S., & Takenaka, H. (2010). Indication for elective neck dissection for N0 carcinoma of the parotid gland: A single institution's 20-year experience. *Acta Oto-Laryngologica*, *130*(2), 286–292. doi:10.3109/00016480903062160 PMID:19544204

Koch, M., Zenk, J., & Iro, H. (2010). Long-term results of morbidity after parotid gland surgery in benign disease. *The Laryngoscope*, *120*(4), 724–730. doi:10.1002/lary.20822 PMID:20205175

Marchese-Ragona, R., Marioni, G., Restivo, D. A., & Staffieri, A. (2006). The role of botulinum toxin in postparotidectomy fistula treatment. A technical note. *American Journal of Otolaryngology*, *27*(3), 221–224. doi:10.1016/j.amjoto.2005.09.009 PMID:16647991

McGurk, M., & Combes, J. (Eds.). (2013). *Controversies in the Management of Salivary Gland Disease*. Oxford: Oxford University Press.

Meier, J. D., Wenig, B. L., Manders, E. C., & Nenonene, E. K. (2006). Continuous intraoperative facial nerve monitoring in predicting postoperative injury during parotidectomy. *The Laryngoscope*, *116*(9), 1569–1572. doi:10.1097/01.mlg.0000231266.84401.55 PMID:16954980

Motamed, M., Laugharne, D., & Bradley, P. J. (2003). Management of chronic parotitis: A review. *The Journal of Laryngology and Otology*, *117*(7), 521–526. doi:10.1258/002221503322112923 PMID:12901804

Reilly, J., & Myssiorek, D. (2003). Facial nerve stimulation and postparotidectomy facial paresis. *Otolaryngology - Head and Neck Surgery*, *128*(4), 530–533. doi:10.1016/S0194-5998(03)00089-5 PMID:12707656

Seethala, R. R., LiVolsi, V. A., & Baloch, Z. W. (2005). Relative accuracy of fine-needle aspiration and frozen section in the diagnosis of lesions of the parotid gland. *Head & Neck*, *27*(3), 217–223. doi:10.1002/hed.20142 PMID:15672359

Sood, A. J., Houlton, J. J., Nguyen, S. A., & Gillespie, M. B. (2015). Facial nerve monitoring during parotidectomy: A systematic review and meta-analysis. *Otolaryngology - Head and Neck Surgery*, *152*(4), 631–637. doi:10.1177/0194599814568779 PMID:25628369

Vargas, H., Galati, L. T., & Parnes, S. M. (2000). A pilot study evaluating the treatment of postparotidectomy sialoceles with botulinum toxin type A. *Archives of Otolaryngology--Head & Neck Surgery*, *126*(3), 421–424. doi:10.1001/archotol.126.3.421 PMID:10722021

Wax, M., & Tarshis, L. (1991). Post-parotidectomy fistula. *The Journal of Otolaryngology*, *20*(1), 10–13. PMID:2030529

Witt, R. L. (1999). Facial nerve function after partial superficial parotidectomy: An 11-year review (1987-1997). *Otolaryngology - Head and Neck Surgery*, *121*(3), 210–213. doi:10.1016/S0194-5998(99)70173-7 PMID:10471859

Witt, R. L. (2002). The significance of the margin in parotid surgery for pleomorphic adenoma. *The Laryngoscope*, *112*(12), 2141–2154. doi:10.1097/00005537-200212000-00004 PMID:12461331

Chapter 17
Frey's Syndrome

ABSTRACT

Frey's syndrome is secondary to sympathetic denervation of sweat glands – reinnervation through the auriculotemporal nerve is a secondary event. The aberrant regeneration theory explains the physiopathology of Frey's syndrome. Frey's syndrome incidence after parotidectomy, without prevention techniques, is 40-80% by clinical questioning and 80–100% by objective testing. It occurs months to years after surgery. A topographic and quantitative testing for Frey's is required prior to its treatment – the iodine-sublimated paper histogram (ISPH) test has the majority of desired features. Intradermic botulinum toxin injection is a well-tolerated and efficient treatment. The recommended dilution is 50 IU/1 ml, inter-injection distance is 1 cm, and injection volume is 0.1 ml. Complications to avoid include (1) facial muscle paralysis (rare and reversible complication; inject only intradermally and avoid injecting toward the midline) and (2) pain during injection (if bothersome could be decreased by the prior application of topical anesthetic cream).

INTRODUCTION

Frey's syndrome is characterized clinically by sweating and flushing of the lateral aspect of the face and upper neck, usually around the parotid region, during meals with no direct relation with chewing (Figure 1) (Frey, 1923). It results from injury to the auriculo-temporal nerve (ATN), a branch of the mandibular division of the trigeminal nerve. Once present, gustatory sweating

DOI: 10.4018/978-1-7998-5603-0.ch017

and flushing remain unchanged; there is no spontaneous resolution, even after numerous years (Balfour & Bloom, 1970).

Despite the fact that similar cases were already reported by *Baillarger* in 1853, Frey's syndrome is named after *Dr. Lucia Frey-Gottesman*; a neurologist at the University of Warsaw, Poland who published a landmark paper entitled "syndrome du nerf auriculotemporal" in 1923 and called it auriculotemporal nerve syndrome (Dulguerov, Marchal, & Gysin, 1999).

Frey's syndrome is also known as *gustatory sweating and flushing syndrome, Baillarger's syndrome, Frey-Baillarger syndrome, Dupuy's syndrome, and auriculotemporal syndrome.*

Figure 1. Frey's syndrome. Note the erythema of the face in the left parotid region (gustatory flushing).

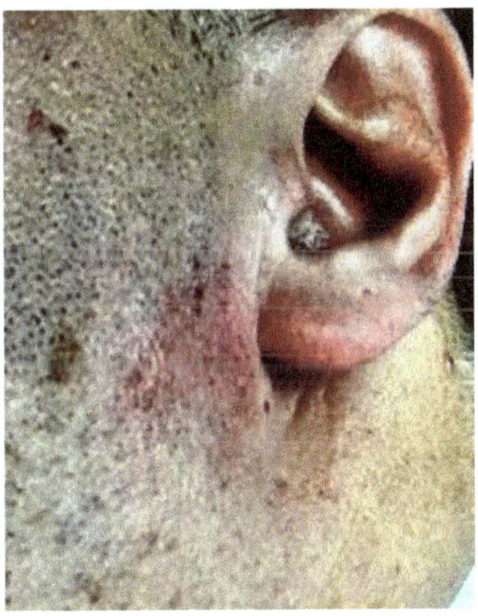

INCIDENCE

The reported incidence of gustatory sweating after parotidectomy is highly variable. (Sood, Quraishi, & Bradley, 1998). In the late 1950s, this problem was seriously studied (Laage-Hellmann, 1957; Laage-Hellmann, 1958a; Laage-Hellmann, 1958b). A group of 123 patients who underwent a parotidectomy was evaluated retrospectively with a questionnaire and clinical testing. On questioning, 62% of the patients complained of problems during eating: 22%

had both sweating and flushing, 26% had sweating only, and 14% had only flushing. When a gustatory stimulus was used, flushing was observed in 92% of patients, and 98% of patients exhibited a positive Minor sweat test. Laage-Hellmann (1957) concluded that gustatory sweating is an unavoidable sequel of parotidectomy that is not overtly symptomatic in all patients. The incidence of clinical and gustatory sweating after parotidectomy in the literature (1958-2000) varies largely between 6%-63% (Allison, 1993; Cavalot, 2000; Dulguerov, 1999; Farrell, 1991; Gordon, 1976; Korblut, 1974; Laage-Hellman, 1957; Laskawi, 1998; Linder, 1997; Nosan, 1991; Yu, 1992).

The *severity* of the gustatory sweating was judged moderate by 58% of patients, important by 15%, and embarrassing by 27% (Laage-Hellman, 1957). Clinical severity has been correlated to the surface involved (Linder, 1997; Laccourreye, 1993) and extent of parotid surgery (superficial versus total) (Gordon, 1976; Laccourreye, 1993; Gavric, 1991). Laage-Hellman (1958a) reported that the minimal delay between parotidectomy and the appearance of gustatory sweating as examined by sequential Minor tests was 5 weeks and the median delay was approximately 8 weeks. In some patients, the test became positive at 9 months and in less than 1% of patients, after 1 year. Clinical gustatory sweating has also been reported to appear up to 8.5 years after parotidectomy (Hays, 1978).

ANATOMY AND PHYSIOLOGY

The Auriculotemporal branch (ATN) of the mandibular division of the Trigeminal nerve carries parasympathetic fibers to the parotid salivary gland and sympathetic fibers to the sweat glands of the scalp.

During eating, a reflex arc is stimulated leading to increased salivary secretion of minor and major salivary glands, including the parotid gland. The origin of the afferent limb is at the level of the gustatory papillae of the oral cavity and oropharynx. The afferent neurons terminate in the nucleus solitarius and project to the inferior salivary nucleus.

Preganglionic parasympathetic efferent fibers leave the inferior salivary nucleus and the brain stem with the glossopharyngeal nerve. After passing through the jugular foramen and the superior and inferior glossopharyngeal ganglions, the parasympathetic fibers follow the *tympanic (Jacobson's) nerve*, which nerve enters the temporal bone on its inferior aspect and travels in the inferior tympanic canaliculus toward the middle ear cavity. A plexus is formed on the promontory, but the parasympathetic fibers not supplying the middle ear unite to form the *lesser superficial petrosal nerve*. This nerve exits the temporal bone and travels on the floor of the middle cranial fossa.

The fibers then exit the skull through the foramen ovale and reach the otic ganglion where they synapse with postganglionic parasympathetic fibers, which then join the ATN and reach the parotid gland through its medial aspect in the para-pharyngeal space. The neurotransmitter of these fibers is acetylcholine. The muscarinic receptors of the parotid gland are of the M3 subtype (Dai, Ambudkar, Horn, & DiJulio, 1991). Secretion of the parotid gland is controlled predominantly by the *parasympathetic* system.

The *sympathetic* fibers for the cutaneous vessels and sweat glands follow the cervical sympathetic chain and a synaptic relay is found in the sympathetic cervical ganglions. The fibers then follow the periarterial plexuses of the internal carotid artery (ICA) and external carotid artery (ECA) and their branches before joining and following the branches of the trigeminal nerve supplying the cutaneous sensation of the skin (List, 1938; Matthews, 1980). Thus, for the *preauricular* skin, these sympathetic fibers also travel within the ATN. The result of sympathetic activation is increased secretion from sweat glands (Sato, 1977) and vasoconstriction (Matthews & Robinson, 1980). A vasodilatation role of the parasympathetic facial system (Chorobski & Penfield, 1932) has been demonstrated (Blair, Glover, Roddie, 1961) and found to follow the facial nerve and then the greater superficial petrosal branch (Lambert, Bogduk, Goadsby, Duckworth, & Lance, 1984). Fibers probably synapse in the sphenopalatine ganglion before joining the corresponding branches of the trigeminal nerve, (Lambert, Bogduk, Goadsby, Duckworth, & Lance, 1984); in this case, the ATN.

Contrary to other post-ganglionic sympathetic fibers, which are adrenergic, sweat glands have acetylcholine as the main neurotransmitter (fox, 1962; Lee, 1954). The cholinergic receptors on sweat glands are muscarinic, predominantly of the M3 subtype, similar to that of parasympathetic salivary gland nerves (Vilches, Navarro, & Verdu, 1995).

PATHOGENESIS

Thomas (1927) and later Ford and Woodhall (1938) postulated that the severed parasympathetic fibers to the parotid gland regenerate along the wrong neurilemmal sheaths of the sectioned cutaneous sympathetic fibers, the so-called *aberrant regeneration theory* (Figure 2), which is supported by several experimental and clinical observations; (1) ATN block by local anesthetics induces a local anesthesia and cessation of gustatory sweating of similar cutaneous distribution (Ford, 1938; Glaister, 1958); (2) stimulation of the tympanic plexus results in sweating in the involved skin area (Ross, 1970); (3) symptoms are unaffected by anesthesia of the stellate ganglion, despite the appearance of a temporary Horner syndrome (Ford, 1938; Glaister, 1958; Drummon, 1995); (4) in the involved area, there is an impairment of the normal sympathetic function, such as reduced thermoregulatory sweating (List, 1938; Ford, 1938; Glaister, 1958; Drummond, 1994; Haxton, 1948) and absence of emotional flushing (List, 1938; Ford, 1938; Drummond, 1994; Haxton, 1948); (5) a latent period (minimum 1-2 months) is present between the initial injury and the appearance of gustatory flushing and sweating (Lindet 1997; List, 1938; Glaister, 1958; Haxton, 1948; Wilson, 1936); (6) Sequential follow-up of patients showed that positivity of the sweat test increases and the involved area progressively increases in size (Linder, Huber, & Schmid, 1997); (7) symptoms can be abolished by local injection of anti-cholinergic substances such as atropine (Ford, 1938; Glaister, 1958), and botulinum toxin; (8) a localized hypersensitivity to cholinergic drugs is described with mecholine (Wilson, 1936), acetylcholine (Ford, 1938; Glaister, 1958), and pilocarpine (Glaister, 1958; Wilson, 1936); and (9) the syndrome appears after various lesions or resections of the homolateral cervical sympathetic chain (List, 1938; Drummond, 1994; Haxton, 1948; Wilson, 1936; Nesathurai, 1995).

The postulated etiology is an aberrant regeneration of the sectioned parasympathetic fibers normally innervating the parotid gland. *The traumatized fibers lose their parotid targets and regenerate to innervate the vessels and sweat glands of the overlying skin.* In order for this aberrant regeneration to occur, the sympathetic fibers to these vessels and sweat glands have to be damaged, a frequent event in either parotid surgery or penetrating parotid trauma. The regular function of the parotid parasympathetic fibers is to increase salivary secretion during eating. The activation following aberrant regeneration produces an activation of the *new targets* during meals, resulting in a local vasodilatation ("gustatory flushing") and localized sweating ("gustatory sweating"). Despite all these convincing arguments, the aberrant regeneration remains a hypothesis until the demonstration of parasympathetic neurons on the re-innervated sweat glands.

Figure 2. Proposed aberrant regeneration mechanism of Frey's syndrome. A, Normal parotid gland and sweat gland parasympathetic and sympathetic innervation. B, Aberrant regeneration of severed parotid postganglionic para-sympathetic nerve fibers to severed sweat gland post-ganglionic sympathetic fibers.

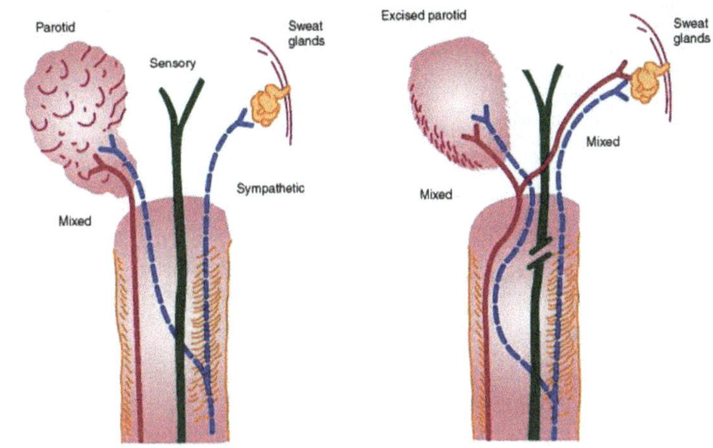

ETIOLOGY

Since Frey, emphasis has been placed on the ATN (Ross, 1970) and the regeneration of the parasympathetic fibers it contains to explain gustatory sweating and flushing (Thomas, 1927; ford, 1938). Although parotidectomy is the most frequent etiology (Dulguerov et al, 1999) the syndrome has been described with other surgical procedures such as mandibular surgery (Kryshtalskyj, 1989; Tuinzing, 1982), drainage of parotid or other local abscesses (Baillarger, 1983; Goatcher, 1954; Morfit, 1961; New, 1922; Payne, 1940; Weber, 1897) and neck dissection (Laskawi, Drobik, & Schonebeck, 1998); together with regional trauma such as mandibular fractures (Zoller, 1993; Gerbino, 1997) or penetrating wounds (Baddour, 1980; Duphenix, 1957; Ottomo, 1980); and with surgery or lesions of the cervical sympathetic chain (List, 1938; Haxton, 1948; Wilson, 1936; Nesathurai, 1995; Ottomo, 1980).

Rare causes of facial gustatory sweating, in single case reports, include herpes simplex of the mandibular division of the trigeminal nerve (Drummond, Boyce, & Lance, 1987), large cerebello-pontine angle tumor (Schnarch & Markitziu, 1990), and "gustatory otorrhea" (Saito, 1999). These cases could also be explained by the aberrant regeneration theory, with the locus of cross-fiber regeneration being at the level of the maxillary division (Schnarch &

Table 1. Causes of gustatory flushing and sweating

Typical Frey's Syndrome Etiologies
1. Trauma in parotid region - Parotidectomy - Other procedures in the parotid region (mandibular surgery, drainage of parotid abscess, neck dissection) - Penetrating trauma in the parotid region - Closed mandibular fractures 2. Trauma to the cervical sympathetic chain - Endoscopic thoracic sympathectomy 3. Other aberrant regeneration locations - Cerebellopontine angle - Middle ear - Otic ganglion 4. Autonomic neuropathies - Diabetic neuropathy
Atypical Variants of Gustatory Sweating
1. Physiological 2. Pediatric gustatory flushing syndrome 3. Gustatory neuralgia

Markitziu, 1990), at the level of the middle ear (Saito, 1999), or in the deep portion of the ATN instead of the parotid space portion of ATN (Drummond, Boyce, & Lance, 1987). A similar explanation, i.e. peripheral para-sympathetic sprouting to degenerated sympathetic fibers, has been offered for the observed facial, and often neck and upper chest, gustatory sweating seen in patients with severe diabetic neuropathy (Freedman, 1973; Hayes, 1982; Janka, 1979; Stuart, 1978; van der Linden, 2000; Watkins, 1973).

"*Physiological*" gustatory sweating and flushing can be induced by certain spicy foods (Lee, 1954). A variation of the threshold of individual cutaneous regions appears to be present, since only certain head and neck areas are found to respond in a given individual (Lee, 1954). Opposite to Frey's syndrome, physiological gustatory sweating and flushing is bilateral and usually symmetrical (Lee, 1954) similar to physiological thermal sweating (Lee, 1954; Randall, 1946).

Few cases of gustatory sweating in the *pediatric age* group have been described (Balfour, 1970; Beck, 1989; Davis, 1981; Feiwel, 1959; Johnson, 1995; Kozma, 1993; Sly, 1981; Zalzal, 1991). The majority are normal children with unilateral (Balfour, 1970; Beck, 1989; Davis, 1981; Feiwel, 1959; Kozma, 1993; Sly, 1981; Zalzal, 1991) or bilateral gustatory facial flushing (Davis, 1981; Johnson, 1995), without any sweating, a hallmark of Frey's syndrome (atypical variant). The term "gustatory flushing syndrome," as proposed by Kozma and Gabriel (1993), might be more appropriate. In addition, a "*gustatory otorrhea*" in a two patients without any previous pathology has been reported (Redlesf, 1993; Sonsale, 1999).

Recently, several cases of facial pain in the territory of the ATN nerve have been described (De Benedittis, 1990; Scrivani, 1998; Sharav, 1991; Truax, 1989) and the name "*gustatory neuralgia*" proposed (Laage-Hellman, 1958b). Other specific characteristics of gustatory neuralgia include an electric, burning (neuralgic) pain, pain distribution in the territory of the ATN, triggering of the pain by eating, numbness in the ATN because of surgery, and lack of response to anticonvulsant medication (Scrivani, Keith, Kulich, & Maciewicz, 1998). Gustatory neuralgia should be differentiated from the classical Frey's syndrome because of the absence of sweating and flushing and because pain is not a symptom in patients with Frey's syndrome (Drummond, 1995; Eckardt, 2003).

SWEATING

Since the most troublesome symptom of Frey's syndrome is sweating, testing for Frey's syndrome has in general been limited to the evaluation of sweating. The major function of sweat glands in humans is thermo-regulation (Sato, Kang, Saga, & Sato, 1989). Sweat is a hypotonic solution that contains mainly sodium chloride, potassium, and bicarbonate, as well as certain inorganic compounds such as lactate, urea, and ammonia (Sato, 1989; Sato, 1977).

Tests of autonomic thermoregulatory function are complex (Low, 2003) and the measure of sweat output is just one of the aspects assessed. Tests of sweat output function measure the production of sweat by a group of sweat glands and these tests could be classified as: (1) topographic, where a chemical reaction provides a view of the anatomic location of sweat secretion; (2) electric, where a change of skin impedance by the humidity of sweat is measured; and (3) thermodynamic, where the skin humidity is evaporated and a "sudometer" measures the thermal mass of the air stream (Low, 2003). Advantages of the electric and thermodynamic tests include the possibility of repeated and dynamic measures, while topographic tests give a better representation of surface and anatomic distribution.

The *ideal test* method for gustatory sweating should provide topographic information and quantification of the amount of sweating. While dynamic measures might be interesting in investigational studies, their use in clinical practice is of limited value. Further characteristics of the test should include: (1) simplicity (one-step); (2) sensitivity; (3) reliability; (4) adequate dynamic range, so that different sweating rates could be appreciated; (5) absence of toxicity and allergenicity of the agents used; (6) easy removal from the skin of the applied agents; and (7) low cost (Dulguerov, 1999; Sato, 1989).

The most frequently used method of sweat secretion assessment for gustatory sweating was originally described by *Victor Minor*, a Russian neurologist (Minor, 1927). The original solution described contains 1.5 g iodine, 10 g castor oil, and 88.5 g of absolute alcohol and is painted on the skin to be tested. Actually, any colored iodine solution used for disinfections, such as Betadine, will work (Glogau, 2004). After drying, the areas are powdered with starch (regular baking corn starch works fine). The water in the sweat

Figure 3. Minor starch-iodine test for diagnosis of Frey's syndrome. Discoloration occurs in the affected area of gustatory stimulation.

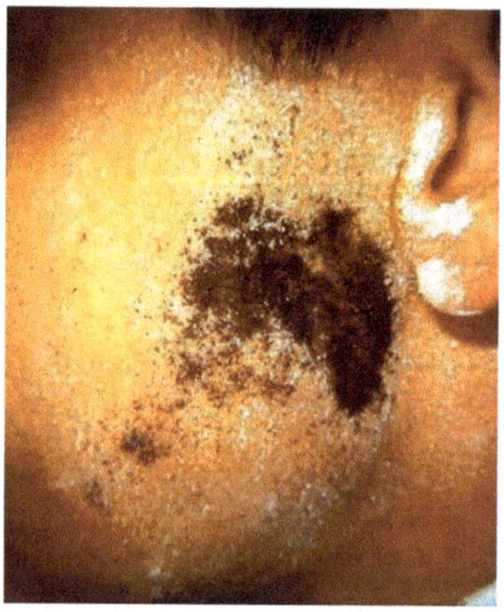

produces blue coloring by a reduction reaction of the iodine-starch mixture. With limited sweat production, the apertures of individual sweat glands are marked as small blue dots, while with larger amounts of sweat secretion the blue dots are larger and eventually become confluent. Therefore, the Minor test is seen as a topographic method allowing accurate mapping of the involved surface (Figure 3).

Disadvantages of the Minor test include the application of several layers of reagents, difficulty of removing the iodine paint, possible allergy to iodine (Sato, Richardson, Timm, & Sato, 1988), and difficulty of using the method with heavy perspiration, since sweat tends to drip down, obscuring assessment of the more dependently located skin (Dulguerov et al., 1999). While it could be seen as objective, it is not a quantitative test and therefore might not be suited for the comparison of two treatments (Dulguerov, 1999; Dulguerov, 2000). Several *modifications* of the Minor test have been proposed but all of these share the inconveniences of the original test (Dulguerov, 1999; Adie,

Figure 4. Simple assessment of Frey's syndrome with facial tissue. The affected area is demarcated by the wet area on the tissue.

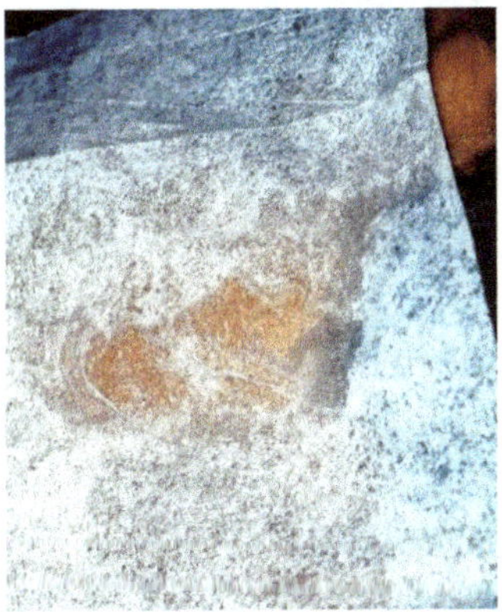

1968). Randall (1946), noting that some papers have starch coatings, modified the method by using paper instead of starch, but continued to paint the skin with the iodine-based mixture. Dole and Thaysen (1953) further simplified the process by the use of paper that was coated with iodine. Unfortunately, this method seems to have been forgotten until recently (Figure 4) (Dulguerov et al., 1999).

Recently, two techniques for the evaluation of gustatory sweating have been reported (Dulguerov et al., 1999). The "*blotting paper method*" simply uses the difference in weight of a piece of blotting paper before and after gustatory stimulation. In the *"iodine-sublimated paper" histogram"* (ISPH) method, regular office paper is sublimated with iodine and acquires the property of changing color when wetted. The paper is than digitized and a histogram algorithm applied to measure the area of color change (Dulguerov et al., 1999). These tests (blotting paper and ISPH) satisfy most of the requirements of an ideal sweat test.

TREATMENT

The treatment modalities proposed for gustatory sweating can be categorized into 5 main groups: (1) external radiotherapy; (2) local or systemic application of anti-cholinergics drugs; (3) section of some portion of the efferent neural arc; (4) interposition of a subcutaneous barrier, as used for Frey's syndrome prevention; and (5) injection of botulinum toxin in the involved skin. Considering that the symptoms are not always very troublesome, it is important that the treatment should be individualized and does not by itself result in more serious side effects.

Radiotherapy (RT)

Needles (1936) was the first scientist to attempt radiotherapy (RT). In Laage-Hellman's studies (1957), irradiated patients had a lower incidence of gustatory sweating, with the involved surface often outside the radiotherapy fields. Similar results were obtained from other publications (Linder, 1997; Dawsn, 1985), indicating that should RT be indicated, the expected incidence and severity of gustatory sweating will be low.

Anti-Cholinergic Medication

Shelley and Horvath showed that *none* of the *systemic* anti-cholinergic substances available could be used in accepted doses to reduce the sweating produced by 0.1 ml intradermal injection of pilocarpine (Shelley & Horvath, 1951). In addition, these authors showed that *local* iontophoresis or application of anti-cholinergics drugs such as scopolamine could be used to reduce sweating (Shelley & Horvath, 1951). Laage-Hellman (1958) was the first to apply *scopolamine* (3% cream) for the treatment of gustatory sweating, with symptom reduction in male and abolition in female patients. The difference was tentatively explained by a thinner female skin.

Double-blind studies have shown *topical glycopyrrolate* (Hays, 1982; May, 1989), *aluminum chloride* (Black, 1990; Hultenbrink, 1986; Schmelzer, 1992), and *diphemanil methylsulfate* (Laccourreye, Bonan, Brasnu, Bonan, 1990) to be superior to placebo. Few patients experienced minor side effects such as dry mouth (Hays, Norvack, & Warsham, 1982). Despite their effectiveness, patients seem in the long run (Linder, Huber, & Schmid, 1997), to abandon the cumbersome daily application requiring skin drying with a hairdryer

Dulguerov, Marchal, & Gysin, 1999). Moreover, skin wounds or infection, and application to the mucosa of the eyes, mouth, and nose result in an enhanced absorption and side effects (Hays, 1978).

Interruption of the Efferent Pathway

Section of the ATN was originally described by Leriche for the treatment of traumatic parotid fistula (Lerishe, 1914). Debets and Munting (1922), and more recently, Coldwater (1954) attempted ATN section, with only partial and temporary improvement of the symptoms (Harrison & Donaldson, 1979). The access to this deeply located region is also complex and carries the risk of injuring several important structures, including the facial nerve. At the other end of the efferent pathway, a division of the intra-cranial portion of the glossopharyngeal nerve was done by Gardner and McCubbin (1956), with a good result lasting 5 years in one patient and a short period of relief in a second one. Because of the extensive surgery, this therapy has *not* been pursued.

Hemenway (1960) suggested interrupting the efferent neuronal pathway at the level of the middle ear, by sectioning the tympanic nerve of Jacobson. The first such procedure for gustatory sweating was carried out on 3 patients with apparently excellent results by Golding-Wood (1962) who named it "*tympanic neurectomy*". Other authors (Hays, 1978; Ross, 1970; Harrison, 1979; Parisier, 1978) reported recurrence of symptoms in most of their patients on long follow-up.

Surgical Interposition

Sessions et al. (1976) pioneered the use of a barrier between the facial skin and the parotid bed in the treatment of established Frey's syndrome. They used the surgical interposition of a *fascia lata graft* in four patients with excellent results. This technique appeared to be effective in the small group of patients reported (Sessions, 1976; Wallis, 1978). Probably a major deterrent of its use is the risk of facial nerve paralysis during reoperation, since the nerve lies just under the skin after superficial or total parotidectomy. A variation of this technique with the use of a *pedicle temporal fascia* has been reported in a case without prior facial nerve dissection (Rubinstein, Rosen, & Leeman, 1999).

Dulguerov et al. (2016) evaluated the difference of the incidence in clinical Frey syndrome in studies comparing classical parotidectomy and parotidectomy with superficial musculo-aponeurotic system (SMAS) flap elevation and suturing through meta-analysis methodology. They reported that SMAS technique is associated with a significant decrease of clinical Frey syndrome.

Botulinum Toxin

The injection of "Botulinum-A toxin" in the skin involved by gustatory sweating was recently proposed by Drobik and Laskawi (1995). Following their case report, the technique has been progressively adopted (Arad-Cohen, 2000; Beerens, 2002; Bjerkhoel, 1977; Cavalot, 2000; Drobik, 1995; Guntinas-Lichius, 2002; Kuttner, 2001; Laccourreye, 1999; Laccourreye, 1988; Naumann, 1997; Quinodoz, 1997). *Advantages* include the following; (1) the substance has been used for a variety of pathologies in the last 3 decades with few side-effects (Jankovic & Hallet, 1994), and (2) its use is simple in the office setting, and avoids complex procedures in the operating room. The only *disadvantage* is the pain associated with the needle sticking and the secondary reluctance of some patients to be stuck, especially on the face.

Mechanism of Botulinum Toxin Action

Eight serotypes (A, B, Cα, Cβ, D, E, F, and G) of Botulinum toxins are produced by different strains of the anaerobic bacteria *Clostridium botulinum* of which only four (A, B, E, and F) are toxic to humans (Kreyden & Scheidegger, 2004). The action of botulinum toxins is that of highly specific endopeptidases that cleave cytosol proteins involved in the fusion of exocytosis vesicles with the cell membrane (Montecucco, Schiavo, Tugnoli, & de Grandis, 1996), with type A toxin acting on synaptosome-associated protein (SNAP)-25 (Blasi et al, 1993) and type B toxin acting on vesicle-associated membrane protein (VAMP) This action is highly specific for cholinergic synapses because the specific membrane proteins required for the internalization of botulinum toxins are found only in the presynaptic endings of cholinergic synapses (Coffield, Considine, & Simpson, 1994). By blocking the exocytosis mechanism of the presynaptic terminal, the release of acetylcholine is inhibited. The synapse remains intact but is non-functional and for neuromuscular junctions results in muscle paralysis. The recovery of function is due to collateral sprouting from the same or other axons and the formation of new synapses.

Practical Aspects

Botulinum toxin A has been approved by the Food and Drug Administration (FDA) since 1989 and is commercially available as Botox (Allergan, Irvine, CA) and Dysport (Speywood Pharmaceuticals, Maidenhead, UK). A Botox vial contains 100 IU of botulinum toxin A, 0.5 mg of human albumin, and 0.9 mg of NaCl as a sterile powder that can remain in a refrigerator for at least 24 months (Dulguerov, Quinodoz, Cosendai, Piletta, Lehmann, 2000).

The practical considerations for botulinum toxin treatment in Frey's syndrome include: (1) Mapping of the facial surface to be treated (Dulguerov, Quinodoz, Cosendai, Piletta, Lehmann, 2000); the contour of the area to be injected is drawn on the patient's face, (2) a grid of 1 cm squares is drawn either physically on the face (Figure 5) or an "imaginary" one is created by the physician, (3) if anesthetic is to be used such as local anesthetic cream (EMLA, Astra, Sweden), it should be applied at this time, (4) the delimited area is injected at sites 1 cm apart, which are infiltrated with 0.1 ml (5 IU) of

Figure 5. Intra-dermal injection of botuluinum toxin for Frey's syndrome. Grid marked across the affected area

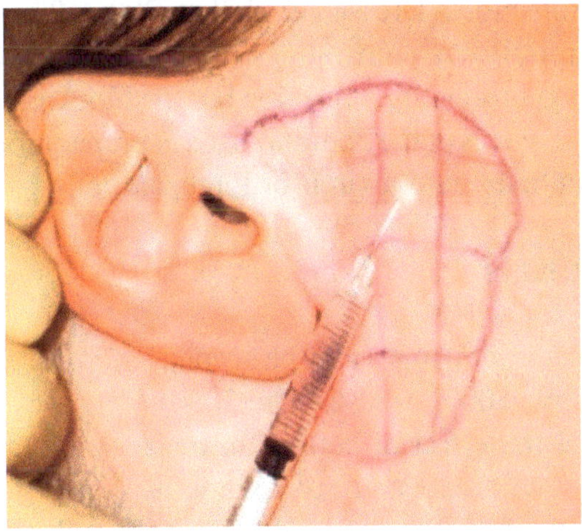

a solution containing botulinum toxin at a concentration of 2.5-5 IU/0.1 ml (2 cc per bottle of Botox powder) (Dulguerov, Quinodoz, Cosendai, Piletta, Lehmann, 2000), (5) the injection should be strictly *intradermal*, rising tiny wheals at each injection site, and (6) a light massage of the area is used for local diffusion.

Side-Effects

Some authors reported temporary *facial paralysis* as a side-effect of the botulinum toxin injection (Beerens, 2002; Bjerkhoel, 1977; Laccourreye, 1999). The most plausible explanation of this rare and partial temporary paresis is an injection deep to the dermis and/or diffusion to facial motor end plates (Beerens & Snow, 2002).

The *pain* associated with the needle injection was reported to be minimal (2/10 on an analog visual pain scale) (Dulguerov, 2000; Bjerkhoel, 1977; Laccourreye, 1999). The use of local anesthetic cream (EMLA, Astra, Sweden) might be tried in the few patients reluctant to undergo this procedure (Bjerkhoel & Trobbe, 1977).

Allergic reaction is surprisingly low. The development of antibodies seems related to the amount of protein load injected and the shortness of the interval between injections (Dressler & Hallett, 2006). The incidence is less than 1% with current Botox preparations (Gressler, 2006; Jankovic, 2003). There is no overt hypersensitivity reaction but the blocking antibodies result in decreased effectiveness of the botulinum toxin preparation. These patients could benefit from botulinum toxin B or F preparations.

Therapeutic Results

Repeat of injections several times may be needed before obtaining a *complete response* (Dulguerov, 2000; Arad-Cohen, 2000).

The duration of the effect of botulinum toxin on gustatory sweating is rather long-lasting, with an average of 15 months (Laskawi, 1998; Beerens, 2002; Laccourreye, 1999). An actuarial estimate puts the clinical gustatory sweating *recurrence* at 1, 2, and 3 years at 27%, 63%, and 92%, respectively (Laccourreye et al, 1999). The severity of the recurrent Frey's syndrome was found to be reduced when compared to that of the initial episode and re-treatment with botulinum toxin was still effective (Laccourreye et al, 1999). A clear explanation for this longer timeframe relative to neuromuscular indications is lacking, but different possibilities have been suggested such as an atrophy of the sweat glands, poor sprouting of autonomic fibers, and increased scarring impeding regenerating axons (Dulguerov, Quinodoz, Cosendai, Piletta, Lehmann, 2000).

REFERENCES

Adie, R. (1968). Gustatory sweating. *The Australian and New Zealand Journal of Surgery, 38*(2), 98–103. doi:10.1111/j.1445-2197.1971.tb05178.x PMID:4302030

Allison, G. R., & Rappaport, I. (1993). Prevention of Frey's syndrome with superficial musculoaponeurotic system interposition. *American Journal of Surgery, 16*(4), 407–410. doi:10.1016/S0002-9610(05)80343-5 PMID:8214303

Arad-Cohen, A., & Blitzer, A. (2000). Botulinum toxin treatment for symptomatic Frey's syndrome. *Otolaryngology - Head and Neck Surgery, 122*(2), 237–240. doi:10.1016/S0194-5998(00)70246-4 PMID:10652397

Baddour, H. M., Ripley, J. F., & Cortez, E. A. (1980). Treatment of Frey's syndrome by an interpositional fascia graft: Report of case. *Journal of Oral Surgery, 38*, 778–781. PMID:6932490

Baillarger, M. (1983). Memoire sur l'obliteration du canal de Stenon. *Gazette Médicale de France (Paris), 23*, 194–197.

Balfour, H. Jr, & Bloom, J. E. (1970). The auriculotemporal syndrome beginning in infancy. *The Journal of Pediatrics, 77*(5), 872–874. doi:10.1016/S0022-3476(70)80251-7 PMID:4323302

Beck, S. A., Burks, A. W., & Woody, R. C. (1989). Auriculotemporal syndrome seen clinically as food allergy. *Pediatrics, 83*, 601–603. PMID:2928001

Beerens, A. J., & Snow, G. B. (2002). Botulinum toxin A in the treatment of patients with Frey syndrome. *British Journal of Surgery, 89*(1), 116–119. doi:10.1046/j.0007-1323.2001.01982.x PMID:11851676

Bjerkhoel, A., & Trobbe, O. (1977). Frey's syndrome: Treatment with botulinum toxin. *The Journal of Laryngology and Otology, 111*(9), 839–844. doi:10.1017/S0022215100138769 PMID:9373550

Black, M. J., & Gunn, A. (1990). The management of Frey's syndrome with aluminium chloride hexahydrate antiperspirant. *Annals of the Royal College of Surgeons of England*, *72*, 49–52. PMID:2301903

Blair, D. A., Glover, W. E., & Roddie, J. C. (1961). Cutaneous vasomotor nerves to the head and trunk. *Journal of Applied Physiology*, *16*(1), 119–122. doi:10.1152/jappl.1961.16.1.119

Blasi, J., Chapman, E. R., Link, E., Link, E., Binz, T., Yamasaki, S., ... Jahn, R. (1993). Botulinum neurotoxin A selectively cleaves the synaptic protein SNAP-25. *Nature*, *365*(6442), 160–163. doi:10.1038/365160a0 PMID:8103915

Cavalot, A. L., Palonta, F., Preti, G., Nazionale, G., Ricci, E., Staffierie, A., ... Corestina, G. (2000). Post-parotidectomy Frey's syndrome. Treatment with botulinum toxin type A. *Acta Otorhinolaryngologica Italica*, *20*, 187–191. PMID:11139877

Chorobski, J., & Penfield, W. (1932). Cerebral vasodilatator nerves and their pathway from the medulla oblongata, with observation on the pial and intracerebral vascular plexus. *Archives of Neurology and Psychiatry*, *28*, 1257–1289. doi:10.1001/archneurpsyc.1932.02240060016002

Coffield, J. A., Considine, R. V., & Simpson, L. L. (1994). The Site and Mechanism of Action of Botulinum Neurotoxin. New York: Marcel Drekker Inc.

Coldwater, K. B. (1954). Surgical treatment of the auriculotemporal syndrome. *American Medical Association Archives of Surgery*, *69*(1), 54–57. doi:10.1001/archsurg.1954.01270010056008 PMID:13170923

Dai, Y. S., Ambudkar, I. S., Horn, V. J., & DiJulio, D. (1991). Evidence that M3 muscarinic receptors in rat parotid gland couple to two second messenger systems. *The American Journal of Physiology*, *261*(6), C1063–C1073. doi:10.1152/ajpcell.1991.261.6.C1063 PMID:1722644

Davis, R. S., & Strunk, R. C. (1981). Auriculotemporal syndrome in childhood. *American Journal of Diseases of Children*, *135*, 832–833. PMID:7282660

Dawson, A. K., & Orr, J. A. (1985). Long-term results of local excision and radiotherapy in pleomorphic adenoma of the parotid. *International Journal of Radiation Oncology, Biology, Physics*, *11*(3), 451–455. doi:10.1016/0360-3016(85)90174-9 PMID:2982770

De Benedittis, G. (1990). Auriculotemporal syndrome (Frey's syndrome) presenting as tic douloureux. Report of two cases. *Journal of Neurosurgery*, *72*(6), 955–958. doi:10.3171/jns.1990.72.6.0955 PMID:1692586

Debets, J. M., & Munting, J. D. (1922). Parotidectomy for parotid tumours: 19-year experience from The Netherlands. *British Journal of Surgery*, *79*(11), 1159–1161. doi:10.1002/bjs.1800791116 PMID:1467891

Dole, V. P., & Thaysen, J. H. (1953). Variation in the functional power of human sweat glands. *The Journal of Experimental Medicine*, *98*(2), 129–144. doi:10.1084/jem.98.2.129 PMID:13069656

Dressler, D., & Hallett, M. (2006). Immunological aspects of Botox, Dysport and Myobloc/NeuroBloc. *European Journal of Neurology*, *13*(suppl 1), 11–15. doi:10.1111/j.1468-1331.2006.01439.x PMID:16417592

Drobik, C., & Laskawi, R. (1995). Frey's syndrome: Treatment with botulinum toxin. *Acta Oto-Laryngologica*, *115*(3), 459–461. doi:10.3109/00016489509139348 PMID:7653272

Drummond, P. D. (1994). Sweating and vascular responses in the face: Normal regulation and dysfunction in migraine, cluster headache and harlequin syndrome. *Clinical Autonomic Research*, *4*(5), 273–285. doi:10.1007/BF01827433 PMID:7888747

Drummond, P. D. (1995). Mechanisms of physiological gustatory sweating and flushing in the face. *Journal of the Autonomic Nervous System*, *52*(2-3), 117–124. doi:10.1016/0165-1838(94)00151-9 PMID:7615894

Drummond, P. D. (1995). Mechanisms of physiological gustatory sweating and flushing in the face. *Journal of the Autonomic Nervous System*, *52*(2-3), 117–124. doi:10.1016/0165-1838(94)00151-9 PMID:7615894

Drummond, P. D., Boyce, G. M., & Lance, J. W. (1987). Postherpetic gustatory flushing and sweating. *Annals of Neurology*, *21*(6), 559–563. doi:10.1002/ana.410210606 PMID:3606044

Dulguerov, N., Makni, A., & Dulguerov, P. (2016). The superficial musculoaponeurotic system flap in the prevention of Frey syndrome: A meta-analysis. *The Laryngoscope*, *126*(7), 1581–1584. doi:10.1002/lary.25895 PMID:26915301

Dulguerov, P., Marchal, F., & Gysin, C. (1999). Frey syndrome before Frey: The correct history. *The Laryngoscope*, *109*(9), 1471–1473. doi:10.1097/00005537-199909000-00021 PMID:10499057

Dulguerov, P., Quinodoz, D., Cosendai, G., Piletta, P., & Lehmann, W. (2000). Frey syndrome treatment with botulinum toxin. *Otolaryngology - Head and Neck Surgery*, *122*(6), 821–827. doi:10.1016/S0194-5998(00)70008-8 PMID:10828793

Dulguerov, P., Quinodoz, D., Cosendai, G., Piletta, P., Marchal, F., & Lehmann, W. (1999). Prevention of Frey syndrome during parotidectomy. *Archives of Otolaryngology--Head & Neck Surgery*, *125*(8), 833–839. doi:10.1001/archotol.125.8.833 PMID:10448728

Dulguerov, P., Quinodoz, D., Vaezi, A., Cosendai, G., Piletta, P., & Lahmann, W. (1999). New objective and quantitative tests for gustatory sweating. *Acta Oto-Laryngologica*, *119*(5), 599–603. doi:10.1080/00016489950180865 PMID:10478603

Duphenix, M. (1957). Observations sur les fistules du canal salivaire de Stenon. Sur une playe compliquee a la joue ou le canal salivaire fut dechire. *Memoires l'Academi royal de Chirugie*, *3*, 431-439.

Eckardt, A., & Kuettner, C. (2003). Treatment of gustatory sweating (Frey's syndrome) with botulinum toxin A. *Head & Neck*, *25*(8), 624–628. doi:10.1002/hed.10262 PMID:12884344

Farrell, M. L., & Kalnins, I. K. (1991). Frey's syndrome following parotid surgery. *The Australian and New Zealand Journal of Surgery*, *61*(4), 295–301. doi:10.1111/j.1445-2197.1991.tb00215.x PMID:2018439

Feiwel, M. (1959). Auriculotemporal syndrome. *Proceedings of the Royal Society of Medicine*, *52*(3), 191. doi:10.1177/003591575905200318 PMID:13633998

Ford, F. R., & Woodhall, B. (1938). Phenomena due to misdirection of regenerating fibers of cranial, spinal, and autonomic nerves: Clinical observations. *Archives of Surgery*, *36*(3), 480–496. doi:10.1001/archsurg.1938.01190210109006

Fox, R. H., Goldsmith, R., & Kidd, D. J. (1962). Cutaneous vasomotor control in the human head, neck and upper chest. *The Journal of Physiology*, *161*(2), 298–312. doi:10.1113/jphysiol.1962.sp006887 PMID:13894392

Freedman, A. (1973). Facial sweating after food in diabetes. *British Journal of Medicine*, *3*(5874), 291. doi:10.1136/bmj.3.5874.291-b PMID:4723474

Frey, L. (1923). Le syndrome du nerf auriculo-temporal. *Revue Neurologique*, *2*, 92–104.

Gardner, W. J., & McCubbin, J. W. (1956). Auriculotemporal syndrome; gustatory sweating due to misdirection of regenerated nerve fibers. *Journal of the American Medical Association*, *160*(4), 272–277. doi:10.1001/jama.1956.02960390022007 PMID:13278188

Gavric, M. (1991). Aurikulotemporalni sindrom kao posledica parotidektomija. *Stomatoloski Glasnik Srbije*, *37*, 385–391. PMID:1664547

Gerbino, G., Roccia, F., Grosso, M., & Regge, D. (1997). Pseudoaneurysm of the internal maxillary artery and Frey's syndrome after blunt facial trauma. *Journal of Oral and Maxillofacial Surgery*, *55*(12), 1485–1490. doi:10.1016/S0278-2391(97)90657-1 PMID:9393413

Glaister, D. H., Hearnshaw, J. R., Heffron, P. F., Peck, A. W., & Patey, D. H. (1958). The mechanism of post-parotidectomy gustatory sweating (the auriculo-temporal syndrome). *British Medical Journal*, *1958*(2), 942–946. doi:10.1136/bmj.2.5102.942 PMID:13584806

Glogau, R. G. (2004). Hyperhidrosis and botulinum toxin A: Patient selection and techniques. *Clinics in Dermatology*, *22*(1), 45–52. doi:10.1016/j.clindermatol.2003.11.007 PMID:15158545

Goatcher, P. D. (1954). The auriculo-temporal syndrome. *British Medical Journal*, *4873*(4873), 1233–1234. doi:10.1136/bmj.1.4873.1233 PMID:13160442

Golding-Wood, P. H. (1962). Tympanic neurectomy. *The Journal of Laryngology and Otology*, *76*(9), 683–693. doi:10.1017/S0022215100059909 PMID:13948738

Gordon, A. B., & Fiddian, R. V. (1976). Frey's syndrome after parotid surgery. *American Journal of Surgery*, *132*(1), 54–58. doi:10.1016/0002-9610(76)90290-7 PMID:952338

Guntinas-Lichius, O. (2002). Increased botulinum toxin type A dosage is more effective in patients with Frey's syndrome. *The Laryngoscope*, *112*(4), 746–749. doi:10.1097/00005537-200204000-00027 PMID:12150533

Harrison, K., & Donaldson, I. (1979). Frey's syndrome. *Journal of the Royal Society of Medicine*, *72*(7), 503–508. doi:10.1177/014107687907200708 PMID:552549

Haxton, H. A. (1948). Gustatory sweating. *Brain*, *71*(1), 16–25. doi:10.1093/brain/71.1.16 PMID:18868742

Hayes, P. C., & Tulloch, J. A. (1982). An unusual case of gustatory sweating. *Postgraduate Medical Journal*, *58*(684), 656–657. doi:10.1136/pgmj.58.684.656 PMID:7177991

Hays, L. L. (1978). The Frey syndrome: A review and double blind evaluation of the topical use of a new anticholinergics agent. *The Laryngoscope*, *88*, 1796–1824. doi:10.1288/00005537-197811000-00010 PMID:362094

Hays, L. L., Novack, A. J., & Worsham, J. C. (1982). The Frey syndrome: A simple, effective treatment. *Otolaryngology - Head and Neck Surgery*, *90*(4), 419–425. doi:10.1177/019459988209000410 PMID:6817270

Hemenway, W. G. (1960). Gustatory sweating and flushing. The auriculotemporal syndrome – Frey's syndrome. *The Laryngoscope*, *70*, 84–90. PMID:14400950

Huttenbrink, K. B. (1986). Die Therapie des gustatorischen Schwitzens nach Parotidektomie. Freysches Syndrom. *Laryngology, Rhinology & Otology (Stuttgart)*, *65*, 135–137.

Janka, H. U., Standl, E., & Mehnert, H. (1979). Clonidine effect on diabetic gustatory sweating. *Annals of Internal Medicine*, *91*(1), 130. doi:10.7326/0003-4819-91-1-130_2 PMID:464437

Jankovic, J., & Hallet, M. (1994). *Therapy with Botulinum Toxin*. New York, NY: Marcel Dekker Inc.

Jankovic, J., Vuong, K. D., & Ahsan, J. (2003). Comparison of efficacy and immunogenicity of original versus current Botulinum toxin in cervical dystonia. *Neurology*, *60*(7), 1186–1188. doi:10.1212/01.WNL.0000055087.96356.BB PMID:12682332

Johnson, I. J., & Birchall, J. P. (1995). Bilatral auriculotemporal syndrome in childhood. *International Journal of Pediatric Otorhinolaryngology*, *32*(1), 83–86. doi:10.1016/0165-5876(94)01903-B PMID:7607824

Kornblut, A. D., Westphal, P., & Miehlke, A. (1974). The effectiveness of a sternomastoid muscle flap in preventing post-parotidectomy occurrence of the Frey syndrome. *Acta Oto-Laryngologica*, *77*(1-6), 368–373. doi:10.3109/00016487409124638 PMID:4835637

Kozma, C., & Gabriel, S. (1993). Gustatory flushing syndrome. A pediatric case report and review of the literature. *Clinical Pediatrics*, *32*(10), 629–631. doi:10.1177/000992289303201013 PMID:8261729

Kreyden, O. P., & Scheidegger, E. P. (2004). Anatomy of the sweat glands, pharmacology of botulinum toxin, and distinctive syndromes associated with hyperhidrosis. *Clinics in Dermatology*, *22*(1), 40–44. doi:10.1016/j.clindermatol.2003.12.029 PMID:15158544

Kryshtalskyj, B., & Weinberg, S. (1989). An assessment for auriculotemporal syndrome following temporomandibular joint surgery through the preauricular approach. *Journal of Oral and Maxillofacial Surgery*, *47*(1), 3–6. doi:10.1016/0278-2391(89)90114-6 PMID:2911055

Kuttner, C., Troger, M., Dempf, R., & Eckardt, A. (2001). Effektivitat von Botulinum-toxin A in der Behandlung des gustatorischen. *Schwitzens Nervenarzt*, *172*, 787–790.

Laage Hellman, J. E. (1957). Gustatory sweating and flushing after conservative parotidectomy. *Acta Oto-Laryngologica*, *48*(3), 234–252. doi:10.3109/00016485709124377 PMID:13469322

Laage-Hellman, J. E. (1958a). Gustatory sweating and flushing: Aetiological implications of response of separate sweat glands to various stimult. *Acta Oto-Laryngologica*, *49*(1), 363–374. doi:10.3109/00016485809134766 PMID:13605714

Laage-Hellman, J. E. (1958b). Gustatory sweating and flushing; aetiological implications of latent period and mode of development after parotidectomy. *Acta Oto-Laryngologica*, *49*(1), 306–314. doi:10.3109/00016485809134759 PMID:13570950

Laccourreye, O., Akl, E., Gutierrez-Fonseca, R., Garcia, D., Brasnu, D., & Bonan, B. (1999). Recurrent gustatory sweating (Frey syndrome) after intracutaneous injection of botulinum toxin type A: Incidence, management, and outcome. *Archives of Otolaryngology--Head & Neck Surgery*, *125*(3), 283–286. doi:10.1001/archotol.125.3.283 PMID:10190799

Laccourreye, O., Bernard, D., de Lacharriere, O., Bazin, R., & Brasnu, D. (1993). Frey's syndrome analysis with biosensor. A preliminary study. *Archives of Otolaryngology--Head & Neck Surgery*, *119*(9), 940–944. doi:10.1001/archotol.1993.01880210028004 PMID:8395192

Laccourreye, O., Bonan, B., Brasnu, D., & Bonan, B. (1990). Treatment of Frey's syndrome with topical 2% diphemanil methylsulfate (Prantal): A double-blind evaluation of 15 patients. *The Laryngoscope*, *100*(6), 651–653. doi:10.1288/00005537-199006000-00019 PMID:2190054

Laccourreye, O., Muscatelo, L., Naude, C., Bonan, B., & Brasnu, D. (1988). Botulinum toxin type A for Frey's syndrome: A preliminary prospective study. *The Annals of Otology, Rhinology, and Laryngology*, *107*(1), 52–55. doi:10.1177/000348949810700110 PMID:9439389

Lambert, G. A., Bogduk, N., Goadsby, P. J., Duckworth, J. W., & Lance, J. W. (1984). Decreased carotid arterial resistance in cats in response to trigeminal stimulation. *Journal of Neurosurgery*, *61*(2), 307–315. doi:10.3171/jns.1984.61.2.0307 PMID:6737055

Laskawi, R., Drobik, C., & Schonebeck, C. (1998). Up-to-date report of botulinum toxin type-A treatment in patients with gustatory sweating (Frey's syndrome). *The Laryngoscope*, *108*(3), 381–384. doi:10.1097/00005537-199803000-00013 PMID:9504611

Lee, T. S. (1954). Physiological gustatory sweating in a warm climate. *The Journal of Physiology*, *124*(3), 528–542. doi:10.1113/jphysiol.1954.sp005126 PMID:13175196

Leriche, R. (1914). Behandlung der permanenten parotis Fisteln durch die Entnervung der Speicheldruse Ausreissen des N. auriculotemporalis. *Zentralblatt für Chirurgie*, *41*, 754–755.

Linder, T. E., Huber, A., & Schmid, S. (1997). Frey's syndrome after parotidectomy: A retrospective and prospective analysis. *The Laryngoscope*, *107*(11), 1496–1501. doi:10.1097/00005537-199711000-00013 PMID:9369396

List, C. F., & Peet, M. M. (1938). Sweat secretion in man: IV. Sweat secretion of the face and its disturbance. *Archives of Neurology and Psychiatry*, *40*(3), 443–470. doi:10.1001/archneurpsyc.1938.02270090037002

Low, P. A. (2003). Testing the autonomic nervous system. *Seminars in Neurology*, *23*(4), 407–421. doi:10.1055-2004-817725 PMID:15088262

Matthews, B., & Robinson, P. P. (1980). The course of post-ganglionic sympathetic fibres distributed with the trigeminal nerve in the cat. *The Journal of Physiology*, *303*(1), 391–401. doi:10.1113/jphysiol.1980.sp013294 PMID:7431241

May, J. S., & McGuirt, W. F. (1989). Frey's syndrome: Treatment with topical glycopyrrolate. *Head & Neck*, *11*(1), 85–89. doi:10.1002/hed.2880110115 PMID:2646246

Minor, V. (1927). Ein neues Verfahren zu der klinischen Untersuchung der Schweissabsonderung. *Deutsche Zeitschrift fur Nervenheilkunde*, *101*(1), 302–308. doi:10.1007/BF01652699

Montecucco, C., Schiavo, G., Tugnoli, V., & de Grandis, D. (1996). Botulinum neurotoxins: Mechanism of action and therapeutic applications. *Molecular Medicine Today*, *2*(10), 418–424. doi:10.1016/1357-4310(96)84845-3 PMID:8897436

Morfit, H. M., & Kramish, D. (1961). Auriculotemporal syndrome (Frey's syndrome) following surgery of parotid tumors. *American Journal of Surgery*, *102*(6), 777–780. doi:10.1016/0002-9610(61)90583-9 PMID:14475945

Naumann, M., Zellner, M., Toyka, K. V., & Reiners, K. (1997). Treatment of gustatory sweating with botulinum toxin. *Annals of Neurology*, *42*(6), 973–975. doi:10.1002/ana.410420619 PMID:9403490

Needles, W. (1936). The auriculotemporal syndrome. With a suggestion regarding therapy. *Archives of Neurology and Psychiatry*, *35*(2), 357–360. doi:10.1001/archneurpsyc.1936.02260020151012

Nesathurai, S., Harvey, D. T., & Schatz, S. W. (1995). Gustatory facial sweating subsequent to upper thoracic sympathectomy. *Archives of Physical Medicine and Rehabilitation*, *76*(1), 104–107. doi:10.1016/S0003-9993(95)80052-2 PMID:7811168

New, G. B., & Bozer, H. E. (1922). Hyperhydrosis of the cheek associated with the parotid region. *Minnesota Medicine*, *5*, 652–657.

Nosan, D. K., Ochi, J. W., & Davidson, T. M. (1991). Preservation of facial contour during parotidectomy. *Otolaryngology - Head and Neck Surgery*, *104*(3), 293–298. doi:10.1177/019459989110400302 PMID:1851274

Ottomo, M., & Heimburger, R. F. (1980). Alternating Horner's syndrome and hyperhidrosis due to dural adhesions following cervical spinal cord injury: Case report. *Journal of Neurosurgery*, *53*(1), 97–100. doi:10.3171/jns.1980.53.1.0097 PMID:7411214

Parisier, S. C., Binder, W. J., Blitzer, A., Friedman, W. F., & Marovitz, W. F. (1978). Evaluation of tympanic neurectomy and chorda tympanectomy for gustatory sweating and benign salivary gland disease. *Ear, Nose, and Throat Journal*, *57*, 213–223. PMID:668593

Payne, R. T. (1940). Pneumococcal parotiditis and antecedent auriculotemporal syndrome. *Lancet*, 634–636. doi:10.1016/S0140-6736(00)61754-3

Quinodoz, D., Dulguerov, P., Cosenday, G., Arechalde, S., & Piletta, P. (1997). Traitement du syndrome de Frey avec la toxine botulinique. *Medecine et Hygiene*, *55*, 2070–2073.

Randall, W. C. (1946). Sweat gland activity and changing patterns of sweat secretion on the skin surface. *The American Journal of Physiology*, *147*(2), 391–398. doi:10.1152/ajplegacy.1946.147.2.391 PMID:21000764

Redleaf, M. I., & McCabe, B. F. (1993). Gustatory otorrhea: Frey's syndrome of the external auditory canal. *The Annals of Otology, Rhinology, and Laryngology*, *102*(6), 438–440. doi:10.1177/000348949310200606 PMID:8512270

Ross, J. A. (1970). The function of the tympanic plexus as related to Frey's syndrome. *The Laryngoscope*, *80*(12), 1816–1833. doi:10.1002/lary.5540801204 PMID:4321509

Rubinstein, R. Y., Rosen, A., & Leeman, D. (1999). Frey syndrome: Treatment with temporoparietal fascia flap interposition. *Archives of Otolaryngology--Head & Neck Surgery*, *125*(7), 808–811. doi:10.1001/archotol.125.7.808 PMID:10406323

Saito, H. (1999). Gustatory otalgia and wet ear syndrome: A possible cross-innervation after ear surgery. *The Laryngoscope*, *109*(4), 569–572. doi:10.1097/00005537-199904000-00009 PMID:10201742

Sato, K. (1977). The physiology, pharmacology, and biochemistry of the eccrine sweat gland. *Reviews of Physiology, Biochemistry and Pharmacology*, *79*, 51–131. doi:10.1007/BFb0037089 PMID:21440

Sato, K. (1977). The physiology, pharmacology, and biochemistry of the eccrine sweat gland. *Reviews of Physiology, Biochemistry and Pharmacology*, *79*, 51–131. doi:10.1007/BFb0037089 PMID:21440

Sato, K., Kang, W. H., Saga, K., & Sato, K. T. (1989). Biology of sweat glands and their disorders. II. Disorders of sweat gland function. *Journal of the American Academy of Dermatology*, *20*(5), 713–726. doi:10.1016/S0190-9622(89)70081-5 PMID:2654213

Sato, K., Kang, W. H., Saga, K., & Sato, K. T. (1989). Biology of sweat glands and their disorders. I. Normal sweat gland function. *Journal of the American Academy of Dermatology*, *20*(4), 537–563. doi:10.1016/S0190-9622(89)70063-3 PMID:2654204

Sato, K. T., Richardson, A., Timm, D. E., & Sato, K. (1988). One-step iodine starch method for direct visualization of sweating. *The American Journal of the Medical Sciences*, *295*(6), 528–531. doi:10.1097/00000441-198806000-00006 PMID:3389391

Schmelzer, A., Rosin, V., & Zur Steinbach, E. (1992). Therapie des Freyschen Syndroms durch ein Anhidrotisches Gel. *Laryngo- Rhino- Otologie*, *71*(01), 59–63. doi:10.1055-2007-997246 PMID:1543523

Schnarch, A., & Markitziu, A. (1990). Dysgeusia, gustatory sweating, and crocodile tears syndrome induced by a cerebellopontine angle meningioma. *Oral Surgery, Oral Medicine, and Oral Pathology*, *70*(6), 711–714. doi:10.1016/0030-4220(90)90005-D PMID:2263327

Scrivani, S. J., Keith, D. A., Kulich, R., & Maciewicz, R. J. (1998). Posttraumatic gustatory neuralgia: A clinical model of trigeminal neuropathic pain. *Journal of Orofacial Pain*, *12*, 287–292. PMID:10425975

Sessions, R. B., Roark, D. T., & Alford, B. R. (1976). Frey's syndrome a technical remedy. *Annals of Otology*, *85*, 734–739.

Sharav, Y., Benoliel, R., Schnarch, A., & Greenberg, L. (1991). Idiopathic trigeminal pain associated with gustatory stimuli. *Pain*, *44*(2), 171–174. doi:10.1016/0304-3959(91)90133-I PMID:2052384

Shelley, W. B., & Horvath, P. N. (1951). Comparative study on the effect of anticholinergic compounds on sweating. *The Journal of Investigative Dermatology*, *16*(4), 267–274. doi:10.1038/jid.1951.34 PMID:14841388

Sly, R. M. (1981). Auriculotemporal syndrome. *Cutis*, *28*, 423–425. PMID:7307560

Sonsale, A., Sharp, J. F., & Johnson, I. J. (1999). Gustatory sweating of the external auditory canal. *The Journal of Laryngology and Otology*, *113*(11), 1000–1001. doi:10.1017/S0022215100145815 PMID:10696379

Sood, S., Quraishi, M. S., & Bradley, P. J. (1998). Frey's syndrome and parotid surgery. *Clinical Otolaryngology*, *23*(4), 291–301. doi:10.1046/j.1365-2273.1998.00154.x PMID:9762489

Stuart, D. D. (1978). Diabetic gustatory sweating. *Annals of Internal Medicine*, *8*(2), 223–224. doi:10.7326/0003-4819-89-2-223 PMID:677588

Thomas, A. (1927). Le double reflexe vaso-dilatateur et sudoral de la face consecutif aux blessures de la loge parotidienne. *Revue Neurologique*, *1*, 447–460.

Truax, B. T. (1989). Gustatory pain: A complication of carotid endarterectomy. *Neurology*, *39*(9), 1258–1260. doi:10.1212/WNL.39.9.1258 PMID:2549453

Tuinzing, D. B., & van der Kwast, W. A. (1982). Frey's syndrome. A complication after sagittal splitting of the *mandibular ramus. International Journal of Oral Surgery*, *11*(3), 197–200. doi:10.1016/S0300-9785(82)80008-2 PMID:6813278

van der Linden, J., Sinnige, H. A., & van den Dorpel, M. A. (2000). Gustatory sweating and diabetes. *The Netherlands Journal of Medicine*, *56*(4), 159–162. doi:10.1016/S0300-2977(00)00004-8 PMID:10727762

Vilches, J. J., Navarro, X., & Verdu, E. (1995). Functional sudomotor responses to cholinergic agonists and antagonists in the mouse. *Journal of the Autonomic Nervous System*, *55*(1-2), 105–111. doi:10.1016/0165-1838(95)00033-T PMID:8690842

Wallis, K. A., & Gibson, T. (1978). Gustatory sweating following parotidectomy: Correction by a fascia lata graft. *British Journal of Plastic Surgery*, *31*(1), 68–71. doi:10.1016/0007-1226(78)90020-6 PMID:623929

Watkins, P. J. (1973). Facial sweating after food: A new sign of diabetic autonomic neuropathy. *British Medical Journal*, *1*(5853), 583–587. doi:10.1136/bmj.1.5853.583 PMID:4144374

Weber, F. P. (1897). Clinical cases V: A case of localized sweating and blushing on eating, possibly due to temporary compression of vasomotor fibers. *Transactions of Clinical Society, London*, *31*, 277–280.

Wilson, W. C. (1936). Observations relating to the innervation of the sweat glands of the face. *Clinical Science*, *2*, 273–286.

Yu, L. T., & Hamilton, R. (1992). Frey's syndrome: Prevention with conservative parotidectomy and superficial musculoaponeurotic system preservation. *Annals of Plastic Surgery*, *29*(3), 217–222. doi:10.1097/00000637-199209000-00005 PMID:1326250

Zalzal, G. H. (1991). Congenital gustatory facial flushing. *Otolaryngology - Head and Neck Surgery*, *104*(6), 878–880. doi:10.1177/019459989110400620 PMID:1908985

Zoller, J., Herrmann, A., & Maier, H. (1993). Frey's syndrome secondary to a subcondylar fracture. *Otolaryngology - Head and Neck Surgery*, *108*(6), 751–753. doi:10.1177/019459989310800620 PMID:8516015

Chapter 18
Extra-Temporal Facial Nerve Reconstruction

ABSTRACT

Hypoglossal-facial anastomosis (HFA) as an end-to-end anastomosis (EEA) has several advantages, and indirect HFA with interposition graft is a safe and excellent method. The extended HFA is the method of choice for all malignant tumors that require extensive resection of the facial plexus, especially when combined with a neck dissection. Facio-facial anastomosis combined with HFA leads to excellent results when resection defect is restricted to the central portion of the facial plexus. Good functional rehabilitation of the musculature of the oral sphincter system is achieved using the hypoglossal nerve. To innervate the musculature of the ocular sphincter system, a facio-facial anastomosis between the nerve trunk and the cranial nerve branches is made using a free nerve transplant. Dynamic reanimation involves nerve repair, nerve transfer, regional muscle transfer, or free-muscle transfer. Dynamic reconstructive techniques can yield improved facial symmetry, spontaneous and symmetrical smile, eye closure and protection, and oral competence.

CONSEQUENCES OF FACIAL NERVE DAMAGE (AXON DEGENERATION)

The facial nerve is the "connecting cable" between the central nervous system (CNS) and the facial muscles. The vital conditions of this threefold system have to be taken into account, especially in cases of delayed reconstruction.

DOI: 10.4018/978-1-7998-5603-0.ch018

As a consequence of any severe facial nerve damage leading to axon degeneration, this degeneration results: a) Centrally, in retrograde changes to the motor neurons and their cellular environment (Blinzinger, 1968; Graeber, 1986; Graeber, 1994; Guntinas-Lichius, 1994a; Guntinas-Lichius, 1994b; Guntinas-Lichius, 2005; Kreutzberg, 1982; Steit, 1994; Tetzlaff, 1986), and b) Peripherally, in the degeneration of muscle fibres (Goebel, 1994; Irintchev, 1994). Reversibility or irreversibility of these degenerative processes depends on the *time* that has elapsed between nerve injury and reinnervation of the musculature.

Facial nerve denervation and paralysis imposes significant psychological and functional impairment. Facial paralysis can inhibit and mar facial expression, communication, symmetrical smile, eye protection, and oral competence. The physician must accurately evaluate and examine the patient and determine the etiology, duration, and the scale of the paralysis.

GOALS AND LIMITATIONS OF RECONSTRUCTION

Reconstructive nerve surgery must be performed as soon as possible, either as a one-stage operation with tumor resection or, if a histopathological analysis of the specimen is necessary, within 10-14 days at most because of the rapid development of scar tissue. Dynamic and static reconstruction procedures are employed for facial reanimation in patients suffering from facial nerve paralysis (Gordin, Lee, Ducic, & Arnaoutakis, 2015). However, dynamic strategies tend to be more successful and fruitful and should be offered to patients considering reconstruction, unless health risk contraindications exist.

The most common approaches for reconstruction are direct facial nerve repair with or without grafting, nerve transfer, cross-facial nerve grafting, and muscle transfer (regional or free) (Gousheh, 2011; Chan, 2011; Robey, 2011; Meltzer, 2010). Understanding facial nerve anatomy with precise assessment of the patient's paralysis and health status dictate the potential for recovery and the appropriate reconstructive scheme.

Goals of Reconstruction

The goals of the reconstruction in facial paralysis include the following:

1. Facial symmetry at rest;
2. Symmetrical smile;
3. Voluntary, coordinated, and spontaneous facial movements;
4. Oral competence and eyelid closure with corneal protection;
5. Absence or limitation of synkinesis and mass movement.

Limitations of Surgery

The facial nerve innervates a total of 23 paired muscles and the orbicular oris, but only 18 of these muscles, working in a delicate balance, produce facial animation and expression. No current reconstructive stratagem can reproduce every facial expression and movement. As part of patient counselling, surgeons need to establish realistic patient expectations and determine whether the patient is willing to expend the time and financial resources required for a successful result.

TIME SCHEDULE FOR FACIAL NERVE REPAIR

Recommendations for the time schedule for facial nerve repair are summarized in Table 1. However, for recovery of facial expression following partial or subtotal resection of the facial nerve and/or the peripheral nerve plexus, an *immediatesurgical reconstruction* should be performed when at all possible for the following reasons:

1. Facial expression plays an extremely important role in the social life and psychology of the patient;
2. Reconstruction should be performed as a one-stage operation together with tumor resection or, if a histological analysis is necessary, within 10-14 days at most, otherwise rapid development of scar tissue may jeopardize the success of this delicate surgery;
3. The general health of the patient is to be considered, since with a reduced tolerance to anesthesia, more complex and therefore longer procedures must be replaced with simpler methods;
4. The patient's age plays a role in the choice of procedure. With advancing age, nerve regeneration diminishes and preference is for procedures that make a safe and fast reinnervation of the paralyzed musculature possible (end-to-end anastomoses);

5. Psychologically unstable patients may find it more difficult to live with a failed procedure than more stable or indifferent individuals;
6. The length of the interposition graft has a substantial influence on the final functional result after reconstruction. The longer the graft, the worse the final outcome will be, particularly if longer than 4-5 cm. The main reason for this is that the axons need more time to penetrate the endoneural tubes, while at the same time, degeneration of the Schwann cells and fibrosis occurs. Penetration of the distal anastomosis will particularly be handicapped through meanwhile development of scar tissue.

Table 1. Time schedule for facial nerve repair

Duration of Paralysis (Years)	Functional Recovery of Facial Musculature
0–1	Absolutely certain
1–2	Expected, therefore recommendable
2–3	Probable, with delay and decrease in function
3–5	Increasingly questionable, patient must be notified
5+	Improbable, therefore not to be recommended.

Main Questions Prior to Delayed Nerve Surgery

The following questions should be addressed before planning surgery for *delayed nerve reconstruction.*

Peripheral Nervous System (Facial Nerve and Plexus)

1. To what extent has the nerve plexus been resected? i.e. is there still enough nerve tissue of the main branches in-situ to perform successful anastomoses?
2. How realistic are the chances of identifying and isolating the branches within the scar tissue from the injury or the previous operation?
3. Is there enough suitable nerve material available for free nerve transplantation?
4. If the hypoglossal nerve (XII) is to be used for anastomosis, are the XIIth and also the Vth cranial nerves (CNs) intact in their extracranial course?
5. In cases of tumor resection, is the remaining facial nerve tissue free from tumor infiltration?

Central Nervous System

1. What is the general condition of the brain? i.e. what is the patient intellectual or emotional status?
2. Are CNs V and XII functioning normally? It is important to note that the function of both motor nerves (VII and XII) depends on the common afferent input from CN V (Kivelitz, 1974; Stennert, 1982).

Musculature

1. Is it still vital enough to regain its contractibility?
2. Is it free from tumor infiltration?
3. Is it free from infection?

ETIOLOGY OF FACIAL PARALYSIS

Etiology is the most important factor in determining the timing and choice of reconstructive technique. A retrospective study of almost 2000 patient records by Hohman and Hadlock (2014) assessing the etiology of facial palsy cases reported *Bell palsy* to be the most common cause of facial paralysis (38%), followed by acoustic neuroma resection (10%), cancer (7%), iatrogenic trauma (7%), varicella zoster (7%), benign lesions (5%), congenital palsy (5%), Lyme disease (4%), and other etiologies (17%). In general, *trauma* is the second most common cause of facial paralysis.

Bell Palsy

Bell palsy is idiopathic. About 80% of patients begin to recover nerve function spontaneously within 3 weeks; 15% do not have any movement for 3-6 months. Peitersen found 94% of patients with *partial* paralysis completely recovered in 1 year without medical or surgical intervention; of those with *complete* paralysis, 71% completely recovered (Peitersen, 1982). Thus, irreversible reconstructive methods are *not* the best in these patients.

Malignancy

Malignancy of the posterior fossa, temporal bone, skull base, or parotid region can present with facial paralysis. If paralysis is caused by a malignancy or its resection, the risk of recurrence and prognosis may influence the choice of reconstruction.

Denervation

The etiology of the denervation dictates the timing of surgical treatment, if any is to be done. In a patient with a paralyzed face secondary to traumatic surgical disruption, the surgeon should initiate reconstruction as soon as possible, generally within the first month. On the other hand, a patient with an intact nerve can be monitored for recovery for up to 12 months. The duration of the facial paralysis is essential.

Extra-Temporal Injury

Extra-temporal injury to the nerve may occur during surgery of the parotid or submandibular gland, temporo-mandibular joint (TMJ) or face-lift procedures, or from traumatic face lacerations. Paralysis of the facial nerve following uncomplicated parotid procedures is reported at a 20% rate of *temporary* palsy, with a 10% rate of *permanent* paresis of temporal or mandibular branches.

Children and patients undergoing total parotidectomy are at a higher risk of facial nerve injury during surgery. If the nerve is resected because of a parotid cancer, histopathological confirmation of clear margins is required prior to repair by EEA or graft. Inadvertent transection during facelift or parotid surgery warrants immediate primary repair. Postoperative paralysis with known facial nerve integrity usually recovers within 6 months. Traumatic transections and division of segmental branches proximal to the lateral canthus should be explored and repaired.

Facial nerve injury following submandibular gland surgery, which usually involves the marginal mandibular branch, is not uncommon. Sacrifice of this branch may be unavoidable because of involvement by the disease process, most commonly chronic infection or tumor.

TMJ procedures may injure the temporal branch or, less commonly, the main trunk of the facial nerve. Facial nerve injury during rhytidectomy is rare, usually temporary and most often involves segmental branches.

DIAGNOSIS OF FACIAL PARALYSIS

Clinical Evaluation

Patient History

A thorough history includes onset, initial degree of paralysis, duration, and associated symptoms. The reconstructive options for acute paralysis, paralysis for less than 18-24 months, and paralysis for greater than 18-24 months differ significantly.

Facial nerve injuries from Bell palsy, trauma, and malignant neoplasm need to be identified, with the reconstructive efforts based on the etiology. For example, a slowly progressive paralysis suggests malignancy, while a sudden onset of complete paralysis suggests Bell palsy.

In addition, the surgical team must investigate previous surgical procedures for reanimation, since these may limit reconstructive options. The patient's overall health, psychological stability, and life expectancy are significant considerations.

Physical Examination

The patient should be scrutinized with the face at rest and during voluntary and reflex emotional movement. The physician must determine the involvement of unilateral or bilateral facial nerves, facial asymmetries, and synkinesis. The degree of brow ptosis, ectropion, lid laxity, and oral competence must also be noted. The surgical team cannot neglect other cranial nerve or neurologic deficits and soft tissue defects in conjunction with the paralysis, in addition to the general condition of the patient.

Investigations

Audiometry

Audiometric testing, including acoustic reflexes and tympanometry, may be useful in identifying the etiology of facial palsy secondary to retrocochlear pathology or mass lesions of the middle ear.

Imaging: CT Scan and MRI

High-resolution CT and MRI scans are essential in *traumatic* facial nerve palsy to delineate features of the temporal bone. Scans are also used to evaluate patients with possible parotid, skull base, temporal bone, intracranial, or extra-temporal tumors.

Electrodiagnostic Tests

Electrodiagnostic tests of facial nerve function include nerve excitability tests (NET), electro-neuronography (ENog), and electromyography (EMG).

Nerve Excitability Testing (NET)

Nerve excitability testing involves percutaneous stimulation of the facial nerve until muscle contraction is observed. The *minimal* NET determines the threshold stimulation required for muscle contraction compared with the unaffected side. The *maximum stimulation test* (MST) is a modification of the NET but is a supra-maximal stimulus compared with the unaffected side, and the stimulus is increased until the patient encounters discomfort. The *subjective* nature of the measurements and lack of recorded data limit both methods, and they do *not* reflect denervation at the moment it is occurring.

Electroneurography (ENog)

ENog is an objective measure of facial nerve function that measures the amplitude of evoked compound muscle action potentials (CMAPs) with electrodes over the skin of the nasolabial fold. The compound action potential is compared between the 2 sides of the face, and the response of the affected side is expressed as a percentage of the response of the unaffected side. A percentage of nerve fiber degeneration is calculated.

A 95% decrease in CMAP compared with the contralateral side signifies a 50% chance that the patient will have unsatisfactory recovery of facial nerve function. Surgery is indicated if a 90% decrease in CMAP is reached within the initial 2 weeks of the onset of paralysis. ENog is *objective* and is the most accurate reproducible test, but it is expensive and time- consuming.

Electromyography (EMG)

EMG is a measure of volitional muscle response. Needle electrodes are used to monitor activity of facial muscles. *Normal* muscle exhibits activity upon needle insertion, electrical silence at rest, and diphasic or triphasic action potentials during voluntary contraction. Fibrillation potentials are observed in the denervated muscle, and polyphasic potentials in muscle undergoing reinnervation. Complete electrical silence is observed in denervated muscle with significant fibrosis.

EMG is useful in evaluating patients with acute or traumatic nerve injury prior to reinnervation procedures. EMG does *not* show any signs until 3 weeks after paralysis and should not be utilized until 3 weeks after paralysis without signs of recovery.

Objective Measures of Facial Motion

These measures include digital photography and video-recording of the patient at rest and during motion. The *maximum static response assay* quantifies facial motion pre- and serially post-operatively. The patient's face is marked and he is asked to perform specific movements (brow lift, eye closure, smiling, frowning, and whistling). Images of the face in repose and the maximum response movements are recorded and processed for computer display. Images are calibrated and normalized, and vectors of movement are determined and measured using a grid and an internal facial coordinate system. Slight improvements in facial movement are detected over the long recovery periods that often accompany facial reanimation procedures.

PRINCIPLES OF NERVE REPAIR

Early Identification and Repair of Nerve Injuries

The most critical factor in achieving good post-operative facial function is early identification and repair of nerve disruption. Several authors reported that earlier repair of the facial nerve produces superior results. Some authors report function in patients who were grafted 18-36 months after injury, but superior results are found with repairs performed within 1 year. Repair within

30 days is preferred based on clinical results and neurobiological investigations that revealed that the regenerative process begins immediately after injury.

Traumatic nerve injuries must be repaired expediently. In the instance of a grossly contaminated wound (eg, shotgun injury), the nerve ends can be tagged and repaired later. Accidental transection during surgery (e.g. face-lift) should be dealt with an end-to-end anastomosis (EEA). If the facial nerve is resected because of tumor involvement, frozen- sections of both ends can be sent for histopathological examination to exclude microscopic invasion before attempting repair. When margins are clear, either EEA or graft repair can be performed immediately.

Evaluation of Nerve Condition

The condition of the nerve depends on the type of injury or trauma. A patient with pre-operative facial palsy secondary to tumor involvement of the facial nerve is unlikely to experience a good result following resection and repair. The amount of functioning nerve fibers existing at the time of surgery does not increase after repair; improved postoperative facial function over preoperative status is not expected.

A sharp facial nerve laceration from glass or a knife should be suitable for EEA. Gunshot wounds, however, either crush or avulse the nerve, which propagates further nerve degeneration/denervation. These injuries should not be repaired in the immediate setting until the extent of the nerve damage has declared itself. In a delayed intervention, scar tissue and neuromas must be removed, and unhealthy nerve ends must be excised. Identifying healthy nerve stumps may necessitate histologic or microscopic confirmation.

Matching of Endoneurial Surfaces

Matching of the endoneurial surfaces is essential in promoting neural regeneration and is more important than a match of the total nerve diameter. The endoneurium is examined more easily by removing the overlying perineurium at the ends of the nerve. Occasionally, a significant mismatch between proximal and distal nerve ends requires a double cable graft (eg, when grafting from the main facial nerve trunk to segmental branches).

Epineural vs. Peri-Neural Suturing

Various neurorrhaphy techniques and adjunctive measures have been investigated in attempts to improve neural regeneration, including epineural versus perineural sutures, tissue adhesives, laser neurorrhaphy, tubulization, and trophic factors. However, the most efficacious method of reapproximation remains unproven, and no specific adjunctive measure has been found to be beneficial. The use of a minimal number (2 or 4) of epineural or perineural sutures, employing a fine monofilament suture under magnification (microscope or loupe) remains the time-tested criterion for nerve repair.

Tension-Free Anastomosis and Nerve Grafts

Any tension on the nerve ends after repair results in the formation of scar tissue and poor neural regeneration. If tensionless nerve repair is not feasible, then a nerve graft (usually the sural nerve) will be interposed between the proximal trunk and distal branches. Mobilization of the nerve may add up to 2 cm of relative length but also may result in devascularization and further neural injury. Any defect greater than 2 cm should be tackled with a nerve graft of adequate length, without any tension and with a small amount of slack.

Cable grafts function as conduits in which sprouting axons from the proximal nerve stump travel to the motor endplates. The graft provides cellular and humoral promoters for neural growth, such as Schwann cells, extracellular matrix, and neurotrophic growth factor.

Success of a nerve graft depends on the following factors:

1. The number of axons remaining in the nerve;
2. The potential for regeneration of axons;
3. The status of the facial muscles – i.e. the more axons that are available, the greater the chance of recovery and a satisfactory result.

Donor Nerves for Facial Nerve Grafting

The great auricular nerve (GAN) and sural nerve are the most commonly selected nerves for facial nerve grafting. *Disadvantages* include a sensory deficit of the earlobe when using the GAN or of the lateral foot when using the sural nerve.

The *GAN* is harvested easily; since it is located near the surgical field, it tends to be a good match in size, and its extensive arborization allows the anastomosis of the proximal facial nerve stump to several segmental branches. However, only 7-10 cm of the great auricular nerve can be harvested safely, which limits its use in extensive repairs. The *sural nerve* is larger, with a greater axonal volume, and up to 35 cm is harvested easily from the posterior lower leg. It is especially useful in cross-facial grafting.

The patient should not expect return of facial function following nerve grafting for 4-6 months, as regenerating axons travel a distance of 1 mm/day. Improvement in function can be expected for up to 2 years. In general, results after nerve grafting are not as good as those observed with primary repair. Spector et al found incomplete reinnervation of facial divisions, decreased voluntary contractions, and more severe synkinesis when comparing cable grafts to direct end-to-end anastomoses (Spector, Lee, Peterein, & Roufa, 1991). However, 92-95% of patients who undergo facial nerve grafting experience some return of facial function, and 72-79% have good functional results.

Rehabilitation

After surgery, rehabilitation of patients with facial paralysis necessitates EMG protocols, behavioral modification, and patient exercises. The patient needs to obtain voluntary control of facial regions. Another adjuvant therapy is the use of percutaneous electrical stimulation to stimulate motor function.

METHODS (TECHNIQUES) OF FACIAL NERVE RECONSTRUCTION

The following methods of extratemporal facial nerve plexus reconstruction are recommended:

1. End-to-end anastomosis (EEA);
2. Free nerve transplantation (interposition graft);
3. Hypoglossal-facial anastomosis (HFA) as EEA;
4. Hypoglossal-facialis jump anastomosis (HFJA) as EEA;
5. Combined approach (facio-facial anastomosis combined with HFA);
6. Cross-facial nerve graft.

In comparison to the overall excellent functional outcome of the above-mentioned techniques that allow a sufficient reanimation of the mimetic musculature in nearly all cases, the *cross-face anastomosis* has several *disadvantages* leading to only suboptimal or bad results:

- The need to harvest the *sural nerve* is time- consuming and leads to decreased sensation at its innervation area;
- Implantation of 2 or 3 transplants across the face are also time-consuming and bothersome to the patient;
- The anastomosis with facial nerve branches of the opposite side destroys healthy structures;
- The long transplants need much more time for reinnervation;
- Long transplants always result in a worse outcome compared to short grafts and especially to EEA.

End-to-End Anastomosis (EEA)

In the majority of cases, trimming of the nerve is unavoidable, which requires a shortening of the nerve endings. Lack of tension in the anastomosis is an important prerequisite for a good, functioning result, and a tension-free suture can only be achieved after mobilization of the central and peripheral nerve stumps.

The possibilities for such a mobilization are limited, and the following procedure is therefore recommended to relieve tension from the anastomosis. Before performing the nerve suture, a 7/0 or 8/0 suture is inserted through the epineurium of one or both of the nerve stumps a few millimeters from the anastomosis to the right and left, and these sutures are gently pulled towards the anastomosis, securing it in the underlying base of the incision. Such a procedure is naturally only possible when the nerve branches are of sufficient size.

Regarding the suture technique for EEA, there are 2 false statements that are frequently found in the literature, supported by unrealistic diagrams (Burgess & Goode, 1994).

First, according to these opinions, the epineurium should be trimmed back at the ends of the fascicles. Although the epineurial sheath is moveable to a certain extent, suture of the epineurium of both nerve endings leads to an additional shortening of this surrounding structure. This can easily lead to an intra-fascicular rejection of the fascicle endings, which in turn prevents correct adaptation of the fascicles. The resultant "bulging" of the fascicles within the anastomosis can often be felt against the bordering nerve section through soft palpation with micro-instruments alone. Conversely, suturing the epineuria that overlap the ends of the fascicles leads to an intra-neural separation, creating an "empty space". Thus, it is recommended that the nerve endings be "cleaned up" by one sharp section through the entire nerve.

Second, claims that a fascicular suture can be performed for facial nerve surgery are particularly unrealistic. This is impossible for three reasons:

1. In contrast to peripheral nerves, which consist of individual fascicles well separated from each other by the perineurium (poly-fascicular form), cranial nerves do not show any clear individual fascicles (mono-fascicular form);
2. Consistency of the alleged fascicles is so soft that they would tear while trying the knot on even the most gentle of sutures;
3. The suture material used for such a technique would shift inward, where it would be perceived as a foreign body and interfere with the healing process by inducing granulation tissue.

Free Nerve Transplantation (Interposition Graft)

As a consequence of resection of malignant parotid tumors, nerve defects arise in the region of the facial nerve plexus (pes anserinus). This has a unique tree-like branching. There are 2 problems encountered when trying to overcome severe material defects in the central region of the nerve plexus (Figure1):

1. Due to the tree-like branching out, there are only a few (or one) central nerve stump(s) compared with numerous peripheral endings, causing a numerical discrepancy;
2. At the same time, the central nerve stumps have a larger diameter than the very thin peripheral nerve endings, causing a size discrepancy.

The extraction of a single graft that imitates this division satisfactorily is only possible in exceptional cases, and one must therefore almost always opt for several individual grafts. Usually nerve transplants cannot imitate the tree-like branching out of the facial fan. The common donor graft is the *greater auricular nerve*, which has two *advantages*:

1. It is easy to extract because it is already within the operative area for the parotid gland surgery;

Figure 1. Two main problems for reconstruction of central parts of the facial nerve plexus with interposition graft(s): numerical discrepancy and discrepancy in size between central and peripheral nerve endings

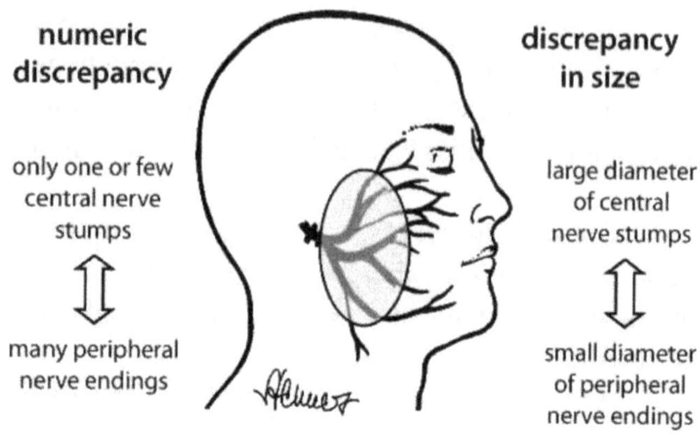

2. Like the facial nerve and its plexus branches, it is mono-fascicular.

As a further possible donor, the *sural nerve* is usually considered, which has two considerable *disadvantages*:

1. Its extraction is very costly;
2. Bifurcations of its nerve branches are very far apart.

Overcoming the Discrepancy in Number and Size by Using Interposition Graft(s)

Excellent functional results have been reported in many cases using the following techniques (Stennert, 1992; Stennert, 2001).

Interventions at the Peripheral Nerve Branches

The ends of the nerve in the region of the peripheral resection are mobilized sufficiently that each of the two neighboring nerve branches can be positioned with their proximal ends about 5 mm alongside each other. If possible, the epineuria at the contact edges are dissected and, finally, the edges are bound together with a 10/0 suture. In this way, a new nerve branch is created from two peripheral nerve branches, now consisting of two fascicles. This allows the number of peripheral branches to be halved, while at the same time doubling their size, resulting in the defect being more easily repairable with a graft (Figure 2). This technique can be taken further when required, using, for example, 3 or 4 neighboring nerve branches to make a new large nerve branch.

Figure 2. Technique for reduction in number and increase in size. After mobilization and adaptation of amputated nerve endings, the epineurium at the site of contact is resected, the edges are bound together with a 10/0 suture and thereby the numbers of peripheral branches are halved, while at the same time doubled in their size.

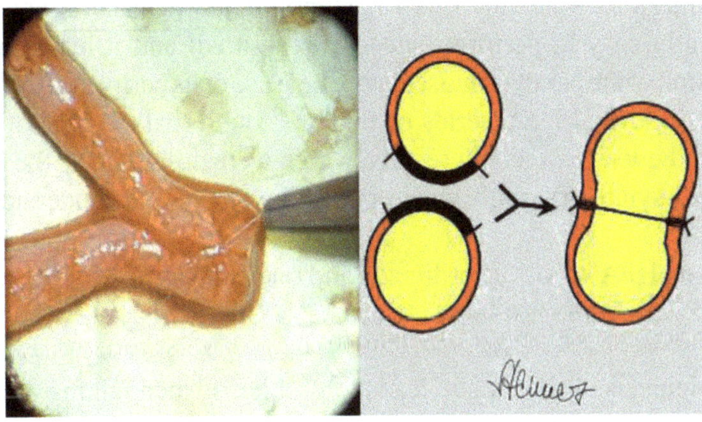

Interventions With the Graft

When a suitable graft is chosen, its peripheral ends can also be split into individual fascicles, which has a branching effect in addition to the interventions taken at the peripheral nerve endings (so-called *diversification*). The combination of both methods results in the most suitable synergistic double-effect: the reduction of number and increase in size of the peripheral nerve structures and the increase in number and reduction of size of the central nerve structures.

Direct Hypoglossal-Facial Nerve Anastomosis (HFA)

Dr. W. Korte, who was at that time head of the ENT Department at the Charite in Berlin, performed this anastomosis in 1901 for the very first time in humans. Two years later, Korte reported unexpectedly good results of this operation. After Bernhard, a neurologist, had critically observed and documented the patient's postoperative course, Korte noted: "It is a most remarkable physiological fact that ganglion cells of the hypoglossal or the accessory nerve nucleus can acquire under voluntary influence the ability to induce contractions of muscles originally innervated from other nerve centers. We cannot yet decide whether there are connections between the two areas of nerve ganglia, or whether by willpower the nerve center can adapt or become accustomed to stimulating a newly acquired muscle system" (Korte, 1903).

Several authors gave answers to Korte's question and could explain the excellent results of this anastomosis (Neiss, 1994; Streppel, 1998; Streppel, 2000; Stennert, 1979; Stennert, 1996). Hypoglossal-facial nerve anastomosis is technically easy to perform; success is assured; and it leads to a rapid reinnervation of the paralytic musculature because of its peripheral localisation. A review of several large series of patients found that 42-65% of patients experienced good to excellent results, which were described as the presence of tone and symmetry, with fair to good movement and moderate to mild synkinesis.

However, HFA was often criticized and rejected, because of the following postulated *disadvantages*:

1. Hemiparesis of the tongue leads to problems when talking and eating;
2. Facial movements are only possible through deliberate movements of the tongue;
3. These deliberate tongue movements lead to uncontrolled grimacing;
4. Spontaneous emotional expression is never regained.

These criticisms are not justified. With respect to the possible *functional results*, experience has shown that:

1. Partial atrophy of the tongue, which varies in degree but is always restricted to the lateral aspect of the involved side, does not lead to substantial problems with talking and eating;
2. Intended movements of facial musculature become independent from deliberate movements of the tongue;
3. Separate activation of different facial muscle groups can be gained, e.g. selective innervation can be achieved;
4. Limited emotional facial expression is possible (e.g. spontaneous smile).

The *quality* of these possible functional results depends on the following factors:

1. The intensity and duration of facial expression rehabilitation by an adequate mimetic training program in order to take advantage of brain plasticity (Beurskens, 2005; Bongers-Janssen, 2005; Coulson, 2005);
2. The vitality of brain function;
3. The duration of denervation (atrophy of facial musculature and retrograde changes in the CNS);
4. The surgical quality of the anastomosis.

Hypoglossal-Facial Nerve Anastomosis (HFA) as End-to-End Anastomosis (EEA)

The classic HFA as EEA between the two cranial nerves is restricted to early tumor infiltration into the nerve stem followed by growth (spreading) proximally into the mastoid, especially in adenoid cystic carcinomas, which develop deep in the parotid gland. A free transplant is required for the reconstruction of the dissected nerve section. Since Wallerian degeneration caused by either the tumor or the surgery extends to the motor end plates, reanimation of the facial musculature can take many months. In such cases, a *direct HFA* as an EEA can be indicated, particularly for older patients with a tendency for rapid drooping of the facial musculature. This is because direct anastomosis is relatively more peripheral, leading to a much quicker reinnervation and thus to a more rapid recovery of muscle tone. Similarly, a direct HFA is indicated in cases where an attempt at rehabilitation using a free graft has failed.

Complications following hypoglossal-to-facial anastomosis include variable degrees of hemi-tongue atrophy and functional disability, including difficulty with chewing, swallowing, and speaking. In general, these impairments improve over time, and many patients report fewer problems chewing post-operatively than pre-operatively. This likely is due to improvement of buccal tone.

Hypoglossal-Facial Nerve Anastomosis With "Jump" Anastomosis (HFJA)

This is a very valuable alternative to the classic HFA. Figure 3 illustrates the procedure. This technique was popularized by May et al., (1991). However, it is worthwhile to note that the first HFA performed by W. Korte in 1901 was also an end-to-side anastomosis (Korte, 1903).

The hypoglossal nerve (CN XII) is exposed in the retro-mandibular fossa and a diagonal incision made into its ventral circumference, half-way through the axons and through the epineurium, leaving an open V-shaped wound. A graft (usually from the greater auricular nerve) is then sutured into this V-shaped incision so that its ends anastomose with the proximal stumps of the dissected axons of the hypoglossal nerve. Finally, the peripheral end of the graft can be sutured with the facial nerve stem as well as with each branch of its plexus. In the plexus region, for overcoming discrepancy in number and size, the same techniques can be used as those described above.

In comparison to direct anastomosis between the two nerve trunks, this technique is more time-consuming and delicate to perform because of the additional need of harvesting and interposing a free nerve graft. However, in the hands of a well-trained micro-surgeon this technique is also a safe method leading to excellent functional results (Manni, 2001; Manni, 2005).

Since the functional deficits of the tongue are negligible, the method is especially indicated for all patients with speech occupation and for rehabilitation of irreversible facial palsy after the removal of an acoustic neurinoma, which might be the first manifestation of a Morbus Recklinghausen (type II) disease and then may later also develop on the contralateral side !!!

Good facial movement and expression were noted in 41% of jump graft patients, and the patients experienced less synkinesis than did the nerve transfer patients. [16] Facial motor function generally is not as strong following a jump graft, and recovery of facial function has been found to take longer in jump grafts.

Extended Hypoglossal-Facial Nerve Anastomosis

This is the method of choice for all tumors that require extensive resection of the facial plexus, which are in general malignant and show a high tendency towards lymphogenous metastasis necessitating simultaneous neck dissection (Stennert, Kisner Jungehulsing, Guntinas-Lichius, & Klussmann, 2003).

For reconstruction of a facial plexus that has been extensively dissected peripherally, HFA offers an ideal solution to many of the problems described above, while at the same time having considerable *advantages*:

Figure 3. Technique of a "hypoglossal-facial jump anastomosis". The hypoglossal nerve is exposed in the retro-mandibular fossa and a diagonal incision is made into half of its ventral circumference. The distal end of the interposed nerve transplant has to be directed towards the proximal stumps of the dissected axons of the hypoglossal nerve.

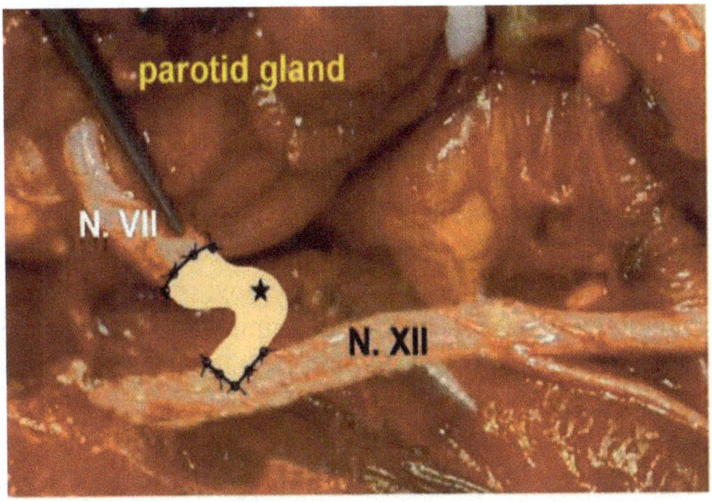

★ interposition graft (greater auricular nerve)

1. The hypoglossal nerve is already exposed within the operative field, especially when combined with a neck dissection i.e. preparation of a nerve transplant from another region of the body is not necessary;
2. The following recommendations are made for preparation of the hypoglossal nerve:
   a. Initially it is exposed to its entrance into the musculature of the floor of the mouth, until its barbarization into peripheral branches can be identified. Beyond this barbarization the nerve is dissected;
   b. With sufficient magnification, stumps of the peripheral branches can be isolated retrograde from connective tissue, and if necessary followed as single fascicles further into the main stem;
   c. This is followed by step-by-step retrograde mobilization of hypoglossal nerve (main trunk) towards the skull base. In the meantime, it is possible to check at which point the resected ends of the transpositioned hypoglossal nerve reach the facial plexus nerve stumps without tension;

d. Separation of the ansa hypoglossi is also necessary when mobilizing the hypoglossal nerve to overcome expansive defects. The ansa should also be separated as far peripherally as possible to be used as a further anastomosis;

3. After such an extensive mobilization, it is possible to twist the hypoglossal nerve ventro-cranially to such an extent that even nerve endings of extremely peripherally located facial branches can be reached;
4. This allows a multiple tension-free end-to-end anastomosis to be made, and guarantees instant axonal growth through the anastomosis (Figure 4);
5. Because the anastomoses are far peripheral, there is rapid reinnervation of the musculature. This is particularly important for malignant tumors with the necessity of additional radiotherapy;
6. This method is much less time-consuming than the removal and transplantation of many individual grafts, and is therefore less of a strain on both patient and surgeon;
7. If necessary, this method can also be combined with the procedure described above to overcome the discrepancy between central and peripheral nerve stumps regarding their number and size by combining the stumps of the facialis branches that remain in situ (Figure 4);
8. Because longer free nerve grafts are avoided and the EEA is far peripheral, post-operative radiotherapy has no negative effect on the functional result.

All above-mentioned points are of particular advantage especially for older patients. As a rule, after 4 months the facial muscle tone is already more balanced in a relaxed state, and within the following 2 months the motor function for intended movements becomes rapidly stronger. This should then be followed by about 2 years of a mimetic training.

Combined Approach (= Diversification Technique = Facio-Facial Anastomosis Combined with HFA)

This method is also considered for patients with total loss of facial expression, but only when the resection defect is restricted to the central portion of the facial plexus i.e. nerve trunk, bifurcation, temporo-facial and cervico-facial main branch and immediately adjacent sections of branches extending from this region. The method pays particular attention to the

Figure 4. Extended HFA for reconstruction of the facial plexus. (a) The situs shows in the upper part the endings of the preserved facial nerve branches, and in the lower part the distal stump of the CN XII resected deep in the floor of the mouth at the beginning of its branching. (b) Same situs after diversification (separation) of CN XII branches. (c) EEAs 1 and 3 are made by combining the facial branches, and anastomosis 3 by additional shortening of the hypoglossal branch. Anastomoses 2 and 4 are made by direct EEAs after shortening of the facial branch in anastomosis 2. (d) End result of the HFA which allowed a large defect of the facial plexus to be bridged over after tumor resection, allowing invariable EEA.

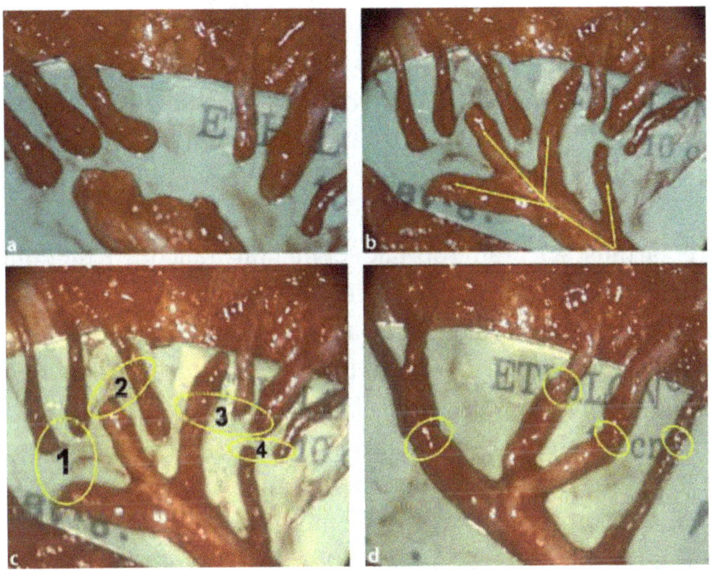

functional anatomy of the facial musculature, which consists of an ocular and oral sphincter system (Stennert, 1982; Stennert, 2005).

Experience with the HFA has shown that good functional rehabilitation of the musculature of the *oral sphincter system* can be achieved using the *hypoglossal* nerve. For this reason, nerve branches that innervate the perioral musculature are supplied either directly or with a jump anastomosis by the hypoglossal nerve.

To innervate musculature of the *ocular sphincter system*, a *facio-facial anastomosis* between the nerve trunk and the cranial nerve branches is made using a free nerve transplant. In this way, the motor neurons (reflex fibers) that are responsible for the blink reflex will have a chance for a more targeted reinnervation of the orbicularis oculi muscle. Here also, the method described for overcoming discrepancy in number and size can be applied for peripheral anastomoses. Using both CNs at the same time leads to a physiologically "diversified" innervation of both independently operating sphincter systems; thus, reducing synkineses, especially in the so-called *mass movements* (Stennert, 2005).

Cross-Facial Nerve Graft

Smith and Scaramella first reported cross-facial nerve grafting in 1971. This technique provides the potential for symmetry and involuntary mimetic function. *Disadvantages* include weakening of the contralateral facial nerve and inadequate power to innervate the ipsilateral musculature.

Cross-face nerve grafting is *indicated* if the proximal ipsilateral facial nerve is not available but the distal stumps are available. *Outcome* of depends on timing and technique and can provide the best facial reanimation scheme if performed on the right patient.

The surgeon must select appropriate segmental branches of the contralateral facial nerve as donors, with the sural nerve serving as a cable graft. Many techniques have been described, such as a single segmental-to – main trunk anastomosis and multiple anastomoses from segmental branches to segmental branches. The grafts are tunneled above the supra-orbital ridge for the orbicularis oculi, the upper lip for the zygomatic and buccal branches, and below the lower lip for the marginal mandibular branch.

Facial muscle movement will not emerge until 9-12 months after the procedure (ie, the allotted time for axonal growth to cross the graft). Cross-facial nerve grafting remains polemic, and many investigators relegate it to serving an adjunctive procedure in combination with other reanimation strategies.

MUSCLE TRANSPOSITION

When facial nerve dysfunction has exceeded 18 months, dynamic slings and free muscle transfers can be executed to restore facial and oral motor function. Severe neurofibrosis and myofibrosis in the distal neuro-muscular unit preclude successful reinnervation. Patients with congenital facial paralyses cannot be reinnervated, since the neuro-muscular units never developed in these individuals. *Regional muscle transposition* and *free-muscle transfer* are the 2 modalities to reanimate the face in this subset of patients.

Regional Muscle Transfer

Regional muscle transfer can reanimate the lower third of the paralyzed face. This new neuro-muscular unit is composed of the transferred muscle (to its new origin) with its original nerve and vascular supply.

Regional muscle transposition is limited by anatomic constraints of size and vectors and often produces results slightly better than static strategies. Regional muscle procedures are appropriate in patients who are in poor health or who will not survive beyond the 12-24 month period of neurotization of a free muscle transfer. Such procedures provide immediate reanimation and are technically less demanding than cross-facial nerve grafting with free muscle transfer.

Temporalis Muscle

The temporalis muscle may improve the symmetry of the commissure of the mouth and re-establish a voluntary smile. The vector of the temporalis muscle resembles that of the zygomaticus major and, thus, results in a lateral smile. Transposition will *not* produce spontaneous mimetic function. Each movement necessitates a specific volitional action, in which the patient must consciously contract the transposed muscle in conjunction with the smiling.

Temporalis muscle transposition can also reanimate the eyelids. However, reanimation of the eye with the temporalis transfer can produce eyelid distortion. To avoid a contour defect, the muscle anterior to the hairline should *not* be used.

The temporalis muscle is harvested through a vertical incision in front of the ear that extends to the scalp. The middle section of the muscle and fascia is elevated and detached superiorly from the skull while the inferior attachments are preserved. Two tongues are created by bisecting the muscle, and the muscle is tunneled through a subcutaneous pocket from the zygomatic arch to the vermillion border. The ends of the temporalis are secured to the orbicularis and the corner of the mouth. The ends should be secured with enough tension to create some level of overcorrection.

The patient initiates a smile by consciously tensing the temporalis muscle. Patients will require therapy to master this technique. In his study, May reported improvement in 95% of patients with temporalis transfer for lower-face reanimation and good to excellent results in 78% of patients. The complication rate was 18%; the most common complications were infection and implant-related complications. Other potential complications include failure of attachment, pulling away of the temporalis muscle from the commissure, and overcorrection of the upper lip. The transfer may also generate excess muscle bulk and a facial deformity, particularly over the zygoma.

Masseter Muscle

The masseter muscle is another muscle used for reanimation of the commissure of the mouth, either alone or in conjunction with the temporalis. Unlike the temporalis, the vector of smile of the masseter muscle is in the buccinator-risorius direction, which produces a less natural smile.

This muscle is elevated by detaching the anterior portion from its mandibular insertion. It is similarly bisected and secured to the modiolus. The muscle is quite bulky and can create facial irregularity or surface deformity, such as a bulge at the commissure. Post-operatively, patients must train the masseter with aggressive physical therapy to learn how to use the transposed masseter to produce a smile (Hontanilla & Rodriguez-Losada, 2001).

Digastric Muscle

Conley developed the modern method of transposing the tendon of the digastric muscle to the orbicularis of the lower lip. The blood supply and nerve to the anterior belly remains intact, and dynamic depression of the lower lip border is achieved. Of 36 patients treated in this manner by Conley, 33 were reported to have satisfactory results. This method is ideal for isolated palsy of the marginal mandibular nerve only, since it can create oral incompetence in patients with more extensive palsy of the lower face.

Depressor muscle function is important to dentured smile, as well as to expressions of sadness, anger, and sorrow. The lower lip is animated by interactions of the orbicularis oris, depressor labii inferioris, depressor anguli oris, mentalis, and platysma. Terzis described a technique to improve this type of smile by transfer either of the anterior belly of the digastric tenor or of the platysma (Terzis & Kalantarian, 2000). Other authors argue that this symmetrical smile could be achieved with less invasive approaches, including Botox injections or myectomy of the depressor labii inferioris.

Free-Muscle Transfer

Principles of Free-Muscle Transfer

Cross-facial nerve grafting with micro-neurovascular muscle transfer is the best strategy for facial reanimation when a patient has long-established facial paralysis (>24 months). Other approaches leave residual asymmetry, an unnatural appearance, and unwanted facial movements while eating.

The advent of micro-surgical technique and free-muscle transfer introduced a new era for facial reconstruction in patients with chronic facial palsy. Free-muscle transfer supplies a new neuro-muscular unit to the face via a free-muscle flap and a grafted donor cranial nerve, usually a cross-facial nerve graft. This modality establishes more precise vectors in addition to spontaneous mimetic facial expression.

Most commonly, the surgeon executes a 2-stage technique of cross-facial nerve graft followed by a delayed free-muscle transfer. The rationale for the delay is to prevent atrophy of the muscle graft while waiting for axons to travel the length of the nerve graft.

Two-Stage Technique

Cross-Facial Nerve Graft

Occasionally, the proximal segment of the ipsilateral facial nerve is available for grafting to innervate a free-muscle transfer. This situation most commonly occurs in the event of a failed interposition nerve graft, resulting in facial musculature that no longer can be reinnervated.

The contralateral facial nerve is chosen as the donor nerve, and a redundant zygomaticus branch is selected for grafting. The hypoglossal nerve also can act as a donor, either by a direct or jump graft alone or in conjunction with a cross-facial graft. The sural nerve is anastomosed to the contralateral facial nerve or substituted cranial nerve and tunneled subcutaneously from the donor nerve to the planned site of free-muscle transfer, and the distal segment of the graft is tagged. The ideal time for the muscle transfer occurs when a Tinel sign is detected in the distal nerve end, indicating completion of axonal growth.

Muscles Suitable for Transfer

Free-muscle transfer is usually performed 9-12 months after nerve graft. A plethora of muscles have been assiduously investigated for free transfer to the paralyzed face, including the gracilis, serratus, pectoralis minor, latissimus dorsi, platysma, rectus abdominis, rectus femoris, and extensor digitorum brevis.

The original report by Harii et al. (1976) of free-muscle transfer for facial paralysis described use of the *gracilis* muscle. It remains the muscle of choice because of its relative ease of dissection, adequate neuro-vascular pedicle, and muscle fiber length, which corresponds to the action of the zygomaticus major muscle. The vascular pedicle is derived from the medial femoral circumflex artery and provides up to 8 cm of length. Innervation of the gracilis is provided by the anterior branch of the obturator nerve, which can be dissected to a length of 10-12 cm.

During the second-stage procedure, the surgeon must identify the distal end of the nerve graft and send a frozen section for confirmation of viable axons. The muscle flap is harvested and transferred to the face. The flap is secured to the periosteum of the zygomatic arch and the modiolus in a vector that corresponds to the smile on the contralateral face. Subsequently, the micro-anastomosis between the flap and recipient vessels is executed, followed by the nerve anastomosis as close to the muscle as possible. Movement can be expected in 6-9 months, with improvement over the following 2-3 years.

Based on their anatomical findings, Lifchez and Gasparri endorse the serratus anterior for free-muscle transfer (Lifchez et al, 2005). Each serratus slip, divided along fascial planes, can generate a distinct force vector for facial reanimation, with a total of 5 slips and 10 subslips. This serratus anterior can, therefore, be used as a single donor muscle with multiple vectors of action and multiple functions (eg, restoration of a symmetrical smile with simultaneous, but independent, eyelid closure).

Terzis and Noah (1997) found no significant effect associated with age, gender, or ischemia time on outcome in their series of 100 free-muscle transfers. They reported moderate or better results in 80% of patients undergoing free-muscle transfer, based on a 5-step scale of judgment. O'Brien et al report "good to excellent" results in 51% of 47 patients treated by micro-vascular free-muscle transfer; the surgeons most commonly used cross-facial nerve grafts and gracilis muscle transfers in their technique (O'Brien, et al, 1990).

One-Stage Free-Muscle Transfer

In their study of 25 patients, Kumar and Hassan (2002) compared single-stage free-tissue transfer with dual-stage free-tissue transfer for facial reconstruction. The gracilis obturator nerve branch can yield a length of 12 cm, which allows primary anastomosis of this nerve to the contralateral facial nerve. However, this technique produces an additional scar on the cheek. The single-stage transfer has fewer complications and a reduced recovery time with decreased rehabilitation, but the dual-stage approach achieves better overall symmetry.

In their investigation of 166 free gracilis transfers, Manktelow and Zuker explored muscle transfer with cross-facial nerve graft versus single-stage transfer to the masseter nerve. The excursion of the free gracilis innervated by the masseter nerves is greater than that of the cross-facial nerve graft. This is probably attributable to the different motor nerve used to reinnervate the muscle. The cross-face nerve graft provides improved spontaneity in terms of movement, which is vital to a normal smile in children. This is a more important characteristic than degree of excursion.

Although use of the masseter nerve with free-tissue transfer was previously explored and considered only in the setting of *Möbius syndrome*, bilateral facial paralysis, and facial paralysis *not* suitable for cross-facial nerve grafting, the masseter nerve's applicability and role has been recently extended to patients with unilateral facial palsy. This one-stage strategy, incorporating the masseter nerve with free tissue transfer, has become a reasonable alternative (and may become the criterion standard) to the dual-stage approach with cross-facial nerve grafting.

The main advantage of the masseter nerve free-tissue transfer technique is that, unlike the cross-facial nerve, the masseter nerve donor produces a movement and muscle excursion (in relation to smile and commissure excursion) in normal range with consistent movement. Also, this technique obviates the need for a second operation.

A study by Liu et al concluded that one-stage reconstruction with free abductor hallucis muscle transfer can effectively restore dynamic facial animation in long-standing, unilateral facial paralysis. The study involved 41 patients who underwent the procedure and were followed up for a mean 54.6-month period. The surgery produced satisfactory results in 37 patients with regard to facial symmetry at rest and voluntary contraction of the transferred muscles; significant increases were achieved in mean values for the Toronto Facial Grading System and the facial nerve function index, at

2-year follow-up, with even greater increases attained at longer-term follow-up. The remaining four patients experienced complications, including infection, hypertrophic scar, hematoma, and muscle loss (Liu et al, 2002).

Revisions

Takushima and Harii determined that predicting muscle bulkiness to obtain symmetry of facial contour is difficult during the initial free-muscle transfer. In their study of a patient population of 486 patients and 183 revisions, Takushima and Harii analyzed excessive muscle bulk and dislocation of the transferred free muscle (Takushima, Harii, Asato, & Momosawa, 2005). Their report illustrated the wide gamut of revisions, including muscle debulking of cheek, adjustment of tension and attachments of transferred free muscle, and lipoinjection to the cheek for better volume symmetry.

Mobius Syndrome

Möbius syndrome involves bilateral facial nerve paralysis and can often attack cranial nerves VI, III, and XII. The syndrome generates psychological disability due to lack of facial animation and lack of emotional expression (immobile face).

The surgical goals for patients with Möbius syndrome are far more modest than and differ from the goals for patients who have unilateral developmental facial paralysis. The restoration of a true smile in these mask-like faces is impossible. Movement can be restored along only 1 vector. A detailed neurological evaluation can identify possible motor donors or residual function, which can be used for additional dynamic restorations. Because of cranial nerve involvement, a thorough clinical and electrophysiological examination is obligatory. Most frequently, the reconstructive surgeon performs free-tissue transfers with bilateral gracilis muscles anastomosed to the masseter nerves on both sides in order to achieve smile restoration.

REFERENCES

Beurskens, C. H. G. (2005). Mime therapy: contents and evidence. In C. H. G. Beurskens, R. S. van Gelder, P. G. Heymans, J. J. Manni, & J.-P. A. Nicolai (Eds.), *The Facial Palsies* (pp. 285–293). Lemma.

Blinzinger, K., & Kreutzberg, G. (1968). Displacement of synaptic terminals from regenerating motor neurons by microglial cells. *Zeitschrift für Zellforschung und Mikroskopische Anatomie*, *85*(2), 145–157. doi:10.1007/BF00325030 PMID:5706753

Bongers-Janssen, H. M. H., Buck, M. J. I., Kleine-Snijders, A. T. H., Neetesen-Lobe, H. J., & Seelen, H. A. M. (2005). Multidisciplinary treatment of patients with a peripheral facial nerve lesion. In C. H. G. Beurskens, R. S. van Gelder, P. G. Heymans, J. J. Manni, & J.-P. A. Nicolai (Eds.), *The Facial Palsies* (pp. 309–320). Lemma.

Burgess, L. P. A., & Goode, R. L. (1994). *Reanimation of the paralyzed Face*. Stuttgart: Thieme.

Chan, J. Y., & Byrne, P. J. (2011). Management of facial paralysis in the 21st century. *Facial Plastic Surgery*, *27*(4), 346–357. doi:10.1055-0031-1283053 PMID:21792778

Coulson, S. E. (2005). Physiotherapy rehabilitation following facial nerve paresis. In C. H. G. Beurskens, R. S. van Gelder, P. G. Heymans, J. J. Manni, & J.-P. A. Nicolai (Eds.), *The Facial Palsies* (pp. 263–274). Lemma.

Goebel, H. H., Schneider, I., Tews, D. S., Gunkel, A., Stennert, E., & Neiss, W. F. (1994). Morphologic studies on human and rodent facial muscles. *European Archives of Oto-Rhino-Laryngology. Supplement*, *§§§*, S24–S27. doi:10.1007/978-3-642-85090-5_6 PMID:10774304

Gordin, E., Lee, T. S., Ducic, Y., & Arnaoutakis, D. (2015). Facial nerve trauma: Evaluation and considerations in management. *Craniomaxillofacial Trauma & Reconstruction*, *8*(1), 1–13. doi:10.1055-0034-1372522 PMID:25709748

Gousheh, J., & Arasteh, E. (2011). Treatment of facial paralysis: Dynamic reanimation of spontaneous facial expression-apropos of 655 patients. *Plastic and Reconstructive Surgery*, *28*(6), 693e–703e. doi:10.1097/PRS.0b013e318230c58f PMID:21841532

Graeber, M. B. (1994). The role of astrocytes in facial nerve regeneration. *European Archives of Oto-Rhino-Laryngology. Supplement*, S75–S77. doi:10.1007/978-3-642-85090-5_21 PMID:10774318

Graeber, M. B., & Kreutzberg, G. W. (1986). Astrocytes increase in glial fibrillary acidic protein during retrograde changes of facial motor neurons. *Journal of Neurocytology, 15*(3), 363–373. doi:10.1007/BF01611438 PMID:3746351

Guntinas-Lichius, O., Gunkel, A., Stennert, E., & Neiss, W. F. (1994a). Astroglial response in facial and hypoglossal-facial anastomoses in the rat. *European Archives of Oto-Rhino-Laryngology. Supplement, §§§*, S557.

Guntinas-Lichius, O., Gunkel, A., Stennert, E., & Neiss, W. F. (1994b). Synaptic stripping in facial and hypoglossal nucleus after hypoglossal-facial anastomoses in the rat. *European Archives of Oto-Rhino-Laryngology. Supplement, §§§*, S558.

Guntinas-Lichius, O., Irintchev, A., Streppel, M., Lenzen, M., Grosheva, M., Wewetzer, K., ... Angelov, D. N. (2005). Factors limiting motor recovery after facial nerve transection in the rat: Combined structural and functional analyses. *The European Journal of Neuroscience, 21*(2), 391–402. doi:10.1111/j.1460-9568.2005.03877.x PMID:15673438

Harii, K., Ohmori, K., & Torii, S. (1976). Free gracilis muscle transplantation, with microneuro-vascular anastomoses for the treatment of facial paralysis. A preliminary report. *Plastic and Reconstructive Surgery, 57*(2), 133–143. doi:10.1097/00006534-197602000-00001 PMID:1250883

Hohman, M. H., & Hadlock, T. A. (2014). Etiology, diagnosis, and management of facial palsy: 2000 patients at a facial nerve center. *The Laryngoscope, 124*(7), E283–E293. doi:10.1002/lary.24542 PMID:24431233

Hontanilla, B., & Rodriguez-Losada, G. (2001). Bilateral reconstruction of smile through muscular transplants neurotized to masseter nerves. *The Journal of Craniofacial Surgery, 22*(3), 1099–1100. doi:10.1097/SCS.0b013e3182107715 PMID:21586953

Irintchev, A., & Wernig, A. (1994). Denervation and reinnervation of muscle: Physiological effects. *European Archives of Oto-Rhino-Laryngology. Supplement*, 28–30. doi:10.1007/978-3-642-85090-5_7 PMID:10774305

Kivelitz, R., Loew, F., & Hubner, H. (1974). Perspectives on the indications and contraindications of various nerve transplant techniques in cases of facial nerve paralysis after pontine angle tumor operations. *Chirurgie Plastische (Berlin)*, *2*, 161–167. doi:10.1007/BF00276613

Korte, W., & Bernhardt, M. (1903). Ein Fall von Nervenpfropfung: Des Nervus facialis auf den Nervus hypoglossus. *Deutsche Medizinische Wochenschrift*, *29*(17), 17. doi:10.1055-0028-1138423

Kreutzberg, G. W. (1982). Acute Neural Reaction to Injury. In Repair and Regeneration of the Nervous System. doi:10.1007/978-3-642-68632-0_5

Kumar, P. A., & Hassan, K. M. (2002). Cross-face nerve graft with free-muscle transfer for reanimation of the paralyzed face: A comparative study of the single-stage and two-stage procedures. *Plastic and Reconstructive Surgery*, *109*(2), 451–462. doi:10.1097/00006534-200202000-00006 PMID:11818819

Lifchez, S. D., Gasparri, M. G., Sanger, J. R., LoGiudice, J. A., Godat, D. M., Tisol, W. B., & Matloub, H. S. (2005). Serratus anterior in vivo contractile force study. *Plastic and Reconstructive Surgery*, *116*(3), 839–845. doi:10.1097/01.prs.0000176254.28792.8c PMID:16141824

Liu, A. T., Lin, Q., Jiang, H., Sun, M. Q., Zhang, J. L., Zhang, Y. F., ... Nagasao, T. (2002). Facial reanimation by one-stage microneurovascular free abductor hallucis muscle transplantation: Personal experience and long-term outcomes. *Plastic and Reconstructive Surgery*, *130*(2), 325–335. doi:10.1097/PRS.0b013e3182589d27 PMID:22842408

Manni, J. J. (2005). Reanimation of the hemiparalysed face with the hypoglossal-facial nerve interpositional graft anastomosis. In C. H. G. Beurskens, R. S. van Gelder, P. G. Heymans, J. J. Manni, & J.-P. A. Nicolai (Eds.), *The Facial Palsies* (pp. 177–185). Lemma.

Manni, J. J., Beurskens, C. H. G., van de Velde, C., & Stokroos, R. J. (2001). Reanimation of the paralyzed face by indirect hypoglossal-facial nerve anastomosis. *American Journal of Surgery*, *182*(3), 268–273. doi:10.1016/S0002-9610(01)00715-2 PMID:11587691

May, M., Sobol, S. M., & Mester, S. J. (1991). Hypoglossal-facial nerve interpositional-jump graft for facial reanimation without tongue atrophy. *Otolaryngology - Head and Neck Surgery*, *104*(6), 818–825. doi:10.1177/019459989110400609 PMID:1908974

Meltzer, N. E., & Alam, D. S. (2010). Facial paralysis rehabilitation: State of the art. *Current Opinion in Otolaryngology & Head & Neck Surgery*, *18*(4), 232–237. doi:10.1097/MOO.0b013e32833bb2d0 PMID:20625293

Neiss, W. F., Schulte, E., Guntinas-Lichius, O., Gunkel, A., & Stennert, E. (1994). Response of Nissl substance in the facial and hypoglossal nucleus after hypoglossal-facial anastomoses in the rat. *European Archives of Oto-Rhino-Laryngology*, (Suppl), S559.

O'Brien, B. M., Pederson, W. C., Khazanchi, R. K., Morrison, W., MacLeod, A., & Kumar, V. (1990). Results of management of facial palsy with microvascular free-muscle transfer. *Plastic and Reconstructive Surgery*, *86*(1), 12–22. doi:10.1097/00006534-199007000-00002 PMID:2359779

Peitersen, E. (1982). The natural history of Bell's palsy. *The American Journal of Otology*, *4*(2), 107–111. PMID:7148998

Robey, A. B., & Snyder, M. C. (2011). Reconstruction of the paralyzed face. *Ear, Nose, and Throat Journal*, *90*(6), 267–275. doi:10.1177/014556131109000608 PMID:21674470

Spector, J. G., Lee, P., Peterein, J., & Roufa, D. (1991). Facial nerve regeneration through autologous nerve grafts: A clinical and experimental study. *The Laryngoscope*, *101*(5), 537–554. doi:10.1288/00005537-199105000-00017 PMID:2030635

Stennert, E. (1979). Hypoglossal facial anastomosis: Its significance for modern facial surgery. II. Combined approach in extratemporal facial nerve reconstruction. *Clinics in Plastic Surgery*, *6*, 471–486. PMID:487711

Stennert, E. (1982). Das Autoparalytische Syndrom – ein Leitsymptom der postparetischen Fazialisfunktion. *Archives of Otorhinolarygology*, *236*(1), 97–114. doi:10.1007/BF00464062 PMID:7126034

Stennert, E. (1992). Prinzipien der Nervenrekonstruktion. In Oto-Rhino-Laryngologie in Klinik und Praxis. Thieme.

Stennert, E. (1996). Neurophysiologische und neuroanatomische Untersuchung zur Hypoglossus-Facialis-Anastomose und ihre klinische Bedeutung. Jahrbuch 1996 der Deutschen Akademie der Naturforscher Leopoldina, Halle/Saale. *Leopoldina (R. 3)*, *42*, 363-385.

Stennert, E. (2005). Synkineses and the Autoparalytic Syndrome. In C. H. G. Beurskens, R. S. van Gelder, P. G. Heymans, J. J. Manni, & J.-P. A. Nicolai (Eds.), *The Facial Palsies* (pp. 117–133). Lemma.

Stennert, E., & Jungehulsing, M. (2001). Chirurgie der Glandula parotis einschlieslich rekonstuktiver Fazialis-Chirurgie: Standard und Qualitatssicherung. *Laryngo- Rhino- Otologie*, *80*(suppl 1), 156–197. doi:10.1055-2001-13922

Stennert, E., Kisner, D., Jungehulsing, M., Guntinas-Lichius, O., & Klussmann, J. P. (2003). High incidence of lymph node metastasis in major salivary gland cancer. *Archives of Otolaryngology--Head & Neck Surgery*, *129*(7), 720–723. doi:10.1001/archotol.129.7.720 PMID:12874071

Stennert, E., & Limberg, C. H. (1982). Central connections between fifth, seventh and twelfth cranial nerves and their clinical significance. In M. D. Graham & W. F. House (Eds.), *Disorders of the Facial Nerve* (pp. 57–65). New York, NY: Raven.

Streit, W. J. (1994). The role of microglia in regeneration. *European Archives of Oto-Rhino-Laryngology. Supplement*, S69–S70. PMID:10774316

Streppel, M., Popratiloff, A., Angelov, D. N., Guntinas-Lichius, O., Hilgers, R. D., Stennert, E., & Neiss, W. F. (1998). Significance of trigeminal sensory input on regrowth of hypoglossal and facial motoneurons after hypoglossal facial anastomosis in rats. *Acta Oto-Laryngologica*, *118*(6), 790–796. doi:10.1080/00016489850182459 PMID:9870621

Streppel, M., Popratiloff, A., Gruart, A., Angelov, D. N., Guntinas-Lichius, O., Delgado-Garcia, J. M., ... Stnnert, E. (2000). Morphological connections between the hypoglossal and facial nerve in the brain stem of the rat. Morphologische Verbindungen zwischen N. hypoglossus und N. facialis im Hirnstamm der Ratte. *HNO*, *48*(12), 911–916. doi:10.1007001060050687 PMID:11196092

Takushima, A., Harii, K., Asato, H., & Momosawa, A. (2005). Revisional operations improve results of neurovascular free muscle transfer for treatment of facial paralysis. *Plastic and Reconstructive Surgery*, *116*(2), 371–380. doi:10.1097/01.PRS.0000169687.94376.78 PMID:16079658

Terzis, J. K., & Kalantarian, B. (2000). Microsurgical strategies in 74 patients for restoration of dynamic depressor muscle mechanism: A neglected target in facial reanimation. *Plastic and Reconstructive Surgery*, *105*(6), 1917–1931. doi:10.1097/00006534-200005000-00001 PMID:10839388

Terzis, J. K., & Noah, M. E. (1997). Analysis of 100 cases of free-muscle transplantation for facial paralysis. *Plastic and Reconstructive Surgery*, *99*(7), 1905–1921. doi:10.1097/00006534-199706000-00016 PMID:9180714

Tetzlaff, W., Graeber, M. B., & Kreutzberg, G. W. (1986). Reactions of motoneurons and their microenvironment to axotomy. *Experimental Brain Research*, *13*(Suppl), 3–8.

About the Author

Mahmoud Sakr, MD, PhD, FACS, Professor of Surgery, graduated in 1981 and had his Master (MS) and Doctorate Degree (PhD) at Alexandria University, Egypt. He had his fellowship in Surgery and Organ Transplantation at University of Pittsburgh School of Medicine, PA, USA. He published 18 books and 105 articles in esteemed journals and is an editorial board member of repute in many international journals.

Index

T

V

X

Z

www.ingramcontent.com/pod-product-compliance
Lightning Source LLC
LaVergne TN
LVHW080904300926
849162LV00003B/543